D1269330

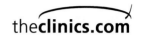

PHYSICAL MEDICINE AND REHABILITATION CLINICS

OF NORTH AMERICA

Dysphagia

GUEST EDITOR
Jeffrey B. Palmer, MD

CONSULTING EDITOR
George H. Kraft, MD, MS

November 2008 • Volume 19 • Number 4

SAUNDERS

An Imprint of Elsevier, Inc.
PHILADELPHIA   LONDON   TORONTO   MONTREAL   SYDNEY   TOKYO

W.B. SAUNDERS COMPANY
A Division of Elsevier Inc.

1600 John F. Kennedy Blvd. • Suite 1800 • Philadelphia, Pennsylvania 19103

http://www.theclinics.com

**PHYSICAL MEDICINE AND REHABILITATION
CLINICS OF NORTH AMERICA**
November 2008
Editor: Debora Dellapena

Volume 19, Number 4
ISSN 1047-9651
ISBN-10: 1-4160-6338-2
ISBN-13: 978-1-4160-6338-4

Reprints. For copies of 100 or more of articles in this publication, please contact the Commercial Reprints Department, Elsevier Inc., 360 Park Avenue South, New York, NY 10010-1710. Tel.: 212-633-3812; Fax: 212-462-1935; E-mail: reprints@elsevier.com.

Physical Medicine and Rehabilitation Clinics of North America (ISSN 1047-9651) is published quarterly by Elsevier Inc., 360 Park Avenue South, New York, NY 10010-1710. Months of publication are February, May, August, and November. Business and Editorial Offices: 1600 John F. Kennedy Blvd., Suite 1800, Philadelphia, PA 19103-2899. Customer Service Office: 11830 Westline Industrial Drive, St. Louis, MO 63146. Periodicals postage paid at New York, NY and additional mailing offices. Subscription price per year is $213.00 (US individuals), $339.00 (US institutions), $107.00 (US students), $259.00 (Canadian individuals), $443.00 (Canadian institutions), $155.00 (Canadian students), $319.00 (foreign individuals), $443.00 (foreign institutions), and $155.00 (foreign students). Foreign air speed delivery is included in all *Clinics* subscription prices. All prices are subject to change without notice. POSTMASTER: Send address changes to *Physical Medicine and Rehabilitation Clinics of North America*, Elsevier Periodicals Customer Service, 11830 Westline Industrial Drive, St. Louis, MO 63146. **Customer Service: 1-800-654-2452 (US). From outside of the United States, call 314-453-7041. Fax: 314-453-5170. E-mail: JournalsCustomerService-usa@elsevier.com (for print support); Journals OnlineSupport-usa@elsevier.com (for online support).**

Physical Medicine and Rehabilitation Clinics of North America is indexed in *Excerpta Medica, MEDLINE/PubMed (Index Medicus), Cinahl,* and *Cumulative Index to Nursing and Allied Health Literature.*

Printed in the United States of America.

CONSULTING EDITOR

GEORGE H. KRAFT, MD, MS, Alvord Professor of Multiple Sclerosis Research; Professor, Rehabilitation Medicine; and Adjunct Professor, Neurology, University of Washington School of Medicine, Seattle, Washington

GUEST EDITOR

JEFFREY B. PALMER, MD, Lawrence Cardinal Shehan Professor and Director, Department of Physical Medicine and Rehabilitation, Johns Hopkins University; Physiatrist-in-Chief, Johns Hopkins Hospital; and Professor, Departments of Otolaryngology–Head and Neck Surgery and Functional Anatomy and Evolution, Johns Hopkins University School of Medicine, Baltimore, Maryland

CONTRIBUTORS

MIKOTO BABA, MD, DMSc, Professor, Faculty of Rehabilitation, School of Health Science, Fujita Health University, Japan

GISELLE CARNABY-MANN, MPH, PhD, Certificate of Clinical Competence in Speech Pathology, Research Scientist, Department of Behavioral Science and Community Health; and Co-Director, Swallowing Research Laboratory, College of Public Health and Health Professions, University of Florida, Gainesville, Florida

MICHELLE R. CIUCCI, PhD, Department of Surgery, Division of Otolaryngology-Head and Neck Surgery, University of Wisconsin School of Medicine and Public Health, Madison, Wisconsin

NADINE P. CONNOR, PhD, Department of Surgery, Division of Otolaryngology-Head and Neck Surgery, University of Wisconsin School of Medicine and Public Health, Madison, Wisconsin

STEPHANIE K. DANIELS, PhD, Research Service, Rehabilitation Research, Michael E. Debakey VA Medical Center, Department of Physical Medicine and Rehabilitation, Baylor College of Medicine, Houston, Texas

MARLÍS GONZÁLEZ-FERNÁNDEZ, MD, PhD, Department of Physical Medicine and Rehabilitation, Johns Hopkins University School of Medicine, Baltimore, Maryland

SHAHEEN HAMDY, PhD, FRCP, Honorary Consultant Physician and Clinical Senior Lecturer in Medicine and Gastrointestinal Sciences, University of Manchester, School of Translational Medicine, Gastrointestinal Sciences; and Faculty of Medical and Human Sciences, Salford Royal NHS Foundation Trust, Salford, United Kingdom

IANESSA A. HUMBERT, PhD, Assistant Professor, Department of Physical Medicine and Rehabilitation, Johns Hopkins University School of Medicine, Baltimore, Maryland

BRONWYN JONES, MBBS, FRACP, FRCR, Professor of Radiology, The Russell H. Morgan Department of Radiology and Radiological Sciences; Director, Johns Hopkins Swallowing Center, The Johns Hopkins Hospital, Baltimore, Maryland; and Editor-in-Chief, Dysphagia, Spring Publishers, New York, New York

ADEYEMI LAWAL, MD, Assistant Professor, Department of Medicine, Division of Gastroenterology and Hepatology, Medical College of Wisconsin, Milwaukee, Wisconsin

STEVEN B. LEDER, PhD, CCC-SLP, Professor, Department of Surgery, Section of Otolaryngology, Yale University School of Medicine, New Haven, Connecticut

MAUREEN A. LEFTON-GREIF, PhD, CCC-SLP, Associate Professor, Department of Pediatrics, Eudowood Division of Pediatric Respiratory Sciences, The Johns Hopkins University School of Medicine, Baltimore, Maryland

KERRY LENIUS, MS, CCC-SLP, Certificate of Clinical Competence in Speech-Language Pathology; Doctoral Candidate, Department of Communication Disorders, Florida State University; and Research Associate, Swallowing Research Laboratory, Department of Behavioral Science and Community Health, University of Florida, Gainesville, Florida

JERI A. LOGEMANN, PhD, CCC-SLP, BRS-S, Ralph and Jean Sundin Professor, Department of Communication Sciences and Disorders, Northwestern University, Evanston; Professor, Department of Neurology, and Professor, Department of Otolaryngology, Head and Neck Surgery, Feinberg School of Medicine, Northwestern University, Chicago, Illinois

BONNIE MARTIN-HARRIS, PhD, SLP, BRS-S, Director, MUSC Evelyn Trammell Institute for Voice and Swallowing; Professor, Department of Otolaryngology-Head and Neck Surgery, Communication Sciences and Disorders, College of Health and Rehabilitation Science, Medical University of South Carolina, Charleston, South Carolina

KOICHIRO MATSUO, DDS, PhD, Assistant Professor, Department of Physical Medicine and Rehabilitation, Johns Hopkins University School of Medicine, Baltimore, Maryland; and Associate Professor, Department of Special Care Dentistry, Matsumoto Dental University, Nagano, Japan

TIMOTHY M. McCULLOCH, MD, Professor and Chairman, Department of Surgery, Division of Otolaryngology-Head and Neck Surgery, University of Wisconsin School of Medicine and Public Health, Madison, Wisconsin

SATISH MISTRY, PhD, Post-Doctoral Research Associate, University of Manchester, School of Translational Medicine, Gastrointestinal Sciences; and Faculty of Medical and Human Sciences, Salford Royal NHS Foundation Trust, Salford, United Kingdom

JOSEPH T. MURRAY, PhD, CCC-SLP, BRS-S, Chief, Audiology/Speech Pathology Service, VA Ann Arbor Healthcare System, Ann Arbor, Michigan

SUMIKO OKADA, SLP, MS, Associate Professor, Faculty of Rehabilitation, School of Health Science, Fujita Health University, Aichi, Japan

JEFFREY B. PALMER, MD, Lawrence Cardinal Shehan Professor and Director, Department of Physical Medicine and Rehabilitation, Johns Hopkins University; Physiatrist-in-Chief, Johns Hopkins Hospital; and Professor, Departments of Otolaryngology, Head and Neck Surgery and Functional Anatomy and Evolution, Johns Hopkins University School of Medicine, Baltimore, Maryland

BARBARA R. PAULOSKI, PhD, CCC-SP, Associate Research Professor, Communication Sciences and Disorders, Northwestern University, Evanston, Illinois

JOANNE ROBBINS, PhD, Professor, Department of Medicine, University of Wisconsin School of Medicine and Public Health; and William S. Middleton Memorial Veterans Hospital, Geriatric Research, Education and Clinical Center, Madison, Wisconsin

EIICHI SAITOH, MD, DMSc, Professor and Chair, Department of Rehabilitation Medicine, School of Medicine, Fujita Health University, Aichi, Japan

REZA SHAKER, MD, Professor and Chief, Department of Medicine, Division of Gastroenterology and Hepatology, Medical College of Wisconsin, Milwaukee, Wisconsin

LIAT SHAMA, MD, Department of Surgery, Division of Otolaryngology-Head and Neck Surgery, University of Wisconsin School of Medicine and Public Health, Madison, Wisconsin

CONTENTS

evolving our understanding and thus ultimately helping to generate novel therapies for the treatment of swallowing problems after cerebral injury, such as stroke. This article provides a general overview of current knowledge of the neural control mechanisms that underlie the coordination of mastication, oral transport, swallowing, and respiration in humans.

implementation of rehabilitation interventions with the goal of promoting safe and efficient swallowing. An overview of the equipment needed for the laryngoscopic evaluation, how to conduct the examination, what can be visualized endoscopically, diagnostic parameters, the implementation of therapeutic strategies, and suggestions for future research are discussed herein.

and dine can have far-reaching implications. With age, the ability to swallow undergoes changes that increase the risk for disordered swallowing, with devastating health implications for older adults. With the growth in the aging population, dysphagia is becoming a national health care burden and concern. Upward of 40% of people in institutionalized settings are dysphagic. There is a need to address dysphagia in ambulatory, acute care, and long-term care settings.

Dysphagia in Stroke and Neurologic Disease 867
Marlís González-Fernández and Stephanie K. Daniels

Dysphagia is a common problem in neurologic disease. The authors describe rates of dysphagia in selected neurologic diseases, and the evaluation and treatment of dysphagia in this population. Applicable physiology and aspects of neural control are reviewed. The decision-making process to determine oral feeding versus alternative means of alimentation is examined.

Rehabilitation of Dysphagia Following Head and Neck Cancer 889
Barbara R. Pauloski

Patients who have cancers of the oral cavity, pharynx, or larynx may be treated with surgery, radiotherapy, chemotherapy, or a combination of these modalities. Each treatment type may have a negative impact on posttreatment swallowing function; these effects are presented in this article. A number of rehabilitative procedures are available to the clinician to reduce or eliminate swallowing disorders in patients treated for cancer of the head and neck. The various procedures—including postures, maneuvers, modifications to bolus volume and viscosity, range-of-motion exercises, and strengthening exercises—and their efficacy in patients treated for head and neck cancer are discussed.

Dysphagia Rehabilitation in Japan 929
Mikoto Baba, Eiichi Saitoh, and Sumiko Okada

This article describes the features of Japanese dysphagia rehabilitation, particularly where it differs from that in the United States. Many kinds of professionals participate in dysphagia rehabilitation; nurses and dental associates take important roles, and the Japanese insurance system covers that. Videofluorography and videoendoscopy are common and are sometimes done by dentists. Intermittent catheterization is applied to nutrition control in some cases. The balloon expansion method is applied to reduce pharyngeal residue after swallowing. If long-term rehabilitation does not work effectively in dysphagia due to brainstem disorder, the authors consider reconstructive surgery to improve function.

Index 939

FORTHCOMING ISSUES

RECENT ISSUES

VISIT OUR WEB SITE

**The Clinics are now available online!
Access your subscription at www.theclinics.com**

ELSEVIER
SAUNDERS

Phys Med Rehabil Clin N Am
19 (2008) xiii–xiv

PHYSICAL MEDICINE
AND REHABILITATION
CLINICS OF
NORTH AMERICA

Foreword

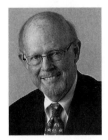

George H. Kraft, MD, MS
Consulting Editor

Dysphagia – [Gr: dys: difficulty + phagia: to eat]

Dysphagia, often confused with dysphasia—impairment of speech—can be a common and often life-threatening problem in disabled patients. The primary consequences of this disorder are: inability to manage secretions satisfactorily; inability to maintain adequate levels of nutritional intake, especially protein; and choking, and its sometimes fatal sequela.

Although an important rehabilitation problem that may be seen in a wide variety of disabilities, ranging from amyotrophic lateral sclerosis (see pages 624–625 in the August, 2008, Volume 19, Number 3 issue of *Physical Medicine and Rehabilitation Clinics*), to muscular dystrophy, stroke, spinal cord injury, multiple sclerosis, degenerative arthritis of the cervical spine, and many to many other disabling conditions, we have never had an issue of these *Clinics* on this specific topic until now.

Therefore, it is a pleasure to offer this issue on dysphagia to the reader of this series. I am very appreciative that Dr Jeffrey Palmer, a world authority on swallowing problems in disabled persons, and the Lawrence Cardinal Shehan professor, Director, Department of Physical Medicine and Rehabilitation, and Physiatrist-in-Chief at the Johns Hopkins Hospital and School of Medicine, agreed to Guest Edit this important issue.

"Dysphagia," the November, 2008 issue, contains 13 excellent articles, starting with the anatomy and physiology of feeding, followed by an article on the neural control of feeding. Next is discussed esophageal dysphagia, followed by three articles on evaluation of swallowing: the bedside examination, videofluoragraphic examination, and fiberoptic endoscopic evaluation.

1047-9651/08/$ - see front matter © 2008 Elsevier Inc. All rights reserved.
doi:10.1016/j.pmr.2008.08.002   *pmr.theclinics.com*

Following these articles on the anatomy, physiology, and evaluation, are a series of articles on management: surgical methods and management in the pediatric population, in the elderly, in stroke, and in head and neck cancer. Finally, the issue concludes with a bonus article on management of dysphagia in another culture: Japan.

This is one terrific volume. I am sure the reader will have it at the ready and frequently refer to it in the management of swallowing problems in disabled patients that she or he is following.

George H. Kraft, MD, MS
Alvord Professor of Multiple Sclerosis Research
Adjunct Professor, Neurology
Professor, Rehabilitation Medicine
University of Washington
1959 NE Pacific Street, Box 356490
Seattle, WA 98195-6490

E-mail address: ghkraft@u.washington.edu

ELSEVIER
SAUNDERS

Phys Med Rehabil Clin N Am
19 (2008) xv–xvi

PHYSICAL MEDICINE
AND REHABILITATION
CLINICS OF
NORTH AMERICA

Preface

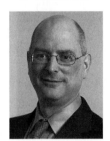

Jeffrey B. Palmer, MD
Guest Editor

I am delighted to present this issue of the *Physical Medicine and Rehabilitation Clinics of North America* dedicated to rehabilitation of dysphagia (abnormal swallowing). This field is my passion and has been the focus of my own research for the past 25 years. I was honored when George Kraft, one of my academic mentors, invited me to serve as guest editor for this issue. We have assembled a truly exceptional and multidisciplinary group of authors for this issue, including many of the leading authorities in dysphagia evaluation and treatment from the fields of speech language pathology, gastroenterology, otolaryngology, radiology, dentistry, and physiatry. I am grateful to these extraordinary people for taking the time to contribute to this volume.

The topics covered include the scientific basis for dysphagia rehabilitation, clinical bedside evaluation of dysphagia, instrumental evaluation (including videofluoroscopy and fiberoptic endoscopic evaluation), and principles of treatment (including rehabilitative and surgical approaches). Articles are devoted to the special problems of dysphagia resulting from head and neck cancer, stroke and neurologic disease, and esophageal disorders. Articles also are devoted to the special issues of dysphagia in children and in the elderly. There are unique efforts in the field of dysphagia rehabilitation in Japan, particularly extensive work on the use of balloon dilatation of the upper esophageal sphincter as a rehabilitation technique. Because of the importance of this work, an entire article is devoted to

Photo by Will Kirk, Homewood Photographic Services

1047-9651/08/$ - see front matter © 2008 Elsevier Inc. All rights reserved.
doi:10.1016/j.pmr.2008.08.001

dysphagia rehabilitation in Japan. Extensive references are provided with each article for further reading and as an evidence base for the authors' recommendations.

I am grateful to my colleagues and mentors for the opportunity to develop my special expertise in swallowing and its disorders. I am grateful to the late Dr. Arthur Siebens, who nurtured my interest in this field, and the late Dr. Karen Hiiemae, who was my partner in research for 15 years. My former students, residents, and fellows have taught me far more than I ever taught them. I am especially grateful to my current and former patients who inspire me to continue this work and move me on a daily basis with their inner strength and determination in the face of adversity. Thanks also go to Debora Dellapena for her excellent job editing each article.

Jeffrey B. Palmer, MD
Department of Physical Medicine and Rehabilitation
Johns Hopkins Hospital, Phipps 160
600 North Wolfe Street
Baltimore, Maryland 21287, USA

E-mail address: jpalmer@jhmi.edu

ELSEVIER
SAUNDERS

Phys Med Rehabil Clin N Am
19 (2008) 691–707

PHYSICAL MEDICINE
AND REHABILITATION
CLINICS OF
NORTH AMERICA

Anatomy and Physiology of Feeding and Swallowing: Normal and Abnormal

Koichiro Matsuo, DDS, PhD[a,b],
Jeffrey B. Palmer, MD[a,c,d,e,*]

[a]Department of Physical Medicine and Rehabilitation, Johns Hopkins University,
Phipps 160 600 North Wolfe Street, Baltimore, MD 21287, USA
[b]Department of Special Care Dentistry, Matsumoto Dental University,
1780 Hirooka Gohara, Nagano, Japan, 399-0781
[c]Johns Hopkins Hospital, Phipps 160, 600 North Wolfe Street, Baltimore, MD 21287, USA
[d]Department of Otolaryngology–Head and Neck Surgery, Johns Hopkins University
School of Medicine, Baltimore, MD, USA
[e]Functional Anatomy and Evolution, Johns Hopkins University School of Medicine,
Baltimore, MD, USA

Anatomy

Anatomy of structures

Understanding the normal physiology and pathophysiology of eating and swallowing is fundamental to evaluating and treating disorders of eating and swallowing and to developing dysphagia rehabilitation programs. Eating and swallowing are complex behaviors that include volitional and reflexive activities involving more than 30 nerves and muscles [1].

Fig. 1 shows the anatomy of the oral cavity, pharynx, and larynx; Table 1 lists the innervation of the major muscles related to swallowing. The tongue has oral and pharyngeal surfaces. The oral cavity is separated from the pharynx by the faucial pillars. The pharynx has a layer of constrictor muscles that originate on the cranium and hyoid bone and the thyroid cartilage anteriorly, and insert on a posterior median raphe. The submental muscles originate on the mandible and attach to the hyoid bone and tongue. The cricopharyngeus muscle is attached to the sides of the cricoid cartilage anteriorly and closes the upper esophageal sphincter (UES) by compressing it

---

* Corresponding author. Department of Physical Medicine and Rehabilitation, Johns Hopkins University, Phipps 160, 600 North Wolfe Street, Baltimore, MD 21287.
E-mail address: jpalmer@jhmi.edu (J.B. Palmer).

1047-9651/08/$ - see front matter © 2008 Elsevier Inc. All rights reserved.
doi:10.1016/j.pmr.2008.06.001

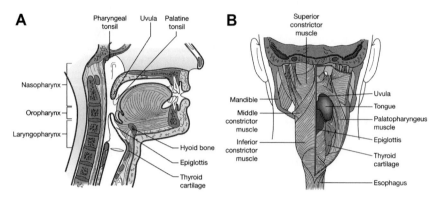

Fig. 1. Anatomy of the oral cavity and pharynx in the lateral (*A*) and posterior view (*B*). (*From* Moses K, Banks JC, Nava PB, et al. Atlas of clinical gross anatomy. Philadelphia: Elsevier; 2005; with permission.)

against the back of the cricoid cartilage. The epiglottis originates in the larynx and is angled upward and backward. It is attached to the hyoid bone anteriorly. The space between the pharyngeal surface of the tongue and the epiglottis is called the valleculae. The larynx includes the true and false vocal folds and the laryngeal surface of the epiglottis. The laryngeal

Table 1
Innervation of major muscles related to swallowing

Cranial nerves	Muscles
Trigeminal nerve (V)	Masticatory muscles
	Mylohyoid
	Tensor veli palatini
	Anterior belly of digastrics
Facial nerve (VII)	Facial muscle
	Stylohyoid
	Posterior belly of digastrics
Glossopharyngeal nerve (IX)	Stylopharyngeus
Vagus nerve (X)	Levator veli palatine
	Palatopharyngeous
	Salpingopharyngeous
	Intrinsic laryngeal muscles
	Cricopharyngeus
	Pharyngeal constrictors
Hypoglossal nerve (XII)	Intrinsic tongue muscles
	Hyoglossus
	Geniohyoid
	Genioglossus
	Styloglossus
	Thyrohyoid

From Palmer JB, Monahan DM, Matsuo K. Rehabilitation of patients with swallowing disorders. In: Braddom R, editor. Physical medicine and rehabilitation. Philadelphia: Elsevier; 2006. p. 6; with permission.

aditus (upper end of the larynx) opens into the lower portion of the pharynx. Lateral to the larynx are two spaces in the pharynx called the pyriform recesses.

Development of anatomy

The anatomy of the head and neck in infants is different from that in adults. In the infant, teeth are not erupted, the hard palate is flatter, and the larynx and hyoid bone are higher in the neck to the oral cavity. The epiglottis touches the back of the soft palate so that the larynx is open to the nasopharynx, but this airway is separated from the oral cavity by a soft tissue barrier (Fig. 2). The anatomy of the pharynx in humans changes with development. As the neck gets longer, the larynx descends to a position lower in the neck. The contact of the soft palate and epiglottis is lost, and the pharynx becomes longer vertically. This change in human development contributes to the development of speech, but because the pharynx becomes part of the food passageway and the airway (see Fig. 2), humans are vulnerable for aspiration.

Physiology

Two paradigmatic models are commonly used to describe the physiology of normal eating and swallowing: the four-stage model for drinking and swallowing liquid and the process model for eating and swallowing solid

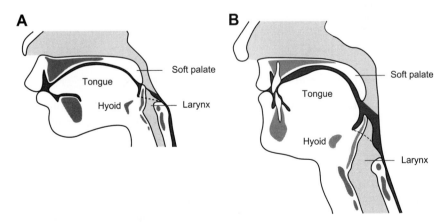

Fig. 2. Sagittal section of the head and neck in an infant (*A*) and an adult (*B*). The food passageway and the airway are shaded in dark gray and light gray, respectively. (*A*) In an infant, the oral cavity is smaller and the tongue and palate are flatter. The epiglottis is almost attached to the soft palate. The airway and food passageway are separated except when swallowing. (*B*) In an adult, the larynx is lower in the neck, and the food passageway and airway cross in the pharynx.

food. The normal swallow in humans was originally described using a three-stage sequential model whereby the swallowing process was divided into oral, pharyngeal, and esophageal stages according to the location of the bolus [2,3]. The oral stage was later subdivided into the oral-preparatory and oral-propulsive stages, thus establishing the four-stage model. Studies based on the four-stage model adequately describe the biomechanics and bolus movement during command swallows of liquids; however, this model cannot represent the bolus movement and the process of eating of solid food. Therefore, the process model of feeding was established to describe the mechanism of eating and swallowing solid food [4,5].

Oral-preparatory stage

After liquid is taken into the mouth from a cup or through a straw, the liquid bolus is held in the anterior part of the floor of the mouth or on the tongue surface against the hard palate surrounded by the upper dental arch (upper teeth). The oral cavity is sealed posteriorly by the contact between the soft palate and the tongue to prevent the liquid bolus from leaking into the oropharynx before the swallow. There may be leakage of liquid into the pharynx when the seal is imperfect, and this leakage increases with aging.

Oral-propulsive stage

During the oral-propulsive stage, the tongue tip rises, touching the alveolar ridge of the hard palate just behind the upper teeth, while the posterior tongue drops to open the back of the oral cavity. The tongue surface moves upward, gradually expanding the area of tongue–palate contact from anterior to posterior, squeezing the liquid bolus back along the palate and into the pharynx. When drinking liquids, the pharyngeal stage normally begins during oral propulsion.

Oral stage in eating solid food (process model of feeding)

The four-stage sequential model has limited utility for describing the process of normal eating in humans, especially that of food transport and bolus formation in the oropharynx [4–6]. When healthy subjects eat solid food, triturated (chewed and moistened) food commonly passes through the fauces for bolus formation in the oropharynx (including the valleculae) several seconds before the pharyngeal stage of a swallow. Additional portions of food can pass into the oropharynx and accumulate there while food remains in the oral cavity and chewing continues. This phenomenon is not consistent with the four-stage model because of the overlap among the oral-preparatory, oral-propulsive, and pharyngeal stages; the observable events during feeding on solid food are better described with the process model of feeding, which has its origin in studies of mammalian feeding [7] and was later adapted to feeding in humans [4].

Stage I transport

When food is ingested into the mouth, the tongue carries the food to the postcanine region and rotates laterally, placing the food onto the occlusal surface of lower teeth for food processing.

Food processing

Food processing immediately follows stage I transport. During food processing, food particles are reduced in size by mastication and are softened by salivation until the food consistency is optimal for swallowing. Chewing continues until all of the food is prepared for swallowing. Cyclic movement of the jaw in processing is tightly coordinated with the movements of the tongue, cheek, soft palate, and hyoid bone (Fig. 3).

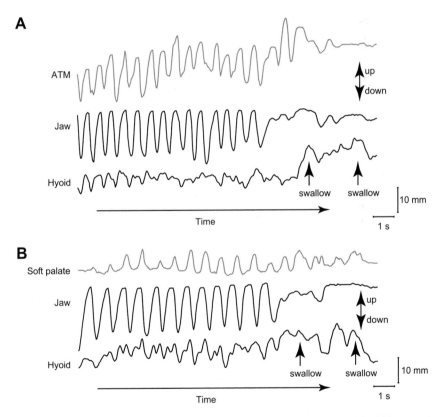

Fig. 3. Movements of (*A*) the anterior tongue marker (ATM), lower jaw, and hyoid bone, and (*B*) the soft palate, lower jaw, and hyoid bone over time, showing the vertical positions in a complete feeding sequence. Movement toward the top of the figure is upward. Positions of the structures are plotted relative to the upper jaw over time. Rhythmic movement of the tongue and soft palate is temporally linked to cyclic jaw movement. The hyoid also moves rhythmically; the amplitude of hyoid motion is greater in swallowing than in processing cycles.

During drinking of liquid, the posterior oral cavity is sealed by tongue–palate contact during the oral-preparatory stage when the bolus is held in the oral cavity. In contrast, during food processing, the tongue and soft palate move cyclically in association with jaw movement, permitting open communication between the oral cavity and pharynx [5,8]. Therefore, there is no sealing of the posterior oral cavity during eating. Movements of the jaw and tongue pump air into the nasal cavity through the pharynx, delivering the food's aroma to chemoreceptors in the nose [9–11].

Cyclic tongue movement during processing is coordinated with jaw movement [12]. Tongue movements during processing are large in the anteroposterior and vertical dimensions; jaw movements are similarly large in the vertical dimension (see Fig. 3A). During jaw opening, the tongue moves forward and downward, reaching its most anterior point in mid to late jaw opening. It then reverses direction and moves backward in late jaw opening, preventing us from biting our tongues when we eat. The tongue also moves medioalaterally and rotates on its long (anteroposterior) axis during chewing [13]. These motions are coordinated with cheek movement to keep food on the occlusal surfaces of the lower teeth. The hyoid bone also moves constantly during feeding, but its motion is more variable than jaw or tongue movements (see Fig 3A and B). The hyoid has mechanical connections to the cranial base, mandible, sternum, and thyroid cartilage by way of the suprahyoid and infrahyoid muscles. With those muscle connections, the hyoid plays an important role in controlling the movements of the jaw and tongue.

Stage II transport

When a portion of the food is suitable for swallowing, it is placed on the tongue surface and propelled back through the fauces to the oropharynx (Fig. 4). The basic mechanism of stage II transport is the same as described for the oral-propulsive stage with a liquid bolus. The anterior tongue surface first contacts the hard palate just behind the upper incisors. The area of tongue–palate contact gradually expands backward, squeezing the triturated food back along the palate to the oropharynx. Stage II transport is primarily driven by the tongue and does not require gravity [14,15]. Stage II transport can be interposed into food processing cycles. The transported food accumulates on the pharyngeal surface of the tongue and in the valleculae. Chewing continues when food remains in the oral cavity, and the bolus in the oropharynx is enlarged by subsequent stage II transport cycles. The duration of bolus aggregation in the oropharynx ranges from a fraction of a second to about 10 seconds in normal individuals eating solid food [5].

Pharyngeal stage

Pharyngeal swallow is a rapid sequential activity, occurring within a second. It has two crucial biologic features: (1) food passage—propelling

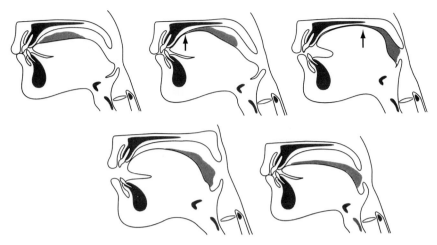

Fig. 4. Diagram of stage II transport based on a videofluorographic recording. The tongue squeezes the bolus backward along the palate, through the fauces, and into the pharynx when the upper and lower teeth are closest together and during early jaw opening phase (*first three frames*). The bolus head reaches the valleculae while food processing continues (*last two frames*).

the food bolus through the pharynx and UES to the esophagus; and (2) airway protection—insulating the larynx and trachea from the pharynx during food passage to prevent the food from entering the airway.

During the pharyngeal stage, the soft palate elevates and contacts the lateral and posterior walls of the pharynx, closing the nasopharynx at about the same time that the bolus head comes into the pharynx (Fig. 5). Soft palate elevation prevents bolus regurgitation into the nasal cavity. The base of the tongue retracts, pushing the bolus against the pharyngeal walls (see Fig. 5). The pharyngeal constrictor muscles contract sequentially from the top to the bottom, squeezing the bolus downward. The pharynx also shortens vertically to reduce the volume of the pharyngeal cavity.

Safe bolus passage in the pharynx without aspirating food is critical in human swallowing. There are several airway protective mechanisms preventing aspiration of the foreign materials to the trachea before or during swallowing. The vocal folds close to seal the glottis (space between the vocal folds), and the arytenoids tilt forward to contact the epiglottic base before opening of the UES [16,17]. The hyoid bone and larynx are pulled upward and forward by contraction of the suprahyoid muscles and thyrohyoid muscle. This displacement tucks the larynx under the base of the tongue. The epiglottis tilts backward to seal the laryngeal vestibule. The mechanism of the epiglottic tilting in human swallowing remains unclear but is probably related to hyolaryngeal elevation, pharyngeal constriction, bolus movement, and tongue-base retraction [18].

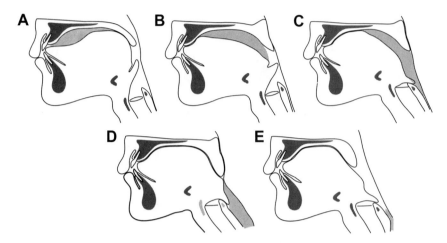

Fig. 5. Diagram of normal swallowing of a liquid bolus based on a videofluorographic record-ing. (*A*) The bolus is held between the anterior surface of the tongue and hard palate, in a "swal-low-ready" position (end of oral-preparatory stage). The tongue presses against the palate in front of and behind the bolus to prevent spillage. (*B*) The bolus is propelled from the oral cavity to the pharynx through the fauces (oral-propulsive stage). The anterior tongue pushes the bolus against the hard palate just behind the upper incisors while the posterior tongue drops away from the palate. (*C–D*) Pharyngeal stage. (*C*) The soft palate elevates, closing off the nasophar-ynx. The area of tongue–palate contact spreads posteriorly, squeezing the bolus into the phar-ynx. The larynx is displaced upward and forward as the epiglottis tilts backward. (*D*) The UES opens. The tongue base retracts to contact the pharyngeal wall, which contracts around the bolus, starting superiorly and then progressing downward toward the esophagus. (*E*) The soft palate descends and the larynx and pharynx reopen. The UES returns to its usual closed state after the bolus passes.

Opening of the UES is essential for the bolus entry into the esophagus. The UES consists of the inferior pharyngeal constrictor muscles, cricopharyn-geous muscle, and the most proximal part of the esophagus. The UES is closed at rest by tonic muscle contraction [19,20]. Three important factors contri-bute to UES opening: (1) relaxation of the cricopharyngeous muscle—this relaxation normally precedes opening of the UES or arrival of the bolus; (2) contraction of the suprahyoid muscles and thyrohyoid muscles—these muscles pull the hyolaryngeal complex forward, opening the sphincter; and (3) the pressure of the descending bolus—this pressure distends the UES, assisting its opening [21]. The most important of these mechanisms is the active opening process, making the opening of the UES different from other sphincters such as the external urethral sphincter, which opens passively (the urethral sphincter relaxes and is pushed open by the descending fluid bolus).

Esophageal stage

The esophagus is a tubular structure running from the lower part of the UES to the lower esophageal sphincter (LES). The LES is also tensioned at rest to prevent regurgitation from the stomach. It relaxes during a swallow and allows bolus passage to the stomach. The cervical esophagus (upper one third) is mainly composed of striated muscle, but the thoracic esophagus (lower two thirds) is smooth muscle. Bolus transport in the thoracic esophagus is different from that in the pharynx because it is true peristalsis regulated by the autonomic nervous system. After the food bolus enters the esophagus, passing the UES, a peristalsis wave carries the bolus down to stomach through the LES. The peristaltic wave consists of two main parts: an initial wave of relaxation that accommodates the bolus, followed by a wave of contraction that propels it. Gravity, in upright positions, assists peristalsis.

Bolus location at swallow initiation in normal swallows

The position of the head of the bolus relative to the time of pharyngeal swallow onset is a measure of swallow elicitation. The point at which the radiographic shadow of the ramus of the mandible crosses the pharyngeal surface of the tongue is commonly used as a marker for this measurement. It was initially thought that the pharyngeal swallow was normally triggered when the bolus head passed the fauces, as observed on videofluoroscopy [3]. When the bolus head passed the lower border of the mandible more than 1 second before the swallow initiation, it was classified as delayed swallow initiation. Delayed swallow initiation is considered an important finding because the airway is open when the bolus approaches the larynx.

Recent studies, however, have revealed that preswallow bolus entry into the pharynx also occurs in healthy individuals when drinking liquids [22–24]. Furthermore, as described previously, during eating of solid food, chewed bolus is aggregated in the oropharynx or valleculae before swallowing. Bolus position at swallow initiation is now known to be variable in normal eating and swallowing. This variability is especially true when consuming a food that has both liquid and solid phases. Saitoh and colleagues [15] demonstrated that in healthy young adults eating a food made up of soft solid and thin liquid components, the leading edge (liquid component) of the food often entered the hypopharynx before swallowing. As seen in Fig. 6, liquid enters the hypopharynx during chewing and approaches the laryngeal aditus at a time when the larynx remains open.

The location of the bolus at swallow initiation is altered by sequential swallowing of liquid [22,25–28]. The bolus head often reaches the valleculae before pharyngeal swallow initiation, especially when the larynx remains closed between swallows.

Coordination among eating, swallowing, and breathing

Eating, swallowing, and breathing are tightly coordinated. Swallowing is dominant to respiration in normal individuals [29–31]. Breathing ceases

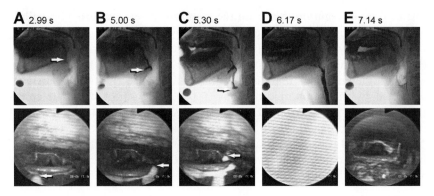

Fig. 6. Images of bolus entry into the pharynx while eating food with liquid and semisolid phases. Selected images from concurrent videofluorographic recordings (*top panel*) and fiberoptic endoscopic examination (*bottom panel*) of a normal subject consuming corned-beef hash and liquid barium. Numbers above the images indicate the time in seconds from the start of the recording. Arrows on the images indicate the leading edge of the barium. The liquid component enters the (*A*) valleculae, (*B*) hypopharynx, and (*C*) piriform sinus before (*D*) swallow initiation while the solid phase is being chewed in the oral cavity. There is no laryngeal penetration or aspiration (*E*).

briefly during swallowing not only because of the physical closure of the airway by elevation of the soft palate and tilting of the epiglottis but also because of neural suppression of respiration in the brainstem [30]. When drinking a liquid bolus, swallowing usually starts during the expiratory phase of breathing. The respiratory pause continues for 0.5 to 1.5 seconds during swallowing, and respiration usually resumes with expiration [32–34]. This resumption is regarded as one of the mechanisms that prevents inhalation of food remaining in the pharynx after swallowing [35]. When performing sequential swallows while drinking from a cup, respiration can resume with inspiration [36].

Eating solid food also alters the respiratory rhythm. The rhythm is perturbed with onset of mastication. Respiratory cycle duration decreases during mastication, but increases with swallowing [31,37,38]. The "exhale—swallow —exhale" temporal relationship persists during eating; however, respiratory pauses are longer, often beginning substantially before swallow onset [11,38,39].

Abnormal eating and swallowing

Dysphagia (abnormal swallowing) can result from a wide variety of diseases and disorders (Box 1) [40,41]. Functional or structural deficits of the oral cavity, pharynx, larynx, esophagus, or esophageal sphincters can cause dysphagia. Dysphagia may lead to serious complications, including dehydration, malnutrition, pneumonia, or airway obstruction. In dysphagia

---

Box 1. Diseases and disorders causing dysphagia

Neurologic disorders and stroke
Cerebral infarction
Brain-stem infarction
Intracranial hemorrhage
Parkinson's disease
Multiple sclerosis
Motor neuron disease
Poliomyelitis
Myasthenia gravis
Dementias

Structural lesions
Thyromegaly
Cervical hypertosis
Congenital web
Zenker's diverticulum
Ingestion of caustic material
Neoplasm

Psychiatric disorders
Psychogenic dysphagia

Connective tissue diseases
Polymyositis
Muscular dystrophy

Iatrogenic causes
Surgical resection
Radiation fibrosis
Medications

From Palmer JB, Monahan DM, Matsuo K. Rehabilitation of patients with swallowing disorders. In: Braddom R, editor. Physical medicine and rehabilitation. Philadelphia: Elsevier; 2006. p. 603; with permission.

---

rehabilitation, clinicians consider how a given abnormality affects bolus passage and airway protection.

Structural abnormalities

Structural abnormalities can be congenital or acquired. Cleft lip and palate is a congenital structural abnormality that hampers labial control for sucking, decreases the oral suction, and causes insufficiency of velopharyngeal closure with nasal regurgitation. Mastication can be impaired by the undergrowth of the maxilla and malalignment of the teeth.

Cervical osteophytes are bony outgrowths from the cervical vertebrae that commonly occurr in the elderly. They may narrow the food pathway and direct the bolus toward the airway (Fig. 7) [42]. Diverticulae can occur in the pharynx or esophagus. Zenker's diverticulum is a pulsion diverticulum of the hypopharynx that occurs at a weak spot in the muscular wall. Its entrance is located just above the cricopharyngeus muscle, but the body of the pouch can extend much lower [43]. The bolus can enter the diverticulum and be regurgitated to the pharynx, which may result in coughing or aspiration.

Webs or strictures may occur in the pharynx, esophagus, or sphincters. These abnormalities can obstruct bolus passage and are usually more symptomatic with solid foods than with liquids. A common site for narrowing is the UES. Failure to open the UES may be structural (due to a web or stricture) or functional (due to weakness of the muscles that open the UES) [44]. It is difficult to differentiate these conditions, and empiric dilatation is recommended. Stricture is common in the body of the esophagus and is often related to gastroesophageal reflux disease. It is important to consider esophageal carcinoma in the differential diagnosis, because this disease is serious and treatment can improve survival and quality of life.

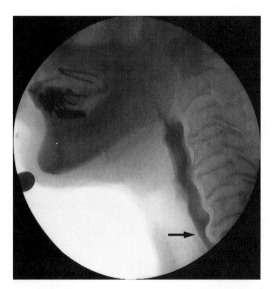

Fig. 7. A partially obstructive C6-7 anterior osteophyte (*arrow*) impinges on the column of barium, narrowing the lumen by more than 50%.

Functional abnormality

Impairments affecting the jaw, lips, tongue, or cheek can hamper the oral phase or food processing. Reduced closing pressure of the lips may lead to drooling. Weak contraction of the tongue and soft palate can cause premature leakage of the bolus into the pharynx, especially with liquids. In weakness of the buccal or labial muscles, food can be trapped in the buccal or labial sulci (between the lower teeth and the cheeks or gums, respectively). Tongue dysfunction produces impaired mastication, bolus formation, and bolus transport, which usually result from tongue weakness or incoordination, but sensory impairments can produce similar effects, including excessive retention of food in the oral cavity after eating and swallowing (Fig. 8).

Loss of teeth reduces masticatory performance. When chewing is prolonged due to missing teeth, particle size of the triturated bolus becomes larger due to lower efficiency of mastication [45]. Xerostomia hampers food processing, bolus formation, and bolus transport during eating. Chemoradiation therapy for head and neck cancer often causes delayed swallow initiation, decreased pharyngeal transport, and ineffective laryngeal protection [46].

Dysfunction of the pharynx can produce impaired swallow initiation, ineffective bolus propulsion, and retention of a portion of the bolus in the pharynx after swallowing. Insufficient velopharyngeal closure may result in nasal regurgitation and reduce pharyngeal pressure in swallow, hampering transport through the UES. Weakness of tongue-base retraction or the pharyngeal constrictor muscles can render inadequate the force of pharyngeal propulsion, resulting in retention of all or part of the bolus in the pharynx (usually the valleculae and pyriform sinuses) after swallowing. Incomplete tilting of the epiglottus may obstruct bolus propulsion, especially with higher viscosity boluses, resulting in retention in the valleculae.

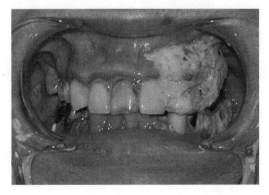

Fig. 8. Food debris retained in the left the buccal sulcus in the mouth due to buccal muscle weakness and sensory deficits caused by a right hemisphere stroke.

Impaired opening of the UES can cause partial or even total obstruction of the food passageway, with retention in the piriform sinuses and hypopharynx, increasing risk of aspiration after the swallow. Insufficient UES opening can be caused by increased stiffness of the UES, as in fibrosis or inflammation, or by failure to relax the sphincter musculature, as noted earlier. Weakness of the anterior suprahyoid muscles can impair opening of the UES, because these muscles normally pull the sphincter open during swallowing.

Esophageal dysfunction is common and often asymptomatic. Esophageal motor disorders include conditions of hyperactivity (eg, esophageal spasm), hypoactivity (eg, weakness), or incoordination of the esophageal musculature [47]. Any of these conditions can lead to ineffective peristalsis, with retention of material in the esophagus after swallowing. Retention can result in regurgitation of material from the esophagus back into the pharynx, with risk of aspirating the regurgitated material. Esophageal motor disorders are sometimes provoked by gastroesophageal reflux disease and, in some cases, can respond to treatment with proton pump inhibitors.

Airway protection—penetration and aspiration

Airway protection is critical to swallowing, and its failure can have serious consequences. Laryngeal penetration occurs when passage of the material transported from the mouth or regurgitated from the esophagus enters the larynx above the vocal folds. In contrast, aspiration is defined as passage of material through the vocal folds (Fig. 9). Laryngeal penetration is sometimes observed in normal individuals. Aspiration of microscopic

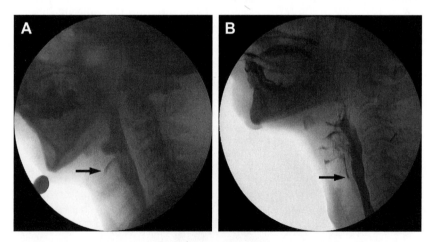

Fig. 9. Videofluorographic images of (*A*) laryngeal penetration and (*B*) aspiration in dysphagic individuals swallowing liquid barium. Arrows indicate the leading edge of the barium in the airway.

quantities also occurs in normal individuals; however, aspiration that is visible on fluoroscopy or endoscopy is pathologic and associated with increased risk of aspiration pneumonia or airway obstruction [48]. Aspiration can occur before, during, or after swallowing. Clinicians should consider the mechanism of aspiration when it is observed on fluoroscopy or endoscopy. Impairments of airway protection can result from reduced hyolaryngeal elevation, impaired epiglottic tilt, incomplete closure of the laryngeal vestibule, or inadequate vocal fold closure due to weakness, paralysis, or anatomic fixation. These impairments can lead to aspiration, usually during the swallow. Aspiration before the swallow is commonly caused by premature entry of liquids into the pharynx (due to impaired containment in the oral cavity) or by delayed onset of laryngeal closure after a bolus is propelled into the pharynx. Aspiration after the swallow is usually due to accumulated residue in the pharynx after the swallow. Material may be inhaled when breathing resumes after the swallow.

The consequences of aspiration are highly variable, ranging from no discernable effect to airway obstruction or severe aspiration pneumonia. The normal response to aspiration is strong reflex coughing or throat clearing; however, laryngeal sensation is often abnormal in individuals who have severe dysphagia [49]. Silent aspiration, or aspiration in the absence of visible response, has been reported in 25% to 30% of patients referred for dysphagia evaluations [49–51]. Several factors determine the effect of aspiration in a given individual, including the quantity of the aspirate, the depth of the aspiration material in the airway, the physical properties of the aspirate (acidic material is most damaging to the lung, producing chemical pneumonitis), and the individual's pulmonary clearance mechanism [52]. Poor oral hygiene can increase the bacterial load in the aspirate, increasing the risk of bacterial pneumonia.

References

[1] Jones B, editor. Normal and abnormal swallowing: imaging in diagnosis and therapy. 2nd edition. New York: Springer-Verlag; 2003.

[2] Dodds WJ, Stewart ET, Logemann JA. Physiology and radiology of the normal oral and pharyngeal phases of swallowing [see comments]. AJR Am J Roentgenol 1990;154(5): 953–63.

[3] Logemann JA. Evaluation and treatment of swallowing disorders. 2nd edition. Austin (TX): Pro-Ed; 1998.

[4] Palmer JB, Rudin NJ, Lara G, et al. Coordination of mastication and swallowing. Dysphagia 1992;7(4):187–200.

[5] Hiiemae KM, Palmer JB. Food transport and bolus formation during complete feeding sequences on foods of different initial consistency. Dysphagia 1999;14(1):31–42.

[6] Dua KS, Ren J, Bardan E, et al. Coordination of deglutitive glottal function and pharyngeal bolus transit during normal eating. Gastroenterology 1997;112(1):73–83.

[7] Hiiemae KM. Feeding in mammals. In: Schwenk K, editor. Feeding: form, function, and evolution in tetrapod vertebrates. 1st edition. San Diego (CA): Academic Press; 2000. p. 411–48.

[8] Matsuo K, Hiiemae KM, Palmer JB. Cyclic motion of the soft palate in feeding. J Dent Res 2005;84(1):39–42.

[9] Buettner A, Beer A, Hannig C, et al. Observation of the swallowing process by application of videofluoroscopy and real-time magnetic resonance imaging—consequences for retronasal aroma stimulation. Chem Senses 2001;26(9):1211–9.

[10] Hodgson M, Linforth RS, Taylor AJ. Simultaneous real-time measurements of mastication, swallowing, nasal airflow, and aroma release. J Agric Food Chem 2003;51(17):5052–7.

[11] Palmer JB, Hiiemae KM. Eating and breathing: interactions between respiration and feeding on solid food. Dysphagia 2003;18(3):169–78.

[12] Palmer JB, Hiiemae KM, Liu J. Tongue-jaw linkages in human feeding: a preliminary video-fluorographic study. Arch Oral Biol 1997;42(6):429–41.

[13] Mioche L, Hiiemae KM, Palmer JB. A postero-anterior videofluorographic study of the intra-oral management of food in man. Arch Oral Biol 2002;47(4):267–80.

[14] Palmer JB. Bolus aggregation in the oropharynx does not depend on gravity. Arch Phys Med Rehabil 1998;79(6):691–6.

[15] Saitoh E, Shibata S, Matsuo K, et al. Chewing and food consistency: effects on bolus transport and swallow initiation. Dysphagia 2007;22(2):100–7.

[16] Shaker R, Dodds WJ, Dantas RO, et al. Coordination of deglutitive glottic closure with oropharyngeal swallowing. Gastroenterology 1990;98(6):1478–84.

[17] Ohmae Y, Logemann JA, Kaiser P, et al. Timing of glottic closure during normal swallow. Head Neck 1995;17(5):394–402.

[18] Logemann JA, Kahrilas PJ, Cheng J, et al. Closure mechanisms of laryngeal vestibule during swallow. Am J Physiol 1992;262(2 Pt 1):G338–344.

[19] Cook IJ, Dodds WJ, Dantas RO, et al. Opening mechanisms of the human upper esophageal sphincter. Am J Physiol 1989;257(5 Pt 1):G748–59.

[20] Ertekin C, Aydogdu I. Electromyography of human cricopharyngeal muscle of the upper esophageal sphincter. Muscle Nerve 2002;26(6):729–39.

[21] Shaw DW, Cook IJ, Gabb M, et al. Influence of normal aging on oral-pharyngeal and upper esophageal sphincter function during swallowing. Am J Physiol 1995;268(3 Pt 1):G389–96.

[22] Daniels SK, Foundas AL. Swallowing physiology of sequential straw drinking. Dysphagia 2001;16(3):176–82.

[23] Martin-Harris B, Brodsky MB, Michel Y, et al. Delayed initiation of the pharyngeal swallow: normal variability in adult swallows. J Speech Lang Hear Res 2007;50(3):585–94.

[24] Stephen JR, Taves DH, Smith RC, et al. Bolus location at the initiation of the pharyngeal stage of swallowing in healthy older adults. Dysphagia 2005;20(4):266–72.

[25] Chi-Fishman G, Stone M, McCall GN. Lingual action in normal sequential swallowing. J Speech Lang Hear Res 1998;41(4):771–85.

[26] Chi-Fishman G, Sonies BC. Motor strategy in rapid sequential swallowing: new insights. J Speech Lang Hear Res 2000;43(6):1481–92.

[27] Chi-Fishman G, Sonies BC. Kinematic strategies for hyoid movement in rapid sequential swallowing. J Speech Lang Hear Res 2002;45(3):457–68.

[28] Daniels SK, Corey DM, Hadskey LD, et al. Mechanism of sequential swallowing during straw drinking in healthy young and older adults. J Speech Lang Hear Res 2004;47(1):33–45.

[29] Nishino T, Yonezawa T, Honda Y. Effects of swallowing on the pattern of continuous respiration in human adults. Am Rev Respir Dis 1985;132(6):1219–22.

[30] Nishino T, Hiraga K. Coordination of swallowing and respiration in unconscious subjects. J Appl Physiol 1991;70(3):988–93.

[31] McFarland DH, Lund JP. Modification of mastication and respiration during swallowing in the adult human. J Neurophysiol 1995;74(4):1509–17.

[32] Selley WG, Flack FC, Ellis RE, et al. Respiratory patterns associated with swallowing: part 1. The normal adult pattern and changes with age. Age Ageing 1989;18(3):168–72.

[33] Klahn MS, Perlman AL. Temporal and durational patterns associating respiration and swallowing. Dysphagia 1999;14(3):131–8.

[34] Martin-Harris B, Brodsky MB, Michel Y, et al. Breathing and swallowing dynamics across the adult lifespan. Arch Otolaryngol Head Neck Surg 2005;131(9):762–70.

[35] Shaker R, Li Q, Ren J, et al. Coordination of deglutition and phases of respiration: effect of aging, tachypnea, bolus volume, and chronic obstructive pulmonary disease. Am J Physiol 1992;263(5 Pt 1):G750–5.

[36] Dozier TS, Brodsky MB, Michel Y, et al. Coordination of swallowing and respiration in normal sequential cup swallows. Laryngoscope 2006;116(8):1489–93.

[37] Smith J, Wolkove N, Colacone A, et al. Coordination of eating, drinking and breathing in adults. Chest 1989;96(3):578–82.

[38] Matsuo K, Hiiemae KM, Gonzalez-Fernandez M, et al. Respiration during feeding on solid food: alterations in breathing during mastication, pharyngeal bolus aggregation and swallowing. J Appl Physiol 2008;104(3):674–81.

[39] Charbonneau I, Lund JP, McFarland DH. Persistence of respiratory-swallowing coordination after laryngectomy. J Speech Lang Hear Res 2005;48(1):34–44.

[40] Kuhlemeier KV. Epidemiology and dysphagia. Dysphagia 1994;9(4):209–17.

[41] Castell DO, Donner MW. Evaluation of dysphagia: a careful history is crucial. Dysphagia 1987;2(2):65–71.

[42] Di Vito J Jr. Cervical osteophytic dysphagia: single and combined mechanisms. Dysphagia 1998;13(1):58–61.

[43] Ferreira LE, Simmons DT, Baron TH. Zenker's diverticula: pathophysiology, clinical presentation, and flexible endoscopic management. Dis Esophagus 2008;21(1):1–8.

[44] Ferguson DD. Evaluation and management of benign esophageal strictures. Dis Esophagus 2005;18(6):359–64.

[45] van der Bilt A, Olthoff LW, Bosman F, et al. The effect of missing postcanine teeth on chewing performance in man. Arch Oral Biol 1993;38(5):423–9.

[46] Eisbruch A, Lyden T, Bradford CR, et al. Objective assessment of swallowing dysfunction and aspiration after radiation concurrent with chemotherapy for head-and-neck cancer. Int J Radiat Oncol Biol Phys 2002;53(1):23–8.

[47] Moayyedi P, Talley NJ. Gastro-oesophageal reflux disease. Lancet 2006;367(9528): 2086–100.

[48] Marik PE. Aspiration pneumonitis and aspiration pneumonia. N Engl J Med 2001;344(9): 665–71.

[49] Garon BR, Engle M, Ormiston C. Silent aspiration: results of 1,000 videofluoroscopic swallow evaluations. J Neurol Rehabil 1996;10(2):121–6.

[50] Leder SB, Sasaki CT, Burrell MI. Fiberoptic endoscopic evaluation of dysphagia to identify silent aspiration. Dysphagia 1998;13(1):19–21.

[51] Smith CH, Logemann JA, Colangelo LA, et al. Incidence and patient characteristics associated with silent aspiration in the acute care setting [see comments]. Dysphagia 1999;14(1): 1–7.

[52] Palmer JB, Drennan JC, Baba M. Evaluation and treatment of swallowing impairments. Am Fam Physician 2000;61(8):2453–62.

ELSEVIER
SAUNDERS

Phys Med Rehabil Clin N Am
19 (2008) 709–728

PHYSICAL MEDICINE
AND REHABILITATION
CLINICS OF
NORTH AMERICA

Neural Control of Feeding and Swallowing

Satish Mistry, PhD*,
Shaheen Hamdy, PhD, FRCP

*University of Manchester, School of Translational Medicine, Gastrointestinal Sciences,
Faculty of Medical and Human Sciences, Clinical Sciences Building, Salford Royal NHS
Foundation Trust, Salford, UK*

Eating and drinking are basic pleasures in life that most of us take for granted, yet the ease with which we perform these tasks belies their complex neurologic system of control. This article provides a general overview of current knowledge of the neural control mechanisms that underlie the coordination of mastication, oral transport, swallowing, and respiration in humans.

Oral feeding

The ability of organisms to maintain adequate energy stores is critical for survival and achieved through feeding. In mammals, this encompasses many factors, including the sight, smell, taste, texture, and temperature of food, all of which involve complex and interrelated neural circuits and responses that have been developed and honed through individual experiences. Some of these homeostatic and hedonistic mechanisms are beyond the remit of this article; feeding is discussed beginning with mastication or chewing.

The masticatory sequence

In humans, the processing of solid ingested material, regardless of size and texture, occurs in a stereotyped manner as categorized by Hiiemae and Palmer [1,2]. This process is termed the masticatory sequence and is composed of four main components.

* Corresponding author. University of Manchester, School of Translational Medicine-Gastrointestinal Sciences, Faculty of Medical and Human Sciences, Clinical Sciences Building, Salford Royal NHS Foundation Trust-Hope Hospital, Stott Lane, Salford, M6 8HD, UK.
 E-mail address: satish.mistry@manchester.ac.uk (S. Mistry).

1047-9651/08/$ - see front matter © 2008 Elsevier Inc. All rights reserved.
doi:10.1016/j.pmr.2008.05.002 *pmr.theclinics.com*

1. Stage I transport, during which food is ingested as a bite-sized portion and positioned on the occlusal surface (between the teeth) for further breakdown if necessary.
2. Processing, during which time trituration occurs. The number of processing cycles depends on how tough the ingested material is to chew.
3. Oropharyngeal accumulation time, during which adequately prepared food, ready for bolus formation, is moved distally through the fauces to the oropharynx (stage II transport) while processing of any remaining food continues.
4. Hypopharyngeal transit time, during which the bolus is swallowed.

The neurophysiology of mastication

Mastication itself is an intermittent, rhythmic process during which the masticatory muscles—tongue, cheeks, lips, palate, and jaw muscles (masseters, temporalis, lateral and medial pterygoids)—coordinate to mechanically break down solid food by way of the teeth into smaller fragments that are mixed with saliva to form a cohesive bolus that can be easily swallowed. Mastication is not a prerequisite of ingestion, because liquid boluses do not require this preswallow step; however, it is the first step of solid bolus digestion and is performed to greatly increase the surface area of ingested foods for more efficient breakdown by digestive enzymes. Until recently this motor task was believed to be solely under reflexive control, but it is now known to be voluntarily controlled through the actions of higher brain centers on the central pattern generator in the brainstem [2]. The fundamental rhythmic pattern of mastication (and therefore the jaw muscles) is controlled by the central pattern generator in the brainstem but is supplemented by the motor cortex, which initiates/stops mastication and also provides preprogrammed movement patterns based on expectations and sensory feedback in conjunction with the basal ganglia. Although under voluntary control, little conscious effort is required once mastication is initiated, with chewing largely occurring automatically. A recent study by Palmer and colleagues [2], however, demonstrated that food processing, transport, and bolus formation can be modified by conscious control. In particular, subjects were able to consciously inhibit stage II transport to the valleculae, thereby indicating a level of cortical control over the brainstem pattern generator. In another recent study by Onozuka and colleagues [3] the authors mapped out regional brain activity seen with functional MRI (fMRI) during gum chewing in healthy volunteers. They demonstrated increased cerebral perfusion bilaterally in the sensorimotor cortex, supplementary motor area, insula, thalamus, and cerebellum, areas also activated during volitional swallowing, implying that there is significant recruitment of cortical regions during chew activity, which overlaps with that seen during the swallowing phase.

The role of sensory feedback in mastication

Peripheral information from receptor systems in the dentures, tongue, cheek, jaw elevator muscles, and temporomandibular joint are also of importance [4–6]. Although they are not necessary during generation of the basic masticatory rhythm, they monitor the progress of chewing and modify commands sent to the appropriate effector muscles by significantly influencing the pattern generator directly and indirectly by descending motor pathways or through jaw reflexes. Degenerative diseases, lesions, infarction, and hemorrhages involving these areas can have profound effects on mastication and mandibular function [7,8]. The modulation of mastication for different foods has been demonstrated by several research groups over the years.

Hiiemae and colleagues [1] using videofluorography demonstrated that soft foods, such as banana and chicken paste, are processed much more quickly than hard foods, such as cookies or peanuts. In a separate study [9], they demonstrated that bite size also varied depending on food type and that food type influenced the parameters of the individual masticatory cycles and the overall duration of processing. Peyron and colleagues [10,11] observed significant differences between males and females chewing standardized artificial but edible foods. Increases were seen in the number of masticatory cycles and the activity in jaw-closing muscles, including the amplitude and velocity of jaw movements, as food hardness progressively increased. The number of masticatory cycles per sequence was also seen to increase gradually with age.

Although other sensory modalities also influence the masticatory sequence, food hardness is the predominant factor making up one of the three major inputs into the central pattern generator. This peripheral feedback system related to food hardness is provided through sensory afferents in muscle spindles and periodontal mechanoreceptors [5,6]. Nerve deafferentation studies in animals removing sensory feedback from periodontal receptors demonstrated reduced facilitation of masseter muscle activity, whereas destruction of spindle cell bodies almost completely removed that facilitation, thereby indicating the importance of these peripheral receptor systems in modulating masticatory muscle motoneuron activity.

Integration of the chemical senses

As mentioned earlier, normal feeding depends on the integration of several systems that include the chemical senses of smell (olfactory) and taste (gustatory). Together they give rise to flavor perception and are accounted for by three sensory systems: olfactory (Fig. 1), gustatory (Fig. 2), and trigeminal chemosensory. Olfactory information can influence feeding behavior, social interactions, and reproduction in many animals. The gustatory system provides information about the quality, quantity, pleasantness,

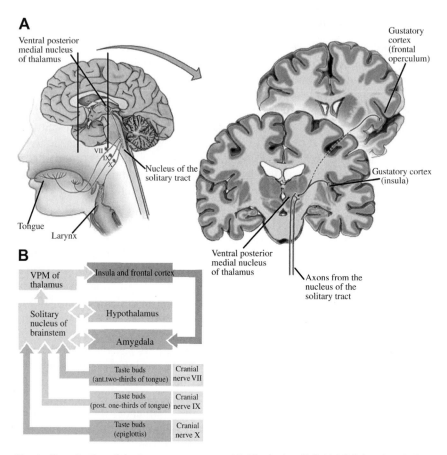

Fig. 1. Organization of the human taste system. (*A*) Illustration (*left*) highlighting the relationship between receptors in the oral cavity and upper alimentary canal with the nucleus tractus solitarius in the medulla. The coronal sections (*right*) show the ventral posterior medial nucleus of the thalamus and its connection with gustatory regions of the cerebral cortex. (*B*) Diagram of the basic pathways for processing taste information. (*Reprinted from* Purves D, Augustine GJ, Fitzpatrick D, et al. Neuroscience, 2nd edition. Sunderland (MA): Sinauer Associates Inc.; 2001; with permission.)

and safety of ingested food, whereas the trigeminal chemosensory system provides information about irritating or noxious stimuli.

Smell

The olfactory epithelium (approximately 10 cm^2 in an average 70-kg male) contains sensory receptors that detect and transduce information about the identity, concentration, and quality of a wide range of chemical stimuli termed odorants. This information is projected directly to neurons in the olfactory bulb by way of cranial nerve I (olfactory), which in turn projects to

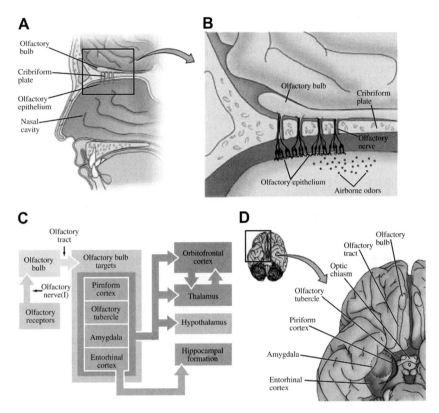

Fig. 2. Organization of the human olfactory system. (*A*). Illustration of the peripheral and central components of the olfactory pathway. (*B*) Enlargement of the region boxed in (*A*) illustrating the relationship between the olfactory epithelium, containing the olfactory receptor neurons, and the olfactory bulb (the central target of olfactory receptor neurons). (*C*) Diagram of the basic pathways for processing olfactory information. (*D*) Central components of the olfactory system. (*Reprinted from* Purves D, Augustine GJ, Fitzpatrick D, et al. Neuroscience, 2nd edition. Sunderland (MA): Sinauer Associates Inc.; 2001; with permission.)

the pyriform cortex (olfactory cortex) in the temporal lobe (see Fig. 1) and other brain regions, such as the amygdala, hypothalamus, and insula [12–16]. The olfactory system is thus unique among the sensory systems in that the thalamus is not involved en route to the primary cortical region processing the sensory information. Projections from the pyriform cortex and other forebrain regions, however, do provide olfactory information to several additional regions of the cerebral cortex (by way of the thalamus), where further processing identifies the odorant and initiates appropriate motor, visceral, and emotional reactions to olfactory stimuli [12,14].

Depending on the origin of the odorant, either from outside (orthonasal) or inside (retronasal) the body, different neuronal processing pathways also exist [17]. Orthonasal stimuli refer to odorants that are sniffed from the environment through the nares and are processed by the olfactory cortex and relayed to the primary olfactory cortex in the orbitofrontal cortex. Retronasal stimuli, however, refer to odorants released through the ingestion and breakdown of foods, causing volatile molecules to move backward from the oral cavity onto the olfactory epithelium through the nasopharynx. This olfactory pathway is only activated during nasal exhalation while masticating or swallowing and additionally incorporates taste, texture, and sound during the sensory processing.

Taste

The human taste system (see Fig. 2) acts in concert with the olfactory and trigeminal chemoreceptive systems to indicate whether or not food should be ingested. Once in the mouth, the chemical constituents of the food interact with (peripheral) taste receptor cells throughout the oral cavity, in lingual and extralingual locations, providing information about the identity (sweet, sour, salty, bitter, and umami), concentration, and pleasant or unpleasant quality [18–20]. This information helps to prepare the rest of the gastrointestinal system to receive food by causing salivation and swallowing, or gagging and regurgitation if the substance is noxious. In humans, two thirds of all taste receptor cells are located in the tongue, with the remaining third being distributed throughout the epiglottis, soft palate, larynx, and oropharynx [21–23]. Information regarding food temperature and texture (including viscosity and fat texture) is also relayed by way of sensory afferents in trigeminal and other sensory cranial nerves. This information is presented to cortical taste areas, such as the insula (primary gustatory cortex) and orbitofrontal cortex (secondary gustatory cortex), by way of the brainstem nucleus tractus solitarius and ventral posterior complex of the thalamus [14]. Projections also connect the nucleus tractus solitarius by way of the pons to the hypothalamus and amygdala, influencing appetite, satiety, and other homeostatic responses associated with eating [24,25]. These regions, also highlighted in human functional brain imaging studies [26–29], have close resemblance to cortical areas activated in human swallowing (see later discussion) and thus imply an important overlap of function.

Swallowing

For most people, swallowing or deglutition is a normal and effortless task, but despite its ease, it is a complex and dynamic sensorimotor activity involving 26 pairs of muscles and five cranial nerves. This complexity emerges as a consequence of the common shared pathway between the respiratory and gastrointestinal tracts and has arisen to avoid the threat of food or liquid entering the airway. Swallowing thus enables the safe delivery of ingested food, as a bolus, from the mouth to the stomach while ensuring protection of the airway. It is an integral component of feeding, learned during gestation, organized at birth [30], and essential for the continuation of life.

Traditionally, swallowing is divided into three conventional phases under volitional and reflexive control. They are the (1) oral, (2) pharyngeal, and (3) esophageal phases. Briefly, mastication and the oral phase refer to the volitional transfer of ingested material, as a prepared bolus, from the mouth into the oropharynx and are controlled by the discrete areas of the cerebral cortex. The pharyngeal phase is the first semi-reflexive component triggered by activation of cortical and subcortical brain regions, mainly the central pattern generator in the brainstem, which subsequently controls muscles in the oropharynx to deliver the bolus from the oropharynx to the relaxed cricopharyngeal muscle. The third and final phase, the esophageal phase, begins following closure of the upper esophageal sphincter. This later reflexive component serves the primary function of transporting food to the stomach by a sequential peristaltic contraction of muscles initiated in the pharynx and relaxation of the lower esophageal sphincter.

The neurophysiology of swallowing

The central neural control of swallowing is described as being "multidimensional in nature" [31] recruiting at all levels of the nervous system, and hypothesized to be organized in a hierarchical manner as shown in Fig. 3 [32]. The brainstem swallowing center, which contains the central pattern generator, is at the core of the system and represents the first level of control. Rostral to this and representing a second level of swallowing control are the subcortical structures, such as the basal ganglia, hypothalamus, amygdala, and tegmental area of the midbrain. Representing a third level of swallowing control are the suprabulbar cortical swallowing centers.

The importance of sensation in swallowing

Appropriate preparation of food relies on the continuous feedback of sensory information from receptors in the tongue, soft palate, floor of mouth, and tooth pulp, which detect the size and texture of the bolus, thereby determining the chewing action required from the muscles of mastication [33,34]. The pharyngeal phase of swallowing also relies on sensory input from the posterior oral regions and pharynx to initiate a response [35]. The intensity of pharyngeal muscle activity and overall duration of the pharyngeal phase of swallowing are not constant; they vary in response to sensory information relayed from afferent receptors about the unique characteristics of the bolus [36]. Anaesthetizing these mucosal regions locally has been shown to increase the time to evoke repeated swallows and may disrupt swallowing modulation, but does not eliminate swallowing completely [37–39].

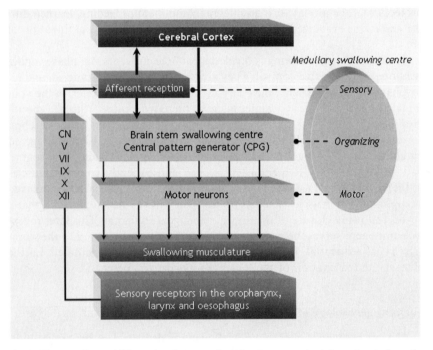

Fig. 3. The complex multidimensional nature of swallowing neurophysiology. Inputs from the periphery and higher brain centers converge onto interneurons in the brainstem swallowing center. The central pattern generator then organizes the sequential excitation of motor neurons controlling swallowing muscles by way of the bulbar nuclei. (*Modified from* Diamant NE. Firing up the swallowing mechanism. Nat Med 1996;2:1190; with permission.)

Sensory input to the swallowing tract therefore has three primary functions (1) to assist in initiating swallowing, (2) to modify the threshold for a pharyngeal swallow, and (3) to alter the level of muscle recruitment during swallowing [40]. Sensory information is carried by three cranial nerves: the trigeminal (V), glossopharyngeal (IX), and vagus (X) [41,42]; however, the most potent stimulus for triggering swallowing is delivered by way of the superior laryngeal nerve, a branch of the vagus nerve.

Innervation of the swallowing musculature

The motor innervation of the different swallowing musculature is provided through five cranial nerves by the release of acetylcholine at neuromuscular junctions. A brief description follows, but for an in-depth review of the deglutitive anatomy and its innervation, the reader is directed to an excellent review by Jonathan Cichero [43].

- Cranial nerve V (trigeminal). Sensory: conveys most sensory modalities (touch, temperature, pressure, and pain), except taste, from the anterior two thirds of the tongue, face, mouth, and mandible. Motor: innervates muscles of mastication and backward bolus propulsion.

- Cranial nerve VII (facial). Special sensory: conveys taste from the anterior two thirds of the tongue and soft palate by way of greater petrosal and chorda tympani, which also stimulates saliva secretion. Mixed-motor: supplies muscles of facial expression, particularly the lips, which prevent spillage during the oral phase of swallowing.

- Cranial nerve IX (glossopharyngeal). General sensory: mediates all sensation from posterior one third of tongue, oropharyngeal mucosal membranes, palatine tonsils, and faucial pillars. According to Zemlin, a lesion affecting this nerve can impair the gag reflex unilaterally [44]. Special sensory: conveys taste from posterior one third of tongue. Motor: in conjunction with the vagus nerve innervates the stylopharyngeus, which elevates and pulls anterior the larynx to aid cricopharyngeal relaxation. Secretomotor: stimulates saliva secretion from parotid gland.

- Cranial nerve X (vagus). Motor: responsible for raising the velum as it innervates the glossopalatine and the levator veli palatine muscles. Together with cranial nerve IX, pharyngeal branch innervates the pharyngeal constrictors and with cranial nerve XI (cranial root of the accessory nerve) innervates intrinsic laryngeal musculature. It is also responsible for vocal fold adduction during swallowing and cricopharyngeal relaxation. Muscles involved in the esophageal stage of swallowing and those that control respiration are also innervated by the vagus. Sensory: superior and recurrent laryngeal nerves carry information from the velum and the posterior and inferior portions of pharynx, and mediate sensation in the larynx. The superior laryngeal nerve is also important for swallowing and has been shown to potentiate the swallow response when combined with cortical stimulation [45,46]. At the thyroid cartilage, it divides into two branches: the internal, which supplies the mucous membrane of the larynx above the vocal cords, and the external, which supplies the inferior pharyngeal constrictor and the cricothyroid muscles.

- Cranial nerve XII (hypoglossal). Motor: innervates all intrinsic and extrinsic tongue muscles (except palatoglossus innervated by cranial nerve XI).

Brainstem control of swallowing

The brainstem swallowing center is located in the upper medullary and pontine areas of the brain and is bilaterally distributed within the reticular formation. This network of neurons is made up of three functional components: an afferent component, an efferent component, and a complex organizing system of interneurons known as the central pattern generator. Although the cortex is recognized to be responsible for the initiation of swallowing [31], the central pattern generator organizes the sequential excitation of motor neurons controlling the swallowing muscles [47]. These interneurons are believed to be organized in a temporal manner and have been referred to as early, late, and very late neurons corresponding with their counterparts in swallowing: the oral cavity, pharynx, and striated esophagus [48]. They are also separated into dorsal and ventral groups. The dorsal neurons lie within the nucleus of the tractus solitarius and the adjacent reticular formation, whereas the ventral neurons lie within the reticular formation and adjacent to the nucleus ambiguus. Dorsal neurons integrate both descending inputs from the cerebral cortex and afferent inputs arriving from cranial nerves V, IX, and X, of which the superior laryngeal branch, the superior laryngeal nerve, is the most important. Stimulation of any of these cranial nerves can initiate or modulate a swallow [47,48]; however, the most potent trigger for stimulating a swallow is carried by the superior laryngeal nerve. This trigger is matched only by direct stimulation of the nucleus of the tractus solitarius, suggesting that the solitary system is the major contributor of swallowing afferent input [47].

The afferent fibers also ascend by way of a pontine relay to the level of the cortex. The dorsal neurons activate the ventral neurons, which in turn activate the motor nuclei of cranial nerves V, VII, and X [47,48], thus triggering the swallowing motor sequence. Concurrent afferent excitation can facilitate swallowing in an intensity- and frequency-dependent manner [45,46,49–51]. Anesthesia of the areas innervated by these afferents disrupts, but does not completely abolish, the ability to swallow, therefore suggesting that sensation from the swallowing tract can have a modulatory effect on swallowing circuitry [39].

Evidence from animal studies suggests a significant role for subcortical structures in the control and modulation of swallowing [52]. These structures in the hindbrain (cerebellum), midbrain (substantia nigra and ventral tegmentum), and basal forebrain (hypothalamus, amygdala, and basal ganglia) have been shown to either induce swallowing or modulate the swallowing sequence after initial triggering by the cortex or superior laryngeal nerve. In humans, supportive evidence from clinical observations in patients who have neurologic disorders or lesions of the basal ganglia, such as in Parkinson's Disease, show marked difficulties in the coordination of oropharyngeal swallowing [53,54] with changes in the neurology of the subcortical structures, which can disrupt the normal feeding process and lead to dysphagia.

The role of the cerebral cortex in swallowing

The importance of the cortex in the control of human swallowing has been recognized for more than a century, dysphagia being first reported by Henry Charlton Bastian (1898) in a patient following hemispheric stroke [55]. Much of our understanding of the central brain control of swallowing has come from invasive animal studies artificially stimulating cortical swallowing areas. In anesthetized animals, electrical microstimulation of either cortical hemisphere is capable of inducing full swallow responses visible to the investigator, providing evidence that swallowing musculature is bilaterally controlled [38,46,56,57]. This evidence may suggest that both hemispheres play an equal role in controlling swallowing [31]. Pathophysiological evidence resulting from cerebral injury, such as stroke, suggests that one hemisphere may be dominant over the other [58].

Neurophysiologic imaging studies of swallowing

Recent advances in technological methodologies have allowed us to probe human swallowing in vivo. These techniques, which include transcranial magnetic stimulation (TMS), positron emission tomography (PET), magnetoencephalography (MEG), and fMRI have been used extensively to study swallowing in vivo.

Transcranial magnetic stimulation

TMS is a safe, non-invasive neurophysiologic tool, which in combination with pharyngeal electromyography (EMG) has been used to map the cortical representation of swallowing musculature in healthy subjects and in stroke patients recovering from dysphagia [59]. Unlike other brain imaging techniques, TMS does not rely on a task being performed; rather, it uses rapidly changing magnetic fields to stimulate neural tissue and elicit EMG motor evoked potential responses to probe cortical pathways from motor cortex to muscles (Fig. 4).

Early mapping studies by Hamdy and colleagues [59] demonstrated that human swallowing musculature is represented on both hemispheres (bilaterally) but one representation tended to be larger than the other (asymmetric in size), confirming the existence of dominant and non-dominant swallowing hemispheres. This finding from a large group of subjects was independent of handedness and discordant in a pair of identical twins, suggesting little genetic contribution to its development. They also demonstrated the different topographic cortical projections to the different groups of swallowing muscles. Esophageal, pharyngeal, and mylohyoid muscles are all discretely represented within the motor cortex, with each muscle group being represented (respectively) more anterolaterally than the previous, beginning most medially with esophageal muscles [59]. Pharyngeal responses evoked through bilateral, almost simultaneous stimulation of each pharyngeal motor cortex are larger and have shorter latencies than those evoked from each hemisphere independently, potentially demonstrating a possible convergence and summation of inputs on shared interneurons within the brainstem [60]. The excitability and representation of swallowing muscles can also be manipulated by performing a simple swallowing task using water [61] or differing flavors [62] by electrically stimulating them [61,63] or by stimulating the motor cortex directly [64,65].

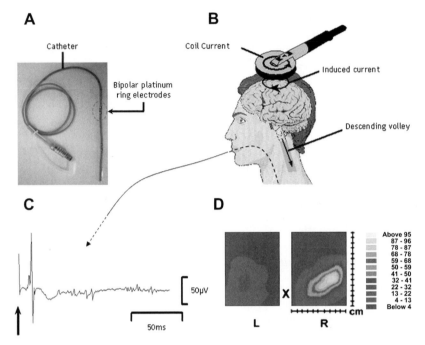

Fig. 4. TMS and recording of pharyngeal motor evoked potentials. (*A*) Intraluminal catheter housing a pair of platinum bipolar ring electrodes is used to record pharyngeal electromyographic responses evoked by performing (*B*) TMS over motor areas of the cortex. (*C*) A typical pharyngeal response elicited by TMS over the swallowing motor cortex. The arrow indicates the start of the TMS pulse. (*D*) TMS-generated pharyngeal representational scalp map as viewed from above, with the position of the cranial vertex marked X. The scale on the right represents the percentage maximum response amplitude across hemispheres. Asymmetry in the pharynx between the hemispheres is shown. (*Part D Reprinted from* Hamdy S, Rothwell JC, Brooks DJ, et al. Identification of the cerebral loci processing human swallowing with $H_2(15)O$ PET activation. J Neurophysiol 1999;81:1917; with permission.)

Although TMS has helped delineate some details of the organization of projections from motor cortex to swallowing and laryngeal muscles [66], this approach does not allow an assessment of cerebral activity associated with functional swallowing. The recent technological advances in functional imaging of the human brain have revolutionized our understanding of how the cerebral cortex operates in processing sensory and motor information. In particular, PET and fMRI have become established as useful methods for exploring the spatial localization of changes in neuronal activity during tasks, within cortical and subcortical structures [67]. PET and fMRI reflect changes in cortical function that are secondary consequences to alterations in regional cerebral blood flow, but have limited temporal resolution (1–2 seconds). MEG is a newer brain imaging modality that has recently overcome its own technical limitations [68] and is now being applied to the study cortical activations during swallowing. MEG is capable of directly recording neural activity within the brain dynamically with a spatial resolution equivalent to PET and fMRI (2 mm) but with a much superior temporal resolution of 1 millisecond [69,70]. All of these techniques have been applied to the study of human swallowing in vivo [63,71–87] and broadly speaking the results (summarized in Table 1) have been similar, confirming that this seemingly simple task recruits multiple discrete regions of the brain.

Positron emission tomography

PET studies using $H_2^{15}O$-labeled water [74,87] and fluorine 18 (F^{18})–labeled fluorodeoxyglucose [75] have shown activations in loci including: right orbitofrontal cortex, left mesial premotor cortex and cingulate, right caudolateral sensorimotor cortex, left caudolateral sensorimotor cortex, right anterior insula, left temporopolar cortex merging with left amygdala, left thalamus, right temporopolar cortex, left medial cerebellum merging across the midline with the right medial cerebellum, and dorsal brainstem. Strongest activations were found to be in the sensorimotor cortices, insula, and cerebellum (Fig. 5). This dominance was unrelated to handedness and correlates well with TMS observations from the same subjects assessing asymmetry of the swallowing musculature in the swallowing motor cortex [74]. These data demonstrate that swallowing recruits multiple cerebral regions, often in an asymmetric manner, particularly in the insula (predominantly activated on the right) and in the cerebellum (mainly on the left).

Table 1
Summary of the main cortical and subcortical activations associated with swallowing identified using different brain imaging modalities

Brain region	PET	fMRI	MEG
Sensorimotor cortex	✔	✔	✔
Insula	✔	✔	
Anterior cingulate	✔	✔	✔
Posterior cingulate		✔	✔
Supplementary motor cortex	✔	✔	✔
Basal ganglia	✔	✔	
Cuneus	✔	✔	
Precuneus	✔	✔	✔
Temporal pole	✔	✔	
Orbitofrontal cortex	✔	✔	
Cerebellum	✔	✔	
Brainstem	✔	✔	

Abbreviations: fMRI, functional MRI; MEG, magnetoencephalography; PET, positron emission tomography.

From Hamdy S. Role of cerebral cortex in the control of swallowing. GI Motility Online 200g. Available at:http://www.nature.com/gimo/contents/pt1/full/gimo8.html. Accessed March 11, 2008.

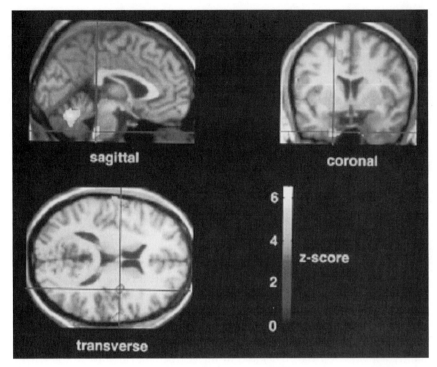

Fig. 5. Brain activations to swallowing as identified using $H_2{}^{15}O$-labeled water and PET. Areas of increased regional cerebral blood flow during swallowing rendered onto normalized T1-weighted MRI brain sections. The colored scale indicates the statistical z-score level of activations. Activations depicted in each of the sections are: cerebellum and dorsal brain stem (sagittal section), right and left sensorimotor cortex and right anterior insula (transverse section), and left mesial frontal and cingulate cortex and left temporal amygdala (coronal section). (*Reprinted from* Hamdy S, Rothwell JC, Brooks DJ, et al. Identification of the cerebral loci processing human swallowing with $H_2(15)O$ PET activation. J Neurophysiol 1999;81:1917; with permission.)

Functional MRI

fMRI has been extensively used to investigate swallowing. Activations seen during fMRI studies [73,76–78,81,82] have been in primary motor cortex, sensory motor cortex, supplementary motor cortex, anterior cingulate, insular cortex, and parietooccipital cortex. Cerebellum and brain stem have also been inconsistently implicated in deglutition; however, using current fMRI techniques, subcortical activations are more difficult to identify. These differences have mainly been attributed to the different swallowing tasks and functional modalities used by the investigating researchers.

Mosier and Bereznaya [82] reported five functional clusters—independent brain regions involved in volitional swallowing—with each area performing a specific role and providing input to the other areas and modulating the performance of deglutition (ie, premotor and parietal cortex supplying primary motor cortex with motor planning information). These areas are:

1. Primary sensorimotor cortex, supplementary motor cortex, and cingulate gyrus
2. Inferior frontal gyrus, secondary sensory cortex, corpus callosum, basal ganglia, and thalamus
3. Premotor cortex and parietal cortex
4. Cerebellum
5. Insula

Kern and colleagues [77] have previously compared cerebral activations during volitional swallowing with those seen during jaw clenching, lip pursing, and tongue rolling, and found that activations were similar, suggesting that some cerebral regions activated during swallowing may not necessarily be specific to deglutition. Cortical and subcortical regions, including primary sensorimotor cortices, are known to be involved in volitional swallowing, whereas reflexive swallowing seems to have (weaker) representation in other sensorimotor cortical regions [37]. The insula and the orbitofrontal cortex are also activated during studies looking at the representation of taste within the brain [26–29,88,89] and regions of the postcentral gyrus are also activated by processing of sensory information during swallowing [90].

Magnetoencephalography

Moving forward, swallowing studies using MEG [68,71,72,83,84,86,91] have been able to further add to our knowledge and compliment existing data from TMS, PET, and fMRI by providing more accurate temporal information about activations within the cortex. Abe and colleagues [91] were able to demonstrate bilateral activity in the anterior cingulate gyrus and supplementary motor areas 1000 to 1500 milliseconds before volitional water swallowing. Dziewas and colleagues [92] used MEG with a new analysis technique known as synthetic aperture magnetometry while subjects performed different swallowing tasks. The authors were able to show bilateral activation of the primary sensorimotor cortex during volitional water swallowing and tongue movements but no activity before reflexive water swallowing. In contrast, strongly lateralized activations of the left midlateral primary sensorimotor cortex were observed during volitional water swallowing, which were less strongly lateralized to the left during reflexive water swallowing and not lateralized at all during tongue movements. Left insula and frontal operculum activity was also observed but only during the preparation and execution of volitional swallowing. Taken together, these new findings suggest a left hemispheric dominance for the cortical control of swallowing in humans, providing further support for the existence of dominant and non-dominant swallowing hemispheres as seen with TMS [59].

Furlong and colleagues [71] dissociated the spatiotemporal cortical neuronal characteristics of volitional swallowing and demonstrated preferential activation in the caudolateral sensorimotor cortex during water infusion into the oral cavity, whereas volitional swallowing and tongue movements strongly activated the superior sensorimotor cortex. Temporal analysis further indicated that sensory input from the tongue simultaneously activated caudolateral sensorimotor and primary gustatory cortex, which seemed to prime the superior sensory and motor cortical areas involved in volitional swallowing. These data support the existence of a temporal synchrony across the whole cortical swallowing network, with sensory input from the tongue being critical. The importance of sensory input for the production of normal swallowing has previously been reported [61,93] and is further supported by Teismann and colleagues [84], who show that topical anesthesia of the oropharynx reduces sensory and motor activations in the brain. In a more recent article by Teismann and colleagues [83], the authors also show sensorimotor activity shifting, but in a time-dependent manner with neural activity moving from left to right sensorimotor cortex during deglutition with left hemispheric dominance in the early stage of volitional swallowing and right hemispheric dominance during its later part.

Integration with respiration

In addition, for individuals to feed orally in a normal manner, several processes must occur simultaneously, thereby requiring the integration of swallowing with several other functions, particularly respiration. Respiration, like swallowing and mastication, is controlled by many of the same neural areas, including the brainstem and cerebral cortex [94]. During a normal swallow, respiration must be temporarily halted, a process termed deglutition apnea. This process is centrally generated and occurs synchronously with but does not depend on laryngeal closure. Exhalation also typically occurs immediately before and after the swallow to prevent accidental inhalation of any bolus remnants. Successful feeding however, also requires effective coughing and intact upper airway reflexes, which includes retching, gagging, vomiting, and reflex swallowing [8].

Summary

The study of the neurologic control mechanisms that underlie the coordination of mastication, oral transport, swallowing, and respiration in humans is an exciting area of research with numerous unanswered questions. In this article we have provided an overview of current knowledge in the field and propose that significant advances in our understanding will still emerge with the application of modern imaging techniques, such as TMS, PET, fMRI, and MEG. As we continue to unravel more and more of these complexities, our expanding knowledge base should ultimately lead to the development of clinically important therapies for the future rehabilitation of patients who have swallowing difficulties.

References

[1] Hiiemae KM, Palmer JB. Food transport and bolus formation during complete feeding sequences on foods of different initial consistency. Dysphagia 1999;14:31–42.

[2] Palmer JB, Hiiemae KM, Matsuo K, et al. Volitional control of food transport and bolus formation during feeding. Physiol Behav 2007;91:66–70.

[3] Onozuka M, Fujita M, Watanabe K, et al. Mapping brain region activity during chewing: a functional magnetic resonance imaging study. J Dent Res 2002;81:743–6.

[4] Lund JP. Mastication and its control by the brain stem. Crit Rev Oral Biol Med 1991;2:33–64.

[5] Lund JP, Kolta A. Generation of the central masticatory pattern and its modification by sensory feedback. Dysphagia 2006;21:167–74.

[6] Turker KS. Reflex control of human jaw muscles. Crit Rev Oral Biol Med 2002;13:85–104.

[7] Bakke M, Moller E, Thomsen CE, et al. Chewing in patients with severe neurological impairment. Arch Oral Biol 2007;52:399–403.

[8] Hughes T. Neurology of swallowing and oral feeding disorders: assessment and management. J Neurol Neurosurg Psychiatr 2003;74(Suppl 3):iii48–52.

[9] Hiiemae K, Heath MR, Heath G, et al. Natural bites, food consistency and feeding behaviour in man. Arch Oral Biol 1996;41:175–89.

[10] Peyron A, Lassauzay C, Woda A. Effects of increased hardness on jaw movement and muscle activity during chewing of visco-elastic model foods. Exp Brain Res 2002;142:41–51.

[11] Peyron MA, Blanc O, Lund JP, et al. Influence of age on adaptability of human mastication. J Neurophysiol 2004;92:773–9.

[12] Cerf-Ducastel B, Murphy C. FMRI brain activation in response to odors is reduced in primary olfactory areas of elderly subjects. Brain Res 2003;986:39–53.

[13] Poellinger A, Thomas R, Lio P, et al. Activation and habituation in olfaction—an fMRI study. Neuroimage 2001;13:547–60.

[14] Rolls ET. Taste, olfactory, and food texture processing in the brain, and the control of food intake. Physiol Behav 2005;85:45–56.

[15] Sobel N, Prabhakaran V, Zhao Z, et al. Time course of odorant-induced activation in the human primary olfactory cortex. J Neurophysiol 2000;83:537–51.

[16] Zald DH, Pardo JV. Emotion, olfaction, and the human amygdala: amygdala activation during aversive olfactory stimulation. Proc Natl Acad Sci U S A 1997;94:4119–24.

[17] Shepherd GM. Smell images and the flavour system in the human brain. Nature 2006;444: 316–21.

[18] Breslin PA, Huang L. Human taste: peripheral anatomy, taste transduction, and coding. Adv Otorhinolaryngol 2006;63:152–90.

[19] Lindemann B. Receptors and transduction in taste. Nature 2001;413:219–25.

[20] Rolls ET. Smell, taste, texture, and temperature multimodal representations in the brain, and their relevance to the control of appetite. Nutr Rev 2004;62:S193–204, discussion S224–41.

[21] Bromley SM, RL D. Taste. In: Ashbury AK, McKhann GM, Ian McDonald W, et al, editors. Diseases of the nervous system—clinical neuroscience and therapeutic principles, 3rd edition. Cambridge (England): Cambridge University Press; 2002, vol. 1. p. 610–20.

[22] Kinnamon SC, Cummings TA. Chemosensory transduction mechanisms in taste. Annu Rev Physiol 1992;54:715–31.

[23] Schiffman SS, Gatlin CA. Clinical physiology of taste and smell. Annu Rev Nutr 1993;13: 405–36.

[24] Rolls ET. Sensory processing in the brain related to the control of food intake. Proc Nutr Soc 2007;66:96–112.

[25] Saper CB, Chou TC, Elmquist JK. The need to feed: homeostatic and hedonic control of eating. Neuron 2002;36:199–211.

[26] O'Doherty J, Rolls ET, Francis S, et al. Representation of pleasant and aversive taste in the human brain. J Neurophysiol 2001;85:1315–21.

[27] Small DM, Zald DH, Jones-Gotman M, et al. Human cortical gustatory areas: a review of functional neuroimaging data. Neuroreport 1999;10:7–14.

[28] Smits M, Peeters RR, van Hecke P, et al. A 3 T event-related functional magnetic resonance imaging (fMRI) study of primary and secondary gustatory cortex localization using natural tastants. Neuroradiology 2006.

[29] Zald DH, Hagen MC, Pardo JV. Neural correlates of tasting concentrated quinine and sugar solutions. J Neurophysiol 2002;87:1068–75.

[30] Hooker D. Early human fetal behavior, with a preliminary note on double simultaneous fetal stimulation. Res Publ Assoc Res Nerv Ment Dis 1954;33:98–113.

[31] Martin RE, Sessle BJ. The role of the cerebral cortex in swallowing. Dysphagia 1993;8: 195–202.

[32] Diamant NE. Firing up the swallowing mechanism. Nat Med 1996;2:1190–1.

[33] Anderson D, Hannam AG, Matthews B. Sensory mechanisms in mammalian teeth and their supporting structures. Physiol Rev 1970;50:171–95.

[34] Luschei ES, Goodwin GM. Patterns of mandibular movement and jaw muscle activity during mastication in the monkey. J Neurophysiol 1974;37:954–66.

[35] Shaker R, Ren J, Zamir Z, et al. Effect of aging, position, and temperature on the threshold volume triggering pharyngeal swallows. Gastroenterology 1994;107:396–402.

[36] Dodds WJ, Man KM, Cook IJ, et al. Influence of bolus volume on swallow-induced hyoid movement in normal subjects. AJR Am J Roentgenol 1988;150:1307–9.

[37] Ertekin C, Aydogdu I. Neurophysiology of swallowing. Clin Neurophysiol 2003;114:2226–44.

[38] Jean A. Brain stem control of swallowing: neuronal network and cellular mechanisms. Physiol Rev 2001;81:929–69.

[39] Mansson I, Sandberg N. Effects of surface anaesthesia on deglutition in man. Laryngoscope 1974;84:427–37.

[40] Miller AJ, Vargervik K, Phillips D. Neuromuscular adaptation of craniofacial muscles to altered oral sensation. Am J Orthod 1985;87:303–10.

[41] Ali GN, Laundl TM, Wallace KL, et al. Influence of mucosal receptors on deglutitive regulation of pharyngeal and upper esophageal sphincter function. Am J Phys 1994;267: G644–9.

[42] Miller AJ. Deglutition. Physiol Rev 1982;62:129–84.

[43] Cichero JA, Murdoch BE. Dysphagia: foundation, theory and practice. Chichester (UK): John Wiley & Sons, Ltd; 2006.

[44] Zemlin WR. Speech and hearing science: anatomy and physiology. Boston: Allyn & Bacon; 1997.

[45] Bieger D, Hockman CH. Suprabulbar modulation of reflex swallowing. Exp Neurol 1976;52: 311–24.

[46] Sumi T. Some properties of cortically-evoked swallowing and chewing in rabbits. Brain Res 1969;15:107–20.

[47] Jean A. Brainstem control of swallowing: localisation and organization of the central pattern generator for swallowing. In: Taylor A, editor. Neurophysiology of the jaws and teeth. London: MacMillan Press; 1990. p. 294–321.

[48] Jean A. Brainstem organization of the swallowing network. Brain Behav Evol 1984;25: 109–16.

[49] Beyak MJ, Collman PI, Valdez DT, et al. Superior laryngeal nerve stimulation in the cat: effect on oropharyngeal swallowing, oesophageal motility and lower oesophageal sphincter activity. Neurogastroenterol Motil 1997;9:117–27.

[50] Jean A, Car A. Inputs to the swallowing medullary neurons from the peripheral afferent fibers and the swallowing cortical area. Brain Res 1979;178:567–72.

[51] Miller AJ. Characteristics of the swallowing reflex induced by peripheral nerve and brain stem stimulation. Exp Neurol 1972;34:210–22.

[52] Hockman CH, Bieger D, Weerasuriya A. Supranuclear pathways of swallowing. Prog Neurobiol 1979;12:15–32.

[53] Bernheimer H, Birkmayer W, Hornykiewicz O, et al. Brain dopamine and the syndromes of Parkinson and Huntington. Clinical, morphological and neurochemical correlations. J Neurol Sci 1973;20:415–55.

[54] Leopold NA, Kagel MC. Pharyngo-oesophageal dysphagia in Parkinsons disease. Dysphagia 1997;12:11–8.

[55] Bastian HC. A treatise on aphasia and other speech defects. London: Lewis; 1898.

[56] Hamdy S, Xue S, Valdez D, et al. Induction of cortical swallowing activity by transcranial magnetic stimulation in the anaesthetized cat. Neurogastroenterol Motil 2001; 13:65–72.

[57] Martin RE, Kemppainen P, Masuda Y, et al. Features of cortically evoked swallowing in the awake primate (Macaca fascicularis). J Neurophysiol 1999;82:1529–41.

[58] Robbins J, Levine RL, Maser A, et al. Swallowing after unilateral stroke of the cerebral cortex. Arch Phys Med Rehabil 1993;74:1295–300.

[59] Hamdy S, Aziz Q, Rothwell JC, et al. The cortical topography of human swallowing musculature in health and disease. Nat Med 1996;2:1217–24.

[60] Hamdy S, Aziz Q, Rothwell JC, et al. Sensorimotor modulation of human cortical swallowing pathways. J Physiol 1998;506(Pt 3):857–66.

[61] Fraser C, Rothwell J, Power M, et al. Differential changes in human pharyngoesophageal motor excitability induced by swallowing, pharyngeal stimulation, and anesthesia. Am J Physiol Gastrointest Liver Physiol 2003;285:G137–44.

[62] Mistry S, Rothwell JC, Thompson DG, et al. Modulation of human cortical swallowing motor pathways after pleasant and aversive taste stimuli. Am J Physiol Gastrointest Liver Physiol 2006;291:G666–71.

[63] Fraser C, Power M, Hamdy S, et al. Driving plasticity in human adult motor cortex is associated with improved motor function after brain injury. Neuron 2002;34:831–40.

[64] Gow D, Rothwell J, Hobson A, et al. Induction of long-term plasticity in human swallowing motor cortex following repetitive cortical stimulation. Clin Neurophysiol 2004;115:1044–51.

[65] Mistry S, Verin E, Singh S, et al. Unilateral suppression of pharyngeal motor cortex to repetitive transcranial magnetic stimulation reveals functional asymmetry in the hemispheric projections to human swallowing. J Physiol 2007;585:525–38.

[66] Rodel RM, Olthoff A, Tergau F, et al. Human cortical motor representation of the larynx as assessed by transcranial magnetic stimulation (TMS). Laryngoscope 2004;114:918–22.

[67] Humbert IA, Robbins J. Normal swallowing and functional magnetic resonance imaging: a systematic review. Dysphagia 2007;22:266–75.

[68] Loose R, Hamdy S, Enck P. Magnetoencephalographic response characteristics associated with tongue movement. Dysphagia 2001;16:183–5.

[69] Gerloff C, Uenishi N, Nagamine T, et al. Cortical activation during fast repetitive finger movements in humans: steady-state movement-related magnetic fields and their cortical generators. Electroencephalogr Clin Neurophysiol 1998;109:444–53.

[70] Nagamine T, Kajola M, Salmelin R, et al. Movement-related slow cortical magnetic fields and changes of spontaneous MEG- and EEG-brain rhythms. Electroencephalogr Clin Neurophysiol 1996;99:274–86.

[71] Furlong PL, Hobson AR, Aziz Q, et al. Dissociating the spatio-temporal characteristics of cortical neuronal activity associated with human volitional swallowing in the healthy adult brain. Neuroimage 2004;22:1447–55.

[72] Gow D, Hobson AR, Furlong P, et al. Characterising the central mechanisms of sensory modulation in human swallowing motor cortex. Clin Neurophysiol 2004;115:2382–90.

[73] Hamdy S, Mikulis DJ, Crawley A, et al. Cortical activation during human volitional swallowing: an event-related fMRI study. Am J Physiol 1999;277:G219–25.

[74] Hamdy S, Rothwell JC, Brooks DJ, et al. Identification of the cerebral loci processing human swallowing with H2(15)O PET activation. J Neurophysiol 1999;81:1917–26.

[75] Harris ML, Julyan P, Kulkarni B, et al. Mapping metabolic brain activation during human volitional swallowing: a positron emission tomography study using [18F]fluorodeoxyglucose. J Cereb Blood Flow Metab 2005;25:520–6.

[76] Hartnick CJ, Rudolph C, Willging JP, et al. Functional magnetic resonance imaging of the pediatric swallow: imaging the cortex and the brainstem. Laryngoscope 2001;111:1183–91.

[77] Kern M, Birn R, Jaradeh S, et al. Swallow-related cerebral cortical activity maps are not specific to deglutition. Am J Physiol Gastrointest Liver Physiol 2001;280:G531–8.

[78] Kern MK, Jaradeh S, Arndorfer RC, et al. Cerebral cortical representation of reflexive and volitional swallowing in humans. Am J Physiol Gastrointest Liver Physiol 2001;280: G354–60.

[79] Martin R, Barr A, Macintosh B, et al. Cerebral cortical processing of swallowing in older adults. Exp Brain Res 2007;176:12–22.

[80] Mosier K, Bereznaya I. Parallel cortical networks for volitional control of swallowing in humans. Exp Brain Res 2001;140:280–9.

[81] Mosier K, Patel R, Liu WC, et al. Cortical representation of swallowing in normal adults: functional implications. Laryngoscope 1999;109:1417–23.

[82] Suzuki M, Asada Y, Ito J, et al. Activation of cerebellum and basal ganglia on volitional swallowing detected by functional magnetic resonance imaging. Dysphagia 2003;18:71–7.

[83] Teismann IK, Dziewas R, Steinstraeter O, et al. Time-dependent hemispheric shift of the cortical control of volitional swallowing. Hum Brain Mapp 2007.

[84] Teismann IK, Steinstraeter O, Stoeckigt K, et al. Functional oropharyngeal sensory disruption interferes with the cortical control of swallowing. BMC Neurosci 2007;8:62.

[85] Toogood JA, Barr AM, Stevens TK, et al. Discrete functional contributions of cerebral cortical foci in voluntary swallowing: a functional magnetic resonance imaging (fMRI) "Go, No-Go" study. Exp Brain Res 2005;161:81–90.

[86] Watanabe Y, Abe S, Ishikawa T, et al. Cortical regulation during the early stage of initiation of voluntary swallowing in humans. Dysphagia 2004;19:100–8.

[87] Zald DH, Pardo JV. The functional neuroanatomy of voluntary swallowing. Ann Neurol 1999;46:281–6.

[88] de Araujo IE, Kringelbach ML, Rolls ET, et al. Representation of umami taste in the human brain. J Neurophysiol 2003;90:313–9.

[89] Ogawa H, Wakita M, Hasegawa K, et al. Functional MRI detection of activation in the primary gustatory cortices in humans. Chem Senses 2005;30(7):583–92.

[90] Martin RE, Goodyear BG, Gati JS, et al. Cerebral cortical representation of automatic and volitional swallowing in humans. J Neurophysiol 2001;85(2):938–50.

[91] Abe S, Wantanabe Y, Shintani M, et al. Magnetoencephalographic study of the starting point of voluntary swallowing. Cranio 2003;21:46–9.

[92] Dziewas R, Soros P, Ishii R, et al. Neuroimaging evidence for cortical involvement in the preparation and in the act of swallowing. Neuroimage 2003;20:135–44.

[93] Chee C, Arshad S, Singh S, et al. The influence of chemical gustatory stimuli and oral anaesthesia on healthy human pharyngeal swallowing. Chem Senses 2005;30:393–400.

[94] Butler JE. Drive to the human respiratory muscles. Respir Physiolo Neurobiol 2007;159: 115–26.

ELSEVIER
SAUNDERS

Phys Med Rehabil Clin N Am
19 (2008) 729–745

PHYSICAL MEDICINE
AND REHABILITATION
CLINICS OF
NORTH AMERICA

Esophageal Dysphagia

Adeyemi Lawal, MD, MBBS, Reza Shaker, MD*

*Medical College of Wisconsin, Department of Medicine,
Division of Gastroenterology and Hepatology, Froedtert East, FEC-4510,
9200 West Wisconsin Avenue, Milwaukee, WI 53226, USA*

Dysphagia is the sensation of food being hindered during the passage from the mouth through the esophagus and into the stomach. Dysphagia is traditionally classified as oropharyngeal or esophageal dysphagia. Oropharyngeal dysphagia is the inability to initiate a swallow or inability to transfer food from the mouth to the upper esophagus whereas esophageal dysphagia is the impedance of food passage through the tubular esophagus once the food has successfully passed into the proximal esophagus.

A variety of mechanical and neuromuscular disorders can impede the passage of the food bolus through the esophagus (Table 1). Patients who have an inflammatory process may have associated odynophagia. Most patients often report food "hanging up" or "sticking" behind the sternum and lump or food being caught at the epigastrium. Patients are able to localize the site correctly in only 70% of cases, with 30% localizing the dysfunction proximally in the esophagus, suprasternal notch, or the throat.

Evaluation of patients with esophageal dysphagia

The importance of detailed medical history cannot be overemphasized in the evaluation of patients presenting with dysphagia [1,2]. Careful history about the type of food that causes symptoms is extremely important as patients may present with solid and/or liquid food dysphagia. Isolated solid food dysphagia suggests a mechanical cause for symptoms whereas both solid and/or liquid food dysphagia points to a neuromuscular etiology. Duration and temporal progression of symptoms are also important; intermittent symptoms may suggest a mechanical cause, such as Schatzki's ring (solid dysphagia) or a neuromuscular disorder, such as esophageal spasm

* Corresponding author.
E-mail address: rshaker@mcw.edu (R. Shaker).

doi:10.1016/j.pmr.2008.07.003
pmr.theclinics.com

Table 1
Etiology of esophageal dysphagia

Mechanical disorders	Neuromuscular disorders	Inflammatory process
Intrinsic causes	a) Achalasia	a) Eosinophilic esophagitis
a) Esophageal rings and webs. eg, Schatzki's ring, Plummer-Vinson, or the Patterson-Kelly syndrome (Iron deficiency anemia and esophageal web)	b) Scleroderma	b) Radiation esophagitis
	c) Nutcracker esophagus	c) Caustic injury
	d) Diffuse esophageal spasm	d) Pill esophagitis
	e) Ineffective esophageal motility disorder	e) Infectious esophagitis: Candidiasis, herpes simplex, cytomegalovirus, or HIV-associated esophagitis
	f) Hypertensive LES	
b) Peptic stricture from gastroesophageal reflux or scleroderma	g) Others: chagas' disease, paraneoplastic syndrome	
c) Carcinoma: Squamous cell cancer and adenocarcinoma		
d) Others: Diverticulae and benign tumors		
e) Post-surgery (laryngeal, esophageal, gastric cancers, fundoplication)		
Extrinsic causes		
Mediastinal mass (lymph nodes, thyromegaly, lung cancer)		
Vascular compression (Enlarged left atrium, aberrant right subclavian artery, or right-sided aorta)		
Cervical spine osteophytes (spurs)		

(solid and liquid dysphagia). A short-duration and rapidly progressive dysphagia is concerning for malignancy. Solid food dysphagia progressing to liquid dysphagia suggests a mechanical problem, which may be benign (peptic stricture) or malignant (adenocarcinoma). Other symptoms such as weight loss, regurgitation of food particles, heartburn, pain during swallowing, or chest pain, as well as medications may give important clues to the etiology of dysphagia. Heartburn symptoms in a patient with dysphagia may suggest complications from acid reflux-induced peptic stricture or adenocarcinoma (solid only or solid progressing to liquid) or scleroderma esophagus (both solid and liquid dysphagia). The caveat is that 25% to 30% of patients presenting with dysphagia due to peptic stricture or adenocarcinoma do not have heartburn at the time of diagnosis [3,4]. An algorithm for evaluating patients with esophageal dysphagia is shown in the following paragraphs (Fig. 1).

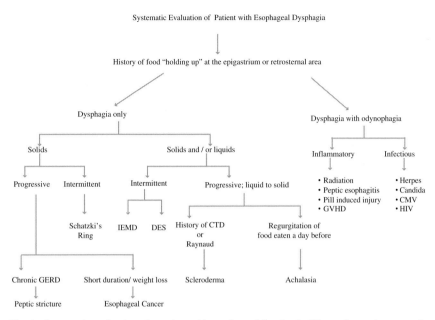

Fig. 1. Systematic evaluation of a patient with esophageal dysphagia. History is very important in elucidating etiology and management. CMV, cytomegalo virus; CTD, connective tissue disease; DES, diffuse esophageal spasm; GERD, gastro esophageal reflux disease; GVHD, graft versus host disease; HIV, human immunodeficiency virus; IEMD, ineffective esophageal motility disorder.

Investigation of patients with esophageal dysphagia should be based on history. If the history is suggestive of a mechanical disorder, upper endoscopy or barium radiography should be requested. However, if history is suggestive of a motility disorder, then manometry is the first diagnostic test. Upper endoscopy is recommended to assess mucosa injury, provide opportunity for biopsy to rule out microscopic disease in a normal appearing esophagus, and to perform therapeutic intervention such as dilatation. Barium radiography with barium-impregnated marshmallow or barium tablet challenge may identify intraesophageal structural abnormalities, site, and length of stricture. High-resolution esophageal manometry is the gold standard for evaluating suspected motility disorder and should be requested if upper endoscopy and radiological studies are negative. The diagnostic algorithm for esophageal dysphagia is shown in Fig. 2.

Epidemiology, etiology, clinical features, and management of differential diagnosis of esophageal dysphagia

Esophageal rings and webs

Esophageal webs are thin mucosal folds that protrude into the lumen and are covered with squamous epithelium. They can be congenital or acquired; congenital webs are rare, seen in pediatrics and usually occur in the middle

Management of Esophageal Dysphagia

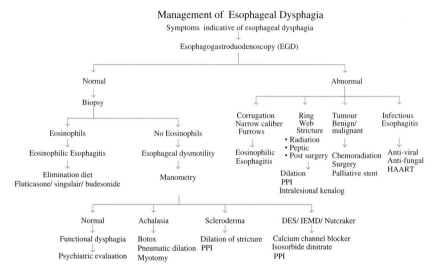

Fig. 2. Management of esophageal dysphagia: Diagnostic approach and treatment. DES, diffuse esophageal spasm; HAART, highly active anti retrovirus therapy; IEMD, ineffective esophageal motility disorder; PPI, proton pump inhibitor.

and lower thirds of the esophagus. They arise from failure of complete coalescence of esophageal vacuoles during embryologic development [5]. Acquired webs are more common than congenital webs and are often located in the cervical esophagus in the post-cricoid region, causing luminal narrowing and dysphagia. Cervical webs are typically diaphragm-like in nature.

Most patients with esophageal webs are asymptomatic and thus the true prevalence of acquired webs is unknown. Esophageal webs are twice as common in women as in men [6], with symptoms occurring more commonly in women than in men. Acquired esophageal webs have been reported in association with gastroesophageal reflux disease [7] and iron-deficiency anemia as in Plummer-Vinson syndrome or Paterson-Kelly syndrome. Others include their association with dermatologic or systemic diseases, such as pemphigus vulgaris [8], epidermolysis bullosa [9], bullous pemphigoid [10], and desquamative esophagitis in chronic graft-versus-host disease [11].

Esophageal rings are usually seen in the lower third of the esophagus. There are two types; A (muscular ring) and B (mucosal ring or Schatzki). Muscular rings are rare and seldom cause dysphagia. They are frequently seen in children undergoing barium study for other reasons. They are located within 2 cm of the squamocolumnar junction and are due to muscular hypertrophy. In contrast, Schatzki's ring is located at the squamocolumnar junction. The upper part is covered with squamous- and the lower part with columnar epithelium. The ring is a thin (<4 mm in axial length) smooth mucosa tissue. It is seen in 6% to 14% of asymptomatic patients during routine barium studies [12]. Schatzki's ring is seen in a quarter of patients with esophageal dysphagia and may be seen in association with patients who have eosinophilic esophagitis [13]. It is more common in older patients (> 40 years) but can also be seen in younger patients. The etiology of esophageal rings is unclear. There are inconclusive evidences implicating gastro esophageal reflux disease (GERD) in the pathogenesis of Schatzki's rings [14–17].

Patients with esophageal web and Schatzki's ring present with episodic solid food dysphagia. This frequently occurs after rapid ingestion of a bolus and when luminal diameter is less than 13 mm. In addition, patients with post-cricoid web may have nasopharyngeal reflux and/or aspiration. The dysphagia is transient, and if the bolus passes, the rest of the meal can be consumed without incident. However, some patients may present with acute bolus impaction. Physical examination may reveal features of associated medical conditions, such as bullous skin lesions and koilonychia in patients with webs. Diagnosis in both disorders is by barium swallow and/or esophagram and upper endoscopy.

Mechanical dilation is the treatment of choice for symptomatic patients. This can be accomplished by using a series of dilators over a guide wire (American dilators) or through scope balloon (controlled radial expansion [CRE]) dilators [18]. Endoscopic incisions of recurring lower esophageal ring have also been reported [19]. In patients with underlying medical conditions, such as eosinophilic esophagitis, GERD, dermatologic or chronic graft-versus-host disease, and iron-deficiency anemia, aggressive treatment of the underlying medical condition should be embarked on, before and after dilatation.

Peptic stricture

This complication is seen in 10% of patients with GERD. Peptic stricture is seen more commonly in patients of older age and male gender, with long-standing heartburn and chronic antacid use [20]. It is associated with the presence of very low lower esophageal sphincter pressure, poor esophageal clearance due to poor motility, and the presence of large hiatal hernia. Other medical conditions that predispose to peptic stricture include scleroderma, post-Heller's myotomy, Zollinger-Ellison syndrome, Schatzki's ring progressing to stricture, and prolonged nasogastric tube placement. The prevalence of peptic stricture has decreased markedly since the introduction of proton pump inhibitors [21]. In addition to pyrosis, patients with peptic stricture present with progressive solid food dysphagia (when luminal diameter is less than 13 mm), with most meals leading to dietary modification (pureed, soft, or liquid) and eventually liquid dysphagia. Up to 25% of patients with peptic stricture do not have reflux- or GERD-associated symptoms, such as water brash, belching, globus sensation, chronic cough, hoarseness, and chest pain.

Upper endoscopy remains the gold standard for diagnosing erosive disease, stricture, and other complications such as Barrett's esophagus and for therapeutic interventions such as dilatation. Peptic stricture usually occurs at the squamocolumnar junction, and is characterized by smooth narrowing that may be difficult to distend with air insufflation. Barium esophagram with barium-soaked marshmallow is complementary to upper endoscopy in patients with complex (tortuous and long stricture) or repeated strictures to reliably localize stricture, approximate length, and diameter of the stricture, in addition to ruling out epiphrenic diverticulum or paraesophageal hernia.

Esophageal peptic strictures are treated with esophageal dilatation, which can be accomplished by using mercury-filled bougies (Hurst or Maloney dilators) or over a guide-wire using either fluoroscopic or endoscopic guidance (Savary dilators) and balloon dilators passed through the endoscope and positioned within the stricture. Most endoscopists use the "rule of threes": Pass no more than three dilators or balloon size at any given time to stretch the stricture. Usually, relief of dysphagia occurs when luminal diameter is greater than 15 mm (45 French). Perforation and bleeding occur post-esophageal dilatation in less than 0.5% of all procedures [22–25]. Endoscopic placements of expandable plastic stent have also been used in recurrent benign severe peptic strictures [26,27]. Aggressive therapy with proton pump inhibitors post-dilatation is mandatory, because this has been shown to improve dysphagia and decrease the need for subsequent esophageal dilatation [21,28,29].

Carcinoma: squamous cell cancer and adenocarcinoma

Esophageal cancer affects older age groups, with a peak incidence in patients between 60 and 70 years old and occurring more commonly in men (Male:Female = 4:1). Squamous cell carcinoma and adenocarcinoma have similar clinical presentations despite different epidemiology. Worldwide, squamous cell cancer is the most common esophageal cancer. Squamous cell carcinoma is associated with tobacco and alcohol abuse, and is common in Asia, particularly in China, where the reported incidence is 131.8 cases per 100,000. In the United States, the reported incidence is 2.6 cases per 100,000. It is prevalent among African American males in the United States. In contrast, adenocarcinoma has a predilection for middle-aged Caucasian males and appears to be related to chronic GERD and underlying Barrett's esophagus. The caveat to this is that 40% of patients with Barrett's esophagus do not have symptoms of GERD. The mid esophagus is the most common site for squamous cell carcinoma whereas adenocarcinoma occurs commonly in the distal esophagus (Fig. 3).

Patients with esophageal carcinoma present with rapidly progressive solid food dysphagia. Ultimately, this progresses to liquid dysphagia and patients may not be able to swallow their saliva. It is often associated with anorexia and significant weight loss. Less commonly, they may present with chest pain, odynophagia, hoarseness from infiltration of the recurrent laryngeal

Barrett's Adeno CA   Squamous Cell CA

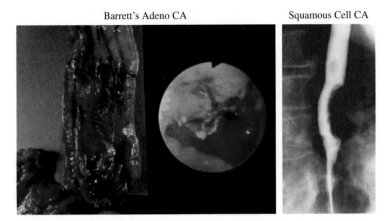

Fig. 3. Surgical specimen showing adenocarcinoma of the distal esophagus. Insert is an endoscopic picture of Barrett's esophagus. Barium radiograph showing squamous cell carcinoma in the mid-esophagus.

nerve, and iron deficiency anemia. Diagnosis is usually by endoscopy and biopsy. After adequate staging with computed tomography (CT) scan and endoscopic ultrasound, surgery is the best chance for long-term disease-free survival. In addition, patients may require presurgery chemoradiation to downstage the tumor in large tumors. In patients with inoperable tumor, placement of an expandable metal stent relieves dysphagia and improves quality of life [30–32].

Achalasia

Achalasia is a relatively uncommon primary esophageal motor disorder involving the smooth muscle segment of the esophagus. This condition is characterized by absence of or incomplete lower esophageal sphincter relaxation and loss of esophageal peristalsis. The etiology of achalasia is unknown and believed to be idiopathic in 98% of cases [33,34]. The incidence is 0.4 to 1.1 cases per 100,000 with a prevalence of 10 cases per 100,000. The incidence increases with age and has been reported in both genders and all ages with peak incidence between 25 to 60 years and nearly equally in all races. Familial clusters have also been described [35–38], suggesting that genetic predisposition probably increases the susceptibility to achalasia.

The cause of initial injury in idiopathic achalasia is thought to be viral in nature. However, this has not been consistently proven [39–42]. The possibility of autoimmune etiology in the pathogenesis of achalasia has been raised because of the high prevalence of the DQw1 antigen particularly those associated with certain human leukocyte antigens (HLAs), such as DQA1 and DQB1 [43]. Anti-myenteric plexus neuronal autoantibodies have also been reported in many achalasia patients. It is believed that achalasia arises from degeneration of intramural myenteric plexus neurons. Degenerative changes in the vagus nerve, including the dorsal motor nucleus, and reduction of vesicles in small intramuscular nerve fibers have also been described.

Other conditions such as achalasia can also present clinically and radiologically and are termed secondary (pseudo-achalasia) achalasia (Table 2). Patients with achalasia present with progressive solid and liquid dysphagia (85%–100%). Various maneuvers such as elevation of the arms above the head, Valsalva, standing up, and shrugging shoulders during meals may be employed by the patients to relieve dysphagia. In addition, heartburn and chest pain are fairly common symptoms in 25% to 50% patients, respectively. Pulmonary symptoms, such as aspiration pneumonia and abscess, are less common. Other symptoms include hiccups, regurgitation, globus sensation, and weight loss.

Diagnosis of achalasia is suspected on the basis of history. Evaluation should include chest X-ray, which may show absence of stomach bubble and air-fluid level in the esophagus. In untreated achalasia, barium esophagram may show a dilated atonic esophagus (sigmoid esophagus in long-standing disease) with classic "bird-peak" smooth narrowing of the gastroesophageal junction (GEJ). These classic findings may be absent in 20% of cases. Upper endoscopy, including retroflexion in the stomach, is usually performed to rule out secondary achalasia, such as carcinoma of the gastric cardia (Fig. 4). This may reveal a dilated esophagus with stasis changes and minimal resistance at the GEJ, and produce a "popping" sound while advancing the endoscope into the stomach. More than minimal resistance and the presence of nodularity of the GEJ on retroflex view may suggest carcinoma of the gastric cardia. Esophageal manometry is performed to confirm diagnosis of achalasia. Manometry documents aperistalsis, elevated intraesophageal pressure, and incomplete lower esophageal sphincter (LES)

Table 2
Types of achalasia

Idiopathic or primary achalasia
Secondary (pesudoachalasia) achalasia
Chagas' disease
Carcinoma of the gastric cardia
Paraneoplastic syndrome from malignancy elsewhere
Amyloidosis
Neuropathic chronic intestinal pseudo-obstruction syndrome
Triple-A syndrome: achalasia, alacrimia, and no response to adrenocorticotrophic hormone
Neurodegenerative disorder with Lewy inclusion bodies, Parkinson's disease, and hereditary cerebella ataxia.
Anderson-Fabry disease
Von Recklinghausen's neurofibromatosis
Post-vagotomy

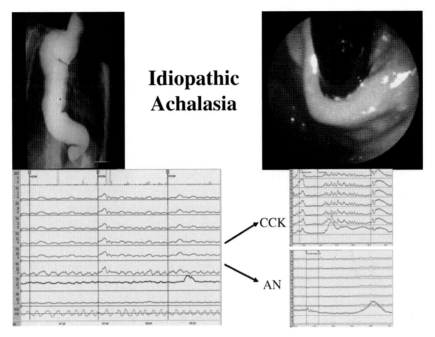

Fig. 4. Barium x-ray showing sigmoid esophagus of end-stage achalasia. In a patient with achalasia, retroflexed view of the stomach was performed during endoscopy to rule out carcinoma of the gastric cardia. This shows absence of abnormalities and the LES snuggly holding the endoscope. Manometry shows aperistalsis with no relaxation of the LES with wet deglutition, relaxation to gastric pressure with amyl nitrite (AN), and a paradoxical increase to cholecystokinin (CCK) challenge.

relaxation and hypertensive LES. It may also show features of vigorous achalasia (High-amplitude simultaneous contraction without peristalsis). Pharmacologic challenge with amyl nitrite and cholecystokinin (CCK) can also be used to define abnormalities of the LES that are not seen in structural disorders of the esophagus, such as peptic stricture or carcinoma of the gastric cardia. Amyl nitrite challenge in achalasia will show relaxation of the LES to almost gastric pressure, confirming smooth muscle dysfunction. CCK challenge in healthy individuals usually results in LES relaxation but paradoxical contraction of the LES and body of the esophagus in patients with achalasia. This positive response is seen in 85% of patients with achalasia (see Fig. 4).

Management of dysphagia in achalasia includes medical, endoscopic, or surgical approach. All of these therapeutic options are palliative and aimed at decreasing the outflow obstruction caused by dysfunctional LES. Medical management involves the use of nitrates, calcium channel blockers, and sildenafil (Viagra). These are given 30 minutes before meals and at bedtime. Pharmacotherapy usually provides temporary relief of symptoms and is useful only in patients who are at high risk for pneumatic dilatation or surgery. Most patients on medication require an additional form of treatment for long-term effect. Endoscopic approach involves injection of botulinum toxin (Botox) into the LES and pneumatic dilatation. The response to Botox is not durable as about 50% of patients remain in remission at 6 months and 30% at 2 years [44–46]. Botox is most effective in elderly patients and is recommended in patients with comorbid illnesses that are high-risk for dilation or surgery. Pneumatic dilation involves forceful dilatation or stretching of the LES using specially designed balloon catheters. It is an effective alternative to surgery, with an immediate response rate reported at 75% to 80% and 50% of patients in clinical remission 15 years after the initial pneumatic dilation [47]. Laparoscopic "Heller" myotomy with antireflux procedure is the most effective means of alleviating dysphagia in ≥90% of patients. Long-term outcomes in these patients range between 80% and 95% in large studies [48,49].

Other esophageal motility disorders

Esophageal motility disorder, affecting the smooth muscle section of the esophagus and the LES, can cause dysphagia to solids and liquids in addition to noncardiac chest pain. This includes diffuse esophageal spasm (DES), nutcracker esophagus, hypertensive LES, ineffective or nonspecific esophageal motility disorders (IEMD or NEMD) and scleroderma.

DES is seen in 3% to 5% patients with unexplained chest pain and dysphagia undergoing esophageal motility testing [50]. It is usually seen in patients older than 50 years but has been described in all ages. Etiology is unknown; it may be due to neuromuscular defect. It can be provoked by GERD, stress, hot or cold food, and rapid eating. About 3% to 5% of these patients may progress to achalasia. Intermittent nonprogressive dysphagia to both solid and liquid occurs in 50% of these patients, and the overall prognosis is excellent as symptoms may spontaneously improve over time [51]. Diagnosis is by manometry, showing simultaneous distal esophageal contractions in more than 20% of wet swallows intermixed with normal peristalsis. In addition, there may be prolonged duration of peristalsis, multi-peaked waves, spontaneous non–swallow-induced contractions, and hypertensive or incomplete LES relaxation. Barium esophagram may show a classic "corkscrew" appearance (Fig. 5). Management includes reassurance, aggressive treatment of reflux, and use of smooth muscle relaxant (isosorbide dinitrate) or calcium channel blocker (diltiazem).

Dysphagia is less common than chest pain in patients with nutcracker esophagus. Nutcracker esophagus is a manometric finding (Fig. 6) of normal peristalsis with increased wave amplitude (more than 180 mmHg) in more than 20% of wet swallows, prolonged duration of contraction (longer than 6 seconds), or hypertensive LES (greater than 45 mmHg). Barium esophagram is normal in these patients. Management is the same as for DES.

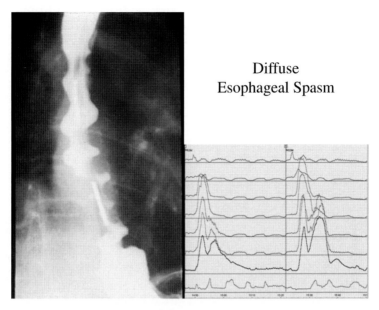

Diffuse
Esophageal Spasm

Fig. 5. Barium radiography showing typical "corkscrew" esophagus and manometry demonstrating simultaneous contractions in patients with DES.

IEMD or NEMD has been associated with dysphagia and is a manometric finding of 30% or more of the distal esophageal amplitudes below 30 mmHg or failed non-transmitted contractions. Most patients with IEMD have associated GERD [52]. Dysphagia is usually mild, and treatment is aimed at the underlying reflux disease.

Esophageal involvement is present in 80% to 90% of patients with scleroderma [53]. The disease process causes secondary fibrosis/sclerosis of the vasculature, innervations, and the smooth muscle of the distal two-thirds of the esophagus. The motility abnormalities in the distal two-thirds of the esophagus include aperistalsis or low-amplitude contractions and low LES pressure (less than 10 mmHg). The striated muscle of the proximal esophagus and UES are spared, exhibiting normal motility. Patients with scleroderma complain of chronic heartburn from severe gastroesophageal reflux disease and esophagitis. They present with dysphagia to both solids and liquids, which may be due to ineffective esophageal motility, peptic stricture, or development of adenocarcinoma arising from Barrett's esophagus.

Inflammatory process associated with dysphagia

Eosinophilic esophagitis

The epidemiology is not well studied. It is seen frequently in children but recently it has become more recognized in adults as a cause of solid food

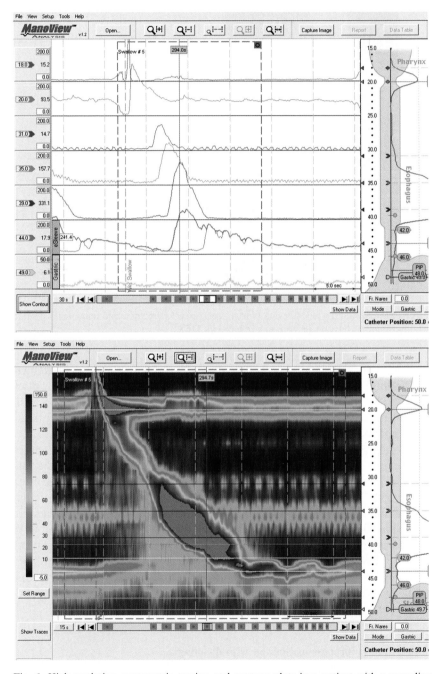

Fig. 6. High-resolution manometric tracing and contour plots in a patient with noncardiac chest pain and intermittent dysphagia to liquid and solid. This shows distal esophageal peristaltic wave amplitude greater than 200 mmHg consistent with nutcracker esophagus (blue tracing 331 mmHg).

dysphagia [54]. It is more common in men between ages of 20 and 40 years. The main presenting symptom is acute or chronic solid food dysphagia, including food impaction. Others include chest pain, allergic symptoms, such as atopy, and environmental and food allergies. This condition may be associated with GERD. Eosinophilic esophagitis is a clinicopathologic diagnosis as these patients commonly have a normal esophagram and upper endoscopy. Thus, biopsy of a normal appearing esophagus cannot be overemphasized in patients with esophageal dysphagia. Other endoscopic findings include edema, erythema, and friability of the mucosa, vertical furrows, white papules, or exudates (eosinophilic microabscess), ringed or corrugated esophagus, Schatzki's ring, and small caliber esophagus (Fig. 7) [55]. Histologic features include greater than 20 eosinophils/HPF and microabscess described as clustering of four or more eosinophils adjacent to each other. Following diagnosis, steps to identify underlying allergic diathesis should be undertaken. Topical steroids, such as fluticasone, budesonide, and leukotriene receptor inhibitor, montelukast are commonly used with varying degrees of success [56–58]. Dilatation should be performed cautiously in these patients because of high risk for perforation.

Radiation esophagitis

Radiation esophagitis occurs in 50% of patients post-radiotherapy for thoracic or head and neck cancer. Symptoms include chest pain, dysphagia,

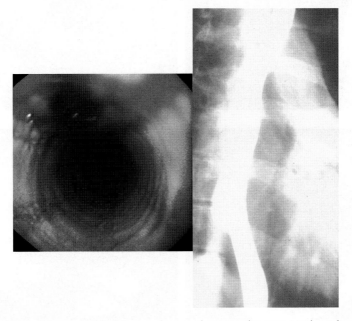

Fig. 7. Eosinophilic esophagitis: Upper endoscopy demonstrating corrugated esophagus with linear furrows and white exudates. There was a big rent following esophageal dilatation. Radiography shows small caliber esophagus.

and odynophagia. Other complications include stricture, perforation, and tracheoesophageal fistula. Diagnosis is based on history, endoscopy, and esophagram. Treatment for acute episodes includes decreasing dose of radiotherapy, symptomatic relief with GI cocktail, and nutritional support. Endoscopic dilatation or placement of percutaneous gastrostomy tube may be required in patients with refractory stricture.

Pill-induced injury

Pill-induced injury is twice as common in women as in men. The risk increases with age, esophageal structural and motility disorder, xerostomia, and use of multiple medications. Many drugs have been associated with esophageal mucosa injury. Common drugs include tetracycline, quinine, alendronate, potassium chloride, and vitamin C. Injury varies from

Dysphagia with Odynophagia

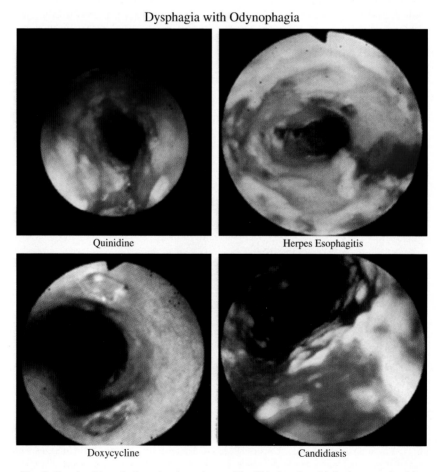

Fig. 8. Esophagitis and ulceration in patients with pill-induced and infectious esophagitis.

self-limited acute ulceration to stricture. Patients typically present with chest pain and odynophagia. Dysphagia indicates inflammatory changes with stricture formation. Pill esophagitis is often suspected on the basis of history and diagnosis is by endoscopy to detect mucosal injury and stricture (Fig. 8). Management is by stopping offending medication, and stricture may require endoscopic dilatation. Prevention is by instructing patients to take medications with at least 150 to 250 mL of water in the upright position and remain upright for at least 30 minutes afterward.

Infectious esophagitis

Infectious esophagitis is more common in immunocompromised patients, for example, AIDS, chemotherapy, and post-transplant patients. Candidiasis, herpes simplex, cytomegalovirus or HIV-associated esophagitis, and acute or chronic graft-versus-host disease can present with chest pain, odynophagia, and dysphagia. Endoscopy is the key to evaluating symptomatic patients (see Fig. 8). Management is tailored to the etiology, and esophageal dilatation may be required in patients with stricture.

References

[1] Castell DO, Donner MW. Evaluation of dysphagia: a careful history is crucial. Dysphagia 1987;2:65–71.
[2] Trate DM, Parkman HP, Fisher RS. Dysphagia: evaluation, diagnosis, and treatment. Prim Care 1996;23:417–32.
[3] Nayyar AK, Royston C, Bardhan KD. Oesophageal acid-peptic strictures in the histamine H2 receptor antagonist and proton pump inhibitor era. Dig Liver Dis 2003;35:143–50.
[4] Lagergren J, Bergstrom R, Lindgren A, et al. Symptomatic gastroesophageal reflux as a risk factor for esophageal adenocarcinoma. N Engl J Med 1999;340:825–31.
[5] Ladd WE. Congenital anomalies of the esophagus. Pediatrics 1950;6:9–19.
[6] Ekberg O, Malmquist J, Lindgren S. Pharyngo-oesophageal webs in dysphageal patients. A radiologic and clinical investigation in 1134 patients. Rofo 1986;145:75–80.
[7] Gordon AR, Levine MS, Redfern RO, et al. Cervical esophageal webs: association with gastroesophageal reflux. Abdom Imaging 2001;26:574–7.
[8] Kaplan RP, Touloukian J, Ahmed AR, et al. Esophagitis dissecans superficialis associated with pemphigus vulgaris. J Am Acad Dermatol 1981;4:682–7.
[9] Ergun GA, Lin AN, Dannenberg AJ, et al. Gastrointestinal manifestations of epidermolysis bullosa. A study of 101 patients. Medicine 1992;71:121–7.
[10] Foroozan P, Enta T, Winship DH, et al. Loss and regeneration of the esophageal mucosa in pemphigoid. Gastroenterology 1967;52:548–58.
[11] McDonald GB, Sullivan KM, Schuffler MD, et al. Esophageal abnormalities in chronic graft-versus-host disease in humans. Gastroenterology 1981;80:914–21.
[12] Goyal RK, Glancy JJ, Spiro HM. Lower esophageal ring. 1. N Engl J Med 1970;282:1298–305.
[13] Mann NS, Leung JW. Pathogenesis of esophageal rings in eosinophilic esophagitis. Med Hypotheses 2005;64:520–3.
[14] Ott DJ, Ledbetter MS, Chen MY, et al. Correlation of lower esophageal mucosal ring and 24-h pH monitoring of the esophagus. Am J Gastroenterol 1996;91:61–4.
[15] Scharschmidt BF, Watts HD. The lower esophageal ring and esophageal reflux. Am J Gastroenterol 1978;69:544–9.

[16] DeVault KR. Lower esophageal (Schatzki's) ring: pathogenesis, diagnosis and therapy. Dig Dis Sci 1996;14:323–9.

[17] Marshall JB, Kretschmar JM, Diaz-Arias AA. Gastroesophageal reflux as a pathogenic factor in the development of symptomatic lower esophageal rings. Arch Intern Med 1990;150:1669–72.

[18] Groskreutz JL, Kim CH. Schatzki's ring: long-term results following dilation. Gastrointest Endosc 1990;36:479–81.

[19] DiSario JA, Pedersen PJ, Bichis-Canoutas C, et al. Incision of recurrent distal esophageal (Schatzki) ring after dilation. Gastrointest Endosc 2002;56:244–8.

[20] Marks RD, Richter JE. Peptic strictures of the esophagus. Am J Gastroenterol 1993;88: 1160–73.

[21] Guda NM, Vakil N. Proton pump inhibitors and the time trends for esophageal dilation. Am J Gastroenterol 2004;99:797–800.

[22] Marshall JB, Afridi SA, King PD, et al. Esophageal dilatation with polyvinyl (American) dilators over a marked guidewire: practice and safety at one center over a 5-yr period. Am J Gastroenterol 1996;91:1503–6.

[23] Scolapio JS, Pasha TM, Gostout CJ, et al. A randomized prospective study comparing rigid to balloon dilators for benign esophageal strictures and rings. Gastrointest Endosc 1999;50:13–7.

[24] Pereira-Lima JC, Ramires RP, Zamin I Jr, et al. Endoscopic dilation of benign esophageal strictures: report of 1043 procedures. Am J Gastroenterol 1999;94:1497–501.

[25] Hernandez LJ, Jacobson JW, Harris MS. Comparison among the perforation rates of Maloney, balloon, and Savary dilation of esophageal strictures. Gastrointest Endosc 2000;51:460–2.

[26] Evrard S, Le Moine O, Lazaraki G, et al. Self-expanding plastic stents for benign esophageal lesions. Gastrointest Endosc 2004;60:894–900.

[27] Garcia-Cano J. Dilation of benign strictures in the esophagus and colon with the polyflex stent: a Case Series Study. Dig Dis Sci 2008;53:341–6.

[28] Barbezat GO, Schlup M, Lubcke R. Omeprazole therapy decreases the need for dilatation of peptic oesophageal strictures. Aliment Pharmacol Ther 1999;13:1041–5.

[29] Swarbrick ET, Gough AL, Foster CS, et al. prevention of recurrence of oesophageal stricture. A comparison of lansoprazole and high-dose ranitidine. Eur J Gastroenterol Hepatol 1996;8:431–8.

[30] Dua KS. New approach to malignant strictures of the esophagus. Curr Gastroenterol Rep 2003;5:198–205 [review].

[31] Power C, Byrne PJ, Lim K, et al. Superiority of anti-reflux stent compared with conventional stents in the palliative management of patients with cancer of the lower esophagus and esophago-gastric junction: results of a randomized clinical trial. Dis Esophagus 2007;20:466–70.

[32] Xinopoulos D, Dimitroulopoulos D, Tsamakidis K, et al. Palliative treatment of advanced esophageal cancer with metal-covered expandable stents. A cost-effectiveness and quality of life study. J BUON 2005;10:523–8.

[33] Mayberry JF. Etiology and demographics of achalasia. Gastrointest Endosc Clin N Am 2001;11:235–48.

[34] Park W, Vaezi MF. Etiology and pathogenesis of achalasia: the current understanding. Am J Gastroenterol 2005;100:1404–14.

[35] Frieling T, Berges W, Borchard F, et al. Family occurrence of achalasia and diffuse spasm of the oesophagus. Gut 1988;29:1595–602.

[36] Stein DT, Knauer CM. Achalasia in monozygotic twins. Dig Dis Sci 1982;27:636–40.

[37] Annese V, Napolitano G, Minervini MM, et al. Family occurrence of achalasia. J Clin Gastroenterol 1995;20:329–30.

[38] Bosher LP, Shaw A. Achalasia in siblings. Clinical and genetic aspects. Am J Dis Child 1981; 135:709–10.

[39] Jones DB, Mayberry JF, Rhodes J, et al. Preliminary report of an association between measles virus and achalasia. J Clin Pathol 1983;36:655–7.

[40] Robertson CS, Martin BA, Atkinson M. Varicella-zoster virus DNA in the oesophageal myenteric plexus in achalasia. Gut 1993;34:299–302.

[41] Niwamoto H, Okamoto E, Fujimoto J, et al. Are human herpes viruses or measles virus associated with esophageal achalasia? Dig Dis Sci 1995;40:859–64.

[42] Birgisson S, Galinski MS, Goldblum JR, et al. Achalasia is not associated with measles or known herpes and human papilloma viruses. Dig Dis Sci 1997;42:300–6.

[43] Wong RK, Maydonovitch CL, Metz SJ, et al. Significant DQw1 association in achalasia. Dig Dis Sci 1989;34:349–53.

[44] Pehlivanov N, Pasricha PJ. Medical and endoscopic management of achalasia. Available at: http://www.nature.com/gimo/index.html. Accessed 2008.

[45] Fishman VM, Parkman HP, Schiano TD, et al. Symptomatic improvement in achalasia after botulinum toxin injection of the lower esophageal sphincter. Am J Gastroenterol 1996;91:1724–30.

[46] Pasricha PJ, Rai R, Ravich WJ, et al. Botulinum toxin for achalasia: long-term outcome and predictors of response. Gastroenterology 1996;110:1410–5.

[47] Karamanolis G, Sgouros S, Karatzias G, et al. Long-term outcome of pneumatic dilation in the treatment of achalasia. Am J Gastroenterol 2005;100:270–4.

[48] Bonatti H, Hinder RA, Klocker J, et al. Long-term results of laparoscopic Heller myotomy with partial fundoplication for the treatment of achalasia. Am J Surg 2005;190:874–8.

[49] Costantini M, Zaninotto G, Guirroli E, et al. The laparoscopic Heller-Dor operation remains an effective treatment for esophageal achalasia at a minimum 6–year follow-up. Surg Endosc 2005;19:345–51.

[50] Katz PO, Dalton CB, Richter JE, et al. Esophageal testing of patients with non-cardiac chest pain and dysphagia. Ann Intern Med 1987;106:593–7.

[51] Spencer HL, Smith L, Riley SA. A questionnaire study to assess long-term outcome in patients with abnormal esophageal manometry. Dysphagia 2006;21:149–55.

[52] Leite LP, Johnston BT, Barrett J, et al. Ineffective esophageal motility (IEM): the primary finding in patients with non-specific esophageal motility disorder. Dig Dis Sci 1997;42:1853–8.

[53] Bassotti G, Baattaglia E, Debernard V, et al. Esophageal dysfunction in scleroderma: relationship with disease subsets. Arthritis Rheum 1997;40:2252–9.

[54] Potter JW, Saeian K, Staff D, et al. Eosinophilic esophagitis in adults: an emerging problem with unique endoscopic features. Gastrointest Endosc 2004;59:355–61.

[55] Croese J, Fairley S, Mansson J, et al. Clinical and endoscopic features of eosinophilic esophagitis in adults. Gastrointest Endosc 2003;58:516–22.

[56] Remedios M, Campbell C, Jones D, et al. Eosinophilic esophagitis in adults: clinical, endoscopic, histologic findings and response to treatment with fluticasone propionate. Gastrointest Endosc 2006;63:3–12.

[57] Aceves SS, Bastian JF, Newbury RO, et al. Oral viscous budesonide: a potential new therapy for eosinophilic esophagitis in children. Am J Gastroenterol 2007;102:2271–9.

[58] Attwood SE, Lewis CJ, Bronder CS, et al. Eosinophilic oesophagitis: a novel treatment using montelukast. Gut 2003;52:181–5.

ELSEVIER
SAUNDERS

Phys Med Rehabil Clin N Am
19 (2008) 747–768

PHYSICAL MEDICINE
AND REHABILITATION
CLINICS OF
NORTH AMERICA

The Bedside Examination in Dysphagia

Giselle Carnaby-Mann, MPH, PhD*, Kerry Lenius, MS, CCC-SLP

*Swallowing Research Laboratory, Department of Behavioral Science & Community Health,
College of Public Health & Health Professions, University of Florida,
101 S. Newel Drive, Gainesville, FL 32610, USA*

Swallowing evaluation

The evaluation of swallowing disorders currently uses a variety of methods. The most common dichotomy is between instrumental and non-instrumental or clinical examinations. Although the specific goals and methods of assessment for dysphagic patients may vary among cases, the most important function of assessment is to understand the physiologic nature of the patient's swallow in relation to the patient's medical history. This understanding is critical for selecting appropriate treatment strategies. The clinical bedside assessment often is considered the mainstay of dysphagia management. As the first line of assessment, it frequently defines the process and requisites of the task. This article reviews the available methods of noninstrumental bedside swallowing assessment and considers the issues surrounding the use of these approaches today.

Noninstrumental clinical assessment: definition and objectives

Swallowing assessment may be defined as an organized, goal-directed evaluation of a variety of interrelated and integrated components of the deglutitive process. It is important to specify the goal of a swallowing assessment to evaluate fully the procedure employed. There are three general possibilities. First, a swallowing evaluation may form part of a medical diagnosis when the practitioner is attempting to determine the underlying pathology. Second, the swallowing evaluation may be conducted to determine the patient's abilities and impairments and the degree to which these

* Corresponding author.
E-mail address: gmann@phhp.ufl.edu (G. Carnaby-Mann).

1047-9651/08/$ - see front matter © 2008 Elsevier Inc. All rights reserved.
doi:10.1016/j.pmr.2008.05.008

impairments can be modified. Third, a clinician may perform a swallowing assessment for a combination of the previous two goals [1]. A swallowing assessment is intended to ascertain the factors related to swallowing function but need not, in itself, be diagnostic of the underlying disease. The information gathered, however, may direct further diagnostic instrumental investigations such as videofluoroscopy, nasendoscopy, manometry, and scintigraphy.

In general, any assessment protocol should reflect an underlying explanatory theory of the relationship between the pathologic mechanisms involved in the disorder. It should not be simply an observational structure used to record behavioral data. Working from a sound theoretic framework can offer direction for diagnosis and therapeutic intervention, further enhancing insights into the swallowing neurophysiology. Although the specific goals and methods of assessment in dysphagic patients may vary among cases, the most important function of an assessment is to enable the clinician to understand the physiologic nature of the patient's swallow in relation to the patient's medical history and thereby select appropriate treatment strategies.

The clinical bedside swallowing assessment

Clinical assessment, or "clinical bedside assessment," as it often is termed, usually includes a history of the patient's swallowing problem, a detailed evaluation of oral, pharyngeal, and laryngeal anatomy, sensory and motor function, behavioral, cognitive, and language abilities, and a trial feeding (if deemed appropriate). Crucial information can be gathered during history taking, such as onset, duration, frequency, and description of swallowing problems. In this early stage, initial hypotheses are formed regarding the location of the problem within the swallowing system. Clinical symptoms such as localization are not always accurate, however. For instance, patients who localize their symptoms to the level of the proximal esophagus frequently are inaccurate; accuracy increases when symptoms are reported at a more distal location [2].

Some investigators divide the clinical examination into a swallowing mechanism examination (oromotor) and a feeding examination [1]. The oromotor examination typically involves the analysis of components of the oral and pharyngeal stages of swallowing. Clinical swallowing examinations that have been proposed range from swallowing as little as 3 oz of water to a series of tasks designed to define the range, rate, coordination, and symmetry of movement of the lips, facial musculature, tongue, and pharynx and larynx and to reflect cranial nerve functioning for swallowing. In addition, most assessments also include activities to determine the patient's language and cognitive abilities in relation to comprehension, attention span, and ability to follow instructions. These cognitive measurements often are limited in scope, however, and the information gathered from these tasks may not be integrated into the resultant analysis of the swallowing examination, except as a review of a patient's "readiness" for assessment.

Ingestion of food or fluid via swallowing trials is not included routinely in a clinical bedside examination. The decision as to which patients will receive routine administration of food or fluid as part of the clinical bedside assessment frequently depends on the clinician's judgment regarding the patient's ability to deal with any aspiration that may occur or go undetected. If ingestion of oral intake is deemed relatively safe, the patient may be observed swallowing either one or more consistencies of food. These swallowing trials enable the clinician to review the swallowing mechanism in action. For instance, specific aspects of the swallow, such as laryngeal elevation, speed of swallow response, and oral clearance, can be evaluated during trial swallows. This information is not available from nonswallowing tasks, and it facilitates recommendations for feeding after completion of the assessment. Furthermore, instrumental tools, such as cervical auscultation and pulse oximetry, can be used during trial swallows in an effort to enhance the detection of penetration/aspiration at bedside [3]. The relative value of incorporating trial swallows into a clinical swallowing evaluation is controversial, however. Because the ingestion of food or fluid brings with it potential risk for a patient suspected of having dysphagia, some authors believe that the risk–benefit ratio for this procedure is poor [1,4,5]. They suggest that complexity of the pharyngeal stage of the swallow makes it impossible to judge the adequacy of the swallow accurately at the bedside. Consequently, the clinician may be left to guess the nature of the impairment, thus placing the patient at undue risk. Therefore some authors consider feeding trials unwarranted and argue that these trials should not be conducted without obtaining further diagnostic information from other instrumental swallowing examinations [5].

Clinical bedside assessment currently is the most widely used form of swallowing assessment. It is used frequently by health professionals as a first-line (and on occasion, as the only) means for investigating a clinical suspicion of a swallowing disorder. It is inexpensive, noninvasive, time efficient, and consumes few resources [6]. It offers important information to help guide the clinician in the evaluation of a patient's swallowing. Although bedside assessment is reported to be less sensitive than alternative instrumental assessment techniques in the identification of dysphagia and aspiration, most authors agree that it does provide valuable information for the prognosis and management of patients who have swallowing impairment [7,8]. Ideally a clinical assessment provides information to help define potential causative factors, formulate a tentative hypothesis regarding the physiologic nature of the patient's swallowing problem, and pinpoint the resultant level of breakdown in the neurophysiologic control system. It can facilitate the development of the preliminary treatment plan and the fabrication of further questions that must be answered to complete a diagnostic work-up. In addition, it may determine a patient's suitability for further instrumental investigations.

Clinical bedside assessment versus videofluoroscopy

During the last decade the development of a variety of instrumental techniques has enabled empiric confirmation of dysphagia and aspiration, thus reducing the potential for intraobserver and interobserver variations. The validity of most clinical bedside techniques for assessing swallowing has been determined through comparison with an instrumental reference test. The most popular has been the videofluoroscopic examination (VFE). This instrumental examination often is considered the reference standard for the evaluation of dysphagia. Several authors have reported that VFE or dynamic imaging studies of the swallowing process provide the only reliable objective measurement of swallowing features and are essential for detecting and localizing abnormalities and/or functional impairments within this process [9–12].

The major advantage of VFE over the traditional clinical ("bedside") swallowing assessment seems to be its ability to view features that are not observable in the clinical examination and therefore must be inferred from symptomatology. Critical information regarding the pharyngeal stage of swallowing is believed to be missing on clinical bedside assessments; thus, aspiration events may go undetected. Splaingard and colleagues [13], in a blinded study comparing observed clinical indicators with videofluoroscopic results, reported clinical signs to be unreliable indicators of the presence or absence of aspiration, identifying only 42% of the subjects who aspirated on VFE. Likewise, Logemann [5], in an unblinded study, found that even expert clinicians failed to identify approximately 40% of aspirating patients on clinical assessment and suggested that silent aspiration (aspiration without cough or any outward sign of difficulty) might be responsible. This author stated that bedside clinical assessment has proven unreliable in defining pharyngeal physiology because of the complexity of pharyngeal motor control during swallowing. Inaccurate clinical evaluation of the degree of aspiration can lead to an understaging of the risk for disability or to life-threatening complications of dysphagia.

Conversely, VFE has been criticized as an expensive and time-consuming procedure that is not commonly available to practicing clinicians [1,3,14]. Although the usefulness of the direct visualization of swallowing is acknowledged, VFE exposes a patient to a degree of irradiation and may provide only a single, perhaps unrealistic, view of a patient's swallowing within an unnatural setting. Lazarus and Logemann [15] reported that many patients who demonstrated observable dysphagic deficits did not aspirate during VFE. Splaingard and colleagues [13] state that the significance of aspiration identified by VFE for each individual patient remains debatable. Radiographic findings cannot necessarily be generalized to a functional situation (ie, a meal). Similarly, the procedural aspects of the technique are highly variable across settings, and the criteria for determining which patients require the procedure and the reliability of results across clinicians remains poor [8,16–18]. Langmore and colleagues [19] state that more research is required to determine the factors resulting in observer variation in video-fluoroscopic diagnoses. Without uniform and accepted procedures for administration and scoring of these examinations, the ability to determine accurately the relative values of VFE or clinical assessments in the diagnosis and management of dysphagia remains dubious.

Currently available clinical bedside assessments

A number of clinical assessment tools have been proposed for the evaluation of swallowing (Table 1). The choice of a clinical assessment method is central to the identification of the disorder and to the clinician's theoretic framework for intervention. Various methods have been used, ranging from checklists to direct administration of food or fluids. Most clinical assessment methods have focused on the identification of symptoms or indicators of impaired swallowing. They can be considered bottom-up assessment models. The principal question that these tools aim to answer is "Does this person aspirate?" The tools used are designed to evaluate the various components of each swallowing phase or other matters considered indicative of the functioning at a particular phase (eg, vocal quality as an indicator of laryngeal function). The clinician then must interpret the information in light of his or her understanding of normal and abnormal swallowing physiology and neurophysiology. The focus of these examinations is primarily at the symptomatic level. Few, if any, clinical assessment methods map assessment findings directly to any model of swallowing neurophysiology. This procedure is left to the individual clinician and thus suggests erroneously that the physiologic organization and control of swallowing is indisputable and that a single theory prevails.

Review of clinical examination methods

Methods used in the clinical evaluation of swallowing fall into two main categories, water-swallow tests and (clinical) swallowing-mechanism examinations/checklists (Table 2). Water-swallow tests require a patient to swallow water, and the effects of this event are recorded. Swallowing-mechanism examinations involve the administration of a series of oromotor/sensory and swallowing tasks designed to evaluate cranial nerve function and swallow physiology. Along with these tasks, some gross cognitive and language measures have been reported, such as the Mini Mental Status examination, the Glasgow Coma scale, and the presence/absence of dysphasia [20].

Table 1
The accuracy of bedside clinical swallowing assessments in detecting aspiration, as defined by videofluoroscopy

Study	No. of patients	Test	Sensitivity (%)	Specificity (%)	Aspiration (%)
Splaingard et al [13]	107	Formal assessment by speech pathologist	42	91	40
Horner et al [45]	70	Weak/absent cough	84	56	49
		Dysphonia	97	29	49
		Reduced gag reflex	67	70	49
DePippo et al [23]	44	3-oz/mL water swallow	76	59	45
Kidd et al [52]	60	50-mL water swallow	80	86	41
Smithard et al [7]	62	Doctors	30	69	25
		Informal assessment by speech pathologist	10	95	
Stanners et al [53]	50	Weak/absent cough	70	78	24
		Dysphonia	60	45	24
		Reduced gag reflex	60	45	24
Mari et al [31]	99	Cough	75	74	46
		90-mL water swallow	52	86	
Daniels et al [44]	59	Two clinical features	92	67	
Mann et al [8]	128	Formal assessment by speech pathologist	93	63	22
Tohara et al [30]	63	3-mL water swallow	70	88	46
		4-g pudding swallow	72	62	
		Radiographs	50	76	
		Combination	90	71	

The water tests

The most commonly reported clinical assessment method used with stroke populations is the water-swallow test [21]. This assessment comes in a variety of forms (eg, the 3-oz water-swallow test, the 50-mL water-swallow test, the 30-mL water-swallow test, the timed test of swallow capacity, and the Burke dysphagia examination). In all these examinations a measured amount of water is administered to the patient. Symptoms of suspected aspiration, such as coughing during consumption or within 1 minute following completion, or the presence of a wet/hoarse vocal quality after swallowing are considered positive signs of swallowing impairment. Most of these methods claim to detect most cases of dysphagia but on videofluoroscopic validation can fail to identify aspiration in 20% to 40% of patients [22].

Numerous investigators have modified the water-swallow protocol in an attempt to improve its sensitivity and specificity [23–28]. One of the initial proponents, DePippo and colleagues [23] validated the original 3-oz water-swallow test on 44 stroke patients admitted to a rehabilitation unit and referred to the study. Although radiographic diagnosis was not reported to be blind to the clinical findings, the authors reported a sensitivity of 76% and specificity of 59% for the identification of aspiration in these patients; however, 34% (15/44) cases were labeled incorrectly by this examination. Most of these events were false negatives, suggesting that a considerable proportion of silent aspiration went undetected. Additionally, confidence intervals around the validity data were not reported. Given the small sample size, it is likely that these intervals were wide, and that the precision of the estimates is poor. Nonetheless, the authors concluded that this test was a sensitive tool for the identification of aspiration after stroke but suggested that it be combined with a clinical symptom checklist.

Since then, other attempts have been made to refine the water-swallow approach further. DePippo and colleagues [24] published the Burke Dysphagia Screening Test (BDST). This examination added a clinical checklist to the previously published water-swallow test. The aim of the examination was to identify patients at greatest risk of dysphagia. The study sample consisted of 139 patients, again in the subacute phase after suffering a stroke. The subjects represented a range of stroke types, and more severe dysphagic cases may have been overrepresented. The data were analyzed by comparing the results of the BDST with the development of pneumonia, upper airway obstruction, and death over an average 2-month admission. The numbers reaching these end points were small, and therefore the statistical power was small also. Fisher's exact tests were used to review statistically the associations between a positive BDST and each outcome event. A secondary analysis to identify which item on the test was the best predictor of dysphagia was conducted also. A significant association was reported between item 4 (coughing associated with feeding or coughing during the 3-oz water test) and all end points. The authors concluded that the BDST identified 92% of patients who developed a negative end point and described the BDST as effective in identifying the patients at greatest risk of medical complications from dysphagia after stroke.

This study highlights the significant methodologic issues associated with most of the water-swallow studies. Inaccurate representation of the dysphagic population in the test samples may lead to an overestimation of the validity of the assessment tool. Although sensitive and specific for the moderate-severity groupings, the results of these studies cannot be generalized widely because the patients are highly selected. The usefulness of these tests in ascertaining either severe and mild cases has yet to be established. Furthermore, the inclusion of different stroke types (eg, first-ever stroke versus multiple strokes; brainstem versus unilateral stroke) may incur differences in risk factors, prognosis, and treatment.

Although this study presented prognostic data to support the validity of the chosen assessment method, the number of outcome events for each end point was relatively small, and consequently the statistical power was low.

Table 2
Comparison of clinical assessment validity studies

Comparison study	DePippo et al [23]	Nathadwarawala et al [25]	Linden et al [32]	Depipo et al [24]	Nathadwarawala et al [29]	Ott et al [41]	Mari et al [31]	Splaingard et al [13]
Year	1992	1992	1993	1994	1994	1996	1997	1988
No. patients	44	81	249	139	90	93	93	107
Diagnosis	rehabilitation neurologic	inpatient neurologic	mixed	rehabilitation neurologic	outpatient neurologic	mixed	in- and outpatients rehabilitation neurologic	adult and child rehabilitation patients
Referral pattern	consecutive admissions	unreported	referred	consecutive admissions	consecutive	referred	consecutive	referred
Variables measured	cough, voice, MBS aspiration	swallow speed, age, sex, perception of diagnosis	demographic and clinical variables, MBS subglottic penetration	demographic variables, diagnosis, cough, feeding time, non-oral feeding, % eaten, pneumonia, aspiration	swallow speed, age, sex, diagnosis perception, cough, clinical variables	demographic, clinical, and radiographic variables	demographic variables, history, clinical cough	demographic, clinical, radiographic variables
Outcome of interest	aspiration	dysphagia	subglottic penetration	aspiration dysphagia	dysphagia	dysphagia	aspiration	aspiration
Study methods	water-swallow test	swallow speed water-swallow test	clinical examination	water-swallow test checklist	water-swallow test checklist	clinical examination	water-swallow test checklist	clinical examination
Reference test	radiographic	patient perception	radiographic	radiographic	clinical examination	radiographic	radiographic	radiographic
Analysis method	sensitivity specificity	sensitivity specificity	chi squared discriminant	relative-risk Fisher's exact tests	t-tests chi squared	% agreement rank order	sensitivity specificity factor analysis	sensitivity/ specificity chi squared t-tests

Table 2
(continued)

Comparison study	Horner et al [45]	Iskander et al [20]	Kidd et al [53]	Garon et al [22]	Smithard et al [7]	Mann et al [8]	Tohara et al [30]
Year	1990	1990	1995	1996	1997	2000	2003
No. patients	70	20	60	100	121	128	63
Diagnosis	bilateral stroke	mixed	first-ever stroke	mixed	first-ever stroke	first-ever stroke	mixed
Referral pattern	referred	referred	consecutive admissions	referred	consecutive admissions	consecutive admissions	referred
Variables measured	retrospective clinical and radiographic variables	demographic clinical and radiographic variables	demographic clinical and radiographic variables	cough, voice quality, radiographic variables	demographic, clinical, and radiographic variables	demographic, clinical, and radiographic variables	demographic, clinical, and radiographic variables
Outcome of interest	aspiration	dysphagia	aspiration	aspiration	aspiration	dysphagia aspiration	aspiration
Study methods	clinical (file audit) retrospective	clinical examination	water-swallow test	water-swallow test	water-swallow test checklist	clinical examination	water-swallow test food test static radiographs
Reference test	radiographic retrospective	radiographic	radiographic	radiographic	radiographic	radiographic	radiographic
Analysis method	chi squared multivariate	Pearson product-moment correlations	chi squared (stratified) t-tests Fisher's exact tests	chi squared Fisher's exact tests	sensitivity/ specificity chi squared multivariate	sensitivity/ specificity chi squared multivariate	sensitivity/ specificity Fisher's exact texts

Abbreviation: MBS, modified barium swallow.

Therefore it is possible that random variation, resulting from the play of chance, accounted for the observed results. The authors based their conclusions on raw correlations of the increased frequency the outcome event in patients who recorded a positive BDST. This univariate analysis describes only the relationship between two variables without taking into account the potential confounding effect of other variables. Consequently, a predictive role may be assigned to factors that actually are merely markers for other factors of greater importance.

Other adaptations of the traditional water-swallow test include timed tests of water swallowing [25,29]. Nathadwarawala and colleagues [25,29] introduced the initial timed test of swallow capacity. These examinations require the patient to swallow 150 mL of water. In addition to the usual water-swallow observations, the time taken to swallow the preparation is recorded, along with the amount of oral residue after the task (for cases in which the test was abandoned). From this information, a ratio of speed (mL/s) by average volume/swallow is generated. In these studies, Nathadwarawala and colleagues [25,29] used a combined measure of patient perception, clinical history, and a swallowing-mechanism examination as the reference test in the examination of a swallow-speed test for dysphagia. The reliability and validity data produced from the timed-swallow studies fare no better under scrutiny than the other water-swallow tests, however. The findings are limited by the use of heterogeneous samples presenting a variety of causes, each potentially incurring a variable aspiration risk, by the questionable validity of the chosen reference tests, by high false-positive rates, and by the limited provision of information concerning the underlying pathologies and their relationship to a positive test result.

Garon and colleagues [22], concerned about physicians using the 3-oz water-swallow test as a replacement for videofluoroscopy, compared the water-swallow test against videofluoroscopy to evaluate swallowing function in 100 patients from multiple neurologic pathology groups. Although using a referred population, this study reported that the 3-oz water-swallow test and a checklist of clinical symptoms identified only 35% of patients aspirating on videofluoroscopy. They concluded that the water-swallow test was less accurate than previously reported and was not a replacement for the precision and accuracy of videofluoroscopy.

Tohara and colleagues [30] also attempted to identify aspiration of various causes in 63 patients, using a combination of the 3-mL water-swallow test, the 4-g pudding-swallow test, and lateral radiographs before and after swallowing 4 mL of liquid barium. These findings were compared with videofluoroscopy with a positive predictive value (PPV) of 83% and negative predictive value (NPV) of 77% for the water-swallow test alone and a PPV of 72% with a NPV of 89% when all three items were combined. The administration and scoring of the three-item battery is lengthy and burdensome when compared with other water-swallow tests, however. Furthermore, the authors suggested this test could be used as a screening or evaluation procedure, but this battery seems to function only as a screening test; a full clinical swallow evaluation is needed if the patient does not meet the acceptable cut-off score. The authors conclude by stating that the test battery is appropriate to use but that videofluorography should be performed to support decision making whenever possible.

Finally Mari and colleagues [31] administered a combination of the 3-oz water-swallow test, a clinical checklist based on a collection of symptoms, and a clinical evaluation of the oropharyngeal swallowing mechanism. The subjects included 93 patients admitted to a rehabilitation clinic with a variety of neurologic disorders. The mean age of the test population was 59.8 years. The presence of symptoms and signs checked for during the clinical examination and positive findings on the 3-oz water-swallow test were compared against videofluoroscopy, and the PPV of each clinical item was assessed. The investigators reported that clinical symptoms of dysphagia showed very poor predictive value for aspiration. The 3-oz water-swallow test demonstrated a higher PPV (76%) than clinical signs, but it had lower sensitivity because patients who had silent aspiration gave negative findings on the 3-oz water-swallow test. Unfortunately, interactions between variables were not reported. Moreover, the authors tended to regard aspiration as synonymous with dysphagia and erroneously described the water-swallow test as a valuable tool for identifying dysphagic patients.

Clinical dysphagia and aspiration batteries

Researchers also have attempted to develop and validate clinical dysphagia batteries that do not include a water-swallow test [20,31]. Linden and colleagues [32] developed the Dysarthria Dysphagia Battery (DDB), which was designed to guide clinical treatment but not to predict the presence or severity of dysphagia. The authors, however, did compare the predictive value of a range of clinical factors thought to be suggestive of subglottic penetration with videofluoroscopic findings. The DDB was administered to 249 patients who had variable neurologic diagnoses, most commonly stroke. Items were evaluated using chi-squared analysis, and significant factors were entered into a discriminant analysis. This investigation found that nine clinical signs, most of which pertained to laryngeal functioning, were associated significantly with subglottic penetration. Overall, subglottic penetration could be predicted 66% of the time using the DDB, and the absence of subglottic penetration could be predicted 67% of the time. Approximately one third of subglottic penetration was not identified by the protocol. This study included a large sample and used more sophisticated statistical analyses, but it relied on data from a doubly referred population of heterogeneous conditions. The time elapsed after the event was not noted, and it was not stated whether the radiologist performing the videofluoroscopy was blind to the clinical examination findings. The predictors of subglottic penetration identified from the analysis also were indefinite. Although items were selected from the univariate analysis and entered into the discriminant analysis in accordance with the author's theoretic rationale, insufficient information was reported to interpret these variables. The reader was given no information about the independent (predictor) variables in terms of the risk of subglottic penetration. In accordance with the findings, the authors concluded that the study results were inadequate for clinical purposes and that the DDB was not a replacement for videofluoroscopy.

Another clinical battery developed in Australia for the assessment of dysphagia in neurologic populations is the Mann Assessment of Swallowing Ability (MASA) [33]. This assessment evaluates 24 skills involved in swallowing, and performance is measured using a 5- and 10-point rating scale. The MASA provides scores for each of the skills identified as well as a composite score (maximum score, 200). Both dysphagia and aspiration are coded as a risk rating. In the initial validation study, Mann and colleagues [8] evaluated the interjudge and intrajudge reliability of this tool by having two judges administer the examination twice on an inception cohort of 128 first-ever stroke subjects admitted to an acute tertiary care facility. The results revealed that more than of 80% of scores were identical and that concordance between speech pathologists was high ($\kappa = 0.82$ for dysphagia; $\kappa = 0.75$ for aspiration). The authors then examined the validity by comparing the results of the MASA with those from blinded VFE ratings completed by a radiologist. The authors reported on sensitivity, specificity, PPV, NPV, and positive likelihood ratios. For both procedures, the investigators found a sensitivity of 73% and a specificity of 89% for the identification of dysphagia (PPV, 92%; NPV, 65%; positive likelihood ratio, 6.6) and a sensitivity of 93% and a specificity of 63% (PPV, 41%; NPV, 97%; positive likelihood ratio, 2.5) for the identification of aspiration. From these measures Mann [33] concluded the MASA has good reliability and validity as a clinical assessment tool. Furthermore other recent studies involving the MASA have found its validity to be comparable to that of other clinical assessment scales [34] and of other instrumental techniques (eg, flexible endoscopic evaluations of feeding) [35]. Although this tool has demonstrated an improvement in the process of evaluation of a bedside examination, and its authors claim that it maps well to an underlying theory of swallowing neurophysiology, the MASA has not been evaluated for predictive ability in the longer term or for use with patients who have non-neurologic dysphagia. Consequently, broad generalization of these findings to dysphagic populations as a whole must be considered with caution.

Methodologic issues in available bedside assessments

Overall, studies using clinical symptom batteries have fared a little better than the water-swallow tests in providing meaningful, valid, data with which to direct diagnosis and treatment. Neither method, however, has proven to have superior validity or reliability. Many studies of clinical assessment methods exhibit large differences and inadequacies in methodology and consequently in results. The major sources of variation hindering the comparison of results are the variations in the diagnosis groups used, in referral patterns, in the time of the examination after onset of the disabling condition, in the outcomes of interest, in the variables measured, in reference tests, in analysis methods, and in the clinical examination method used.

Diagnosis

The prevalence and severity of dysphagia and consequently the risks for both dysphagia and aspiration will vary in patients identified at different stages of disease or from different diagnostic groups. Because of the variety of diagnoses included in the study samples, some assessment methods may seem more sensitive than they actually are. Some investigations have included subjects from acute inpatient hospitals, whereas others have used only patients in the subacute phase after disease (eg, stroke) onset [23,24]. Some investigations have included a mixture of diseases, of which stroke constituted the majority [13,22–25,29,36–38]. Still others have limited examination to first-ever stroke populations [7,39].

Referral patterns

The methods by which subject were recruited to the various studies have contributed to a potential selection bias toward including only subjects who have more obvious deficits. Most studies have used hospital-based populations, but some have been retrospective and have used records from patients previously referred for swallowing review by a specialist [32,40]. There will be systematic differences in patient type and consequently a different prevalence of disorders in patients referred to a center or a specialist service [23,24,31]. For example, patients referred to a rehabilitation center may tend to be younger or to have a better prognosis for functional recovery. Patients referred for specialist swallowing review and videofluoroscopy are more likely to have significant swallowing difficulties that are obvious to the referring agent [32,41]. Patients who have more subtle swallowing deficits may go unnoticed and not be referred for review.

Time from onset

Swallowing difficulties following certain acute disorders (eg, stroke) are thought to diminish considerably in the first few weeks after onset [21,40]. Nonetheless, many assessment studies have examined subjects at a mean of 4 to 5 weeks after insult [23,24]. Subjects presenting with dysphagia at this point are more likely to be those who have significant impairment and whose problem has not resolved or responded to treatment. Assessment methods validated in these populations may not be sensitive enough to identify swallowing difficulties in more acute patients. Therefore, the ability to generalize examination results to other populations is less reliable.

Outcomes of interest

Several studies have attempted to correlate findings on clinical examination only with the occurrence of aspiration [23,31,32]. Others have used dysphagia (defined as abnormal swallowing) as the variable of interest [24,25,29,41]. This variability leads to uncertainty in the interpretation of these results. Aspiration is only one component of dysphagia. Furthermore, it is not an obligatory symptom of dysphagia, and it may be present intermittently in many dysphagic individuals. The sensitivity and specificity of a diagnostic examination in predicting aspiration may be different from that in predicting dysphagia alone. This consideration is particularly important, because there often is a trade-off between sensitivity and specificity: when a test is more sensitive, it tends to be less specific, and vice versa. The consequences resulting from a diagnosis of aspiration versus dysphagia are different also. A sensitive test (ie, one that usually is positive in the presence of disease) is of most benefit when there is an important penalty or negative outcome for missing a disease case [42]. For example, in the case of aspiration, raising the sensitivity of the test (and thereby increasing the false-positive rate) may result in the unnecessary introduction of non-oral feeding methods, the use of chest radiographs, or recommendations for an alternative diet. For dysphagia, increasing the false-positive rate may have similar but less stringent effects. Alternatively, maximizing the specificity of a test of aspiration may have more dangerous effects, because increasing the false-negative rate may result in serious complications associated with aspiration such as pneumonia and death. Again, the effect for dysphagia may be less dire. Clearly identifying the relative validity of a diagnostic clinical examination for both swallowing outcomes, dysphagia and aspiration, is crucial.

Variables measured

One of the greatest sources of variation among the published studies of the validity of clinical assessments is the type of variables included in the various assessment protocols. Variables included for analysis range from oromotor measures to the percentage of a meal eaten [24]. Some studies have included only variables associated with a specific test (eg, cough on or after swallowing, voice quality) [23]. In other studies, the clinical examination result may be only part of the information used to make a diagnosis [24–26,29,31]. The results of the clinical test may have been interpreted by taking other information, such as premorbid vocal quality, into account; this approach presents a source of considerable bias. In addition, many studies do not report whether the person conducting/scoring the reference test was blinded to the results of the clinical examination. Radiographic examinations often are plagued with this source of bias (diagnostic suspicion bias and expectation bias), because radiographic interpretation is subjective and is influenced easily by clinical information. These biases tend to increase the agreement between an examination and the reference standard of validity, so that the clinical test seems to be more useful than it actually is.

Reference test

Most studies of clinical examination validity have used videofluoroscopy as the reference test for the diagnosis of dysphagia or aspiration, but the reference test itself may be an imperfect standard. Given the previous uncertainty regarding the validity of VFE, the use of this test as the reference standard is questionable. Another issue relates to the interpretation of the reference test. The design of the standard measure in the Nathadwarawala study [25,29] suggested the use of multiple tests rather than a single examination, because each section of the total examination supplied very different information. Consequently these tests would be interpreted better as a series rather than as a single result. If conducted in parallel, such multiple testing may result in a more sensitive diagnostic strategy, at the expense of specificity.

When comparing a new test against any standard measure, one must remain aware of the potential paradox that can arise if the standard method, although accepted, is inaccurate. If a new test is compared with an old but inaccurate standard, the new test may seem worse when it actually is better [43]. For example, if a new test is more sensitive than the reference test, the additional patients identified by the new test will be considered false positives in relation to the standard. The opposite is true when the new test presents negative results: they will be considered false negatives compared with the standard. Thus, an inaccurate standard of validity will result in the new examination performing no better than the standard, and the new examination may seem inferior even though it performs better.

Analysis methods

A variety of statistical methods have been used to support the findings of clinical examination validity. Most investigators attempting to predict aspiration or dysphagia have used small numbers of subjects and have interpreted only first-order effects. Some authors have reported sensitivity and specificity ratios, but few, if any, have included an examination of the trade-off between the two measures using a receiver operator characteristic curve. They have discussed clinical data as a dichotomous choice rather than as reflecting a range of values. Clinically, terms that reflect the risk and likelihood of the presence of a disease or disorder may be more meaningful than the rigid present/absent dichotomy. Few investigators have addressed this situation. Even fewer have provided likelihood ratios that make it easier to go beyond the simple dichotomous classification of a test result as either normal or abnormal, as usually is done when describing the accuracy of a diagnostic test only in terms of sensitivity and specificity at a single cut-off point. Likelihood ratios permit a summary of information at different levels of disorder. In this way, information about the degree of abnormality, rather than just the crude presence or absence of abnormality, can be reported.

To investigate the relative contribution of the various clinical variables to the prediction of dysphagia or aspiration, most investigators have used simple methods that do not describe adequately the potential interaction of factors that are likely to influence decisions. Few authors have made adjustments for such confounding factors in the prediction of aspiration or dysphagia. In clinical situations, many factors act together to produce effects, and associations among factors often are complex. The failure to adjust for potential confounding factors may result in a stronger predictive role being assigned to factors that are only markers for other more important components. Most studies have used simple univariate measures of association as evidence that a variable has a predictive role in diagnosis.

Multivariate statistical methods can be used to adjust for the confounding effects of many variables to determine the independent effects of one of them. From a large set of variables, a smaller subset is selected that independently and significantly contributes to the overall variation in the outcome. Overall, multivariate statistical methods have not been used widely in studies of clinical bedside assessments [32]. Multiple regression and logistic regression analysis have been reported in few studies [7,8,32,44,45]. More widespread use of these higher-order multivariate methods would help strengthen analyses of future bedside assessment tools significantly.

The clinical bedside assessment as a screening tool

The process of screening for disease has a long tradition within health care. The screening of patients for preclinical disease is well established within medical practice, and its principles are accepted within most health fields. Indeed, a substantial body of evidence exists regarding the accepted definitions and the utility of such procedures.

Within the field of oropharyngeal dysphagia, the clinical bedside or non-instrumented swallowing examination recently has attracted considerable attention as a potential screening practice for this disorder. The degree to which either the instrumented or noninstrumented swallowing assessments can be abbreviated or incorporated as screening tools remains controversial. In 2000, Martino and colleagues [46] completed a systematic review of the evidence for swallowing screening in patients who had experienced a stroke and included accepted clinical assessments as potential screening tools in their paper, indirectly supporting this position.

The concept that swallowing disorders are preventable if they are recognized early and managed appropriately underlies much of what often is termed "screening" for dysphagia. Although most investigators support the notion of making informed judgments on health status from physical examination, the description of this form of evaluation for dysphagia as "screening" remains controversial. Differences in the definition of dysphagia, in the methods used to assess swallowing function, in the timing of those assessments, and in the benefit derived from swallowing treatment all weigh into the confusion surrounding this issue. Clearly, the definition and function of a screening tool and its utility in the area of dysphagia require closer inspection within the context of the current health care environment.

"Screening" has been defined by the World Health Organization as "an activity in which a previously asymptomatic population is reviewed to identify those individuals requiring further diagnostic evaluation" [47]. The discriminating point in this definition lies in a tool's ability to identify disease/illness in individuals previously not known to have the disease. "Early detection" refers to the process of identifying a disease before obvious signs or symptoms appear. The definition of "diagnosis" encompasses the process of confirming disease in symptomatic individuals; therefore diagnosis is considered different from "screening."

Early identification of dysphagia by formal screening has been reported to decrease the incidence of pneumonia in patients hospitalized with acute stroke [48]. This finding has elevated the importance of early identification of dysphagia in health care organizations, as emphasized recently by the American Stroke Association and the Joint Commission on Accreditation of Health care Organizations [49]. These organizations now have outlined standardized measures for stroke care that include the use of a formal dysphagia screening by centers seeking certification and accreditation as a primary stroke center [49,50]. Although early identification of dysphagia following stroke potentially can reduce lethal comorbidities, adequate screening methods to detect patients at risk for dysphagia have not been delineated clearly.

The primary purpose of a screening protocol is to identify individuals who require further evaluation for a specific problem [47]. Pertaining to dysphagia, a screening protocol should be applied to all patients to identify selectively those who require further diagnostic evaluation of swallowing deficits. Thus, screening protocols, by nature, are different from comprehensive clinical evaluations, which characterize the signs and symptoms of identified dysphagia with the goal of designing interventions. Screening protocols are driven in part by the concept that early identification results in more effective clinical management.

Caution must be used in considering the clinical bedside assessment as a potential swallowing screen. Because a screening test must be inexpensive and easy to perform, it usually is not the most valid diagnostic method for a disease. In addition to sensitivity and specificity, the performance of a test is measured by its predictive ability. Although some information regarding the sensitivity and specificity of this type of tool is available [51], the evidence supporting the notion that early detection of swallowing disorders using clinical bedside assessment techniques prevents long-term negative outcomes is scarce. Similarly, few data exist to confirm that dysphagia can be identified reliably by using this method in asymptomatic individuals.

A clinical dysphagia examination may possess a high PPV for identifying swallowing problems in symptomatic individuals, but if the examination is used to screen asymptomatic people, most positive results may be false. In addition, because the average benefit to an individual from a screening examination is usually smaller than from interventions in response to symptoms, screening tests need to be safer than those used in normal clinical practice. Even a very small risk of complications from the screening examination may outweigh the benefits of early diagnosis. Given the reported level of silent aspiration missed on clinical examination methods, it seems reasonable to question the risk/benefit ratio of this procedure as a screening method alone.

Finally, screening is worthwhile only if a satisfactory diagnostic test is available. A satisfactory test must detect cases in sufficient numbers and at an acceptable cost and must not carry side effects that outweigh the benefits of screening. Evidence supporting the accuracy, safety, simplicity, acceptability, labeling effects, and financial costs of either method of swallowing evaluation (clinical bedside evaluation or VFE) currently are unavailable.

Summary

To date, many of the proposed forms of clinical bedside assessment lack validity and rigor in the evaluation of the various components of their design. The lack of a specific theoretic framework underlying the proposed assessment methods has resulted in symptom-driven assessment tools that prevent the identification of the breakdown in the swallowing process as a whole and do not account for the variability noted in its performance. In addition, the wide variation in sample size, type, methodology, and analysis methods reported has led to inconclusive results that cannot be interpreted or compared meaningfully. Consequently, attempts at establishing the immediate and predictive validity of such measures has resulted in a disparity between measures and measurements.

Currently, the most popular clinical methods for bedside assessment for dysphagia are either informal or nonvalidated, based on examinations of aspiration only, or derived from observational checklists or retrospective analyses of medical notes. In clinical reality the understanding of conditions frequently is unclear, and diagnoses of dysphagia often are vague or consist of a mere description of a set of manifestations. Conversely, with videofluoroscopy the biologic understanding of the condition may be comprehensive, but the measurement of signs or symptoms is imprecise. Before these methods can be considered for comprehensive assessment or screening, more detailed information is needed regarding their performance across diagnostic groups and at various time points in recovery from illness.

Within the field of dysphagia, there is an urgent need for a standardized and accepted clinical assessment tool, grounded in current neurophysiologic swallowing theory, that reflects both dysphagia and aspiration outcomes and has been evaluated through rigorous research design. The use of such an examination would provide a cogent foundation for future research and for clinical management. Because the final purpose of any assessment is to improve patient management and outcome, the traditional paradigm of test accuracy studies will be useful only if a true reference standard is chosen that has either a strong association with patient outcome or a direct relationship with patient management. High sensitivity and specificity alone cannot guarantee an improvement in patient outcome. Currently, the lack of a true reference standard and confusion surrounding the differences between swallowing screening and swallowing assessment measures limit the clinical value of these tests. One proposal to address this dilemma is the development of randomized, controlled trials to compare different assessment strategies. When a unanimously accepted reference standard is lacking, as is the case in swallowing disorders, randomized, controlled trials may be more appropriate than studies of test accuracy to determine the usefulness of a proposed diagnostic test. Although randomized, controlled trials often are undertaken to investigate issues in therapy and prevention, they also could be used to resolve difficulties in diagnosis and monitoring.

For the practicing clinician, data on how test results affect clinical judgment or on how test results are used in making patient-management decisions may be more pertinent. Unfortunately in the arena of swallowing research, comprehensive data on how the results from the various assessment forms affect outcome are not yet available. In the absence of such hard data, clinicians should consider using methods that match the primary objective of the given evaluation. For example, if the aim is to determine swallowing safety, then a water-swallow screen may suffice; however, if the aim is to develop ongoing treatment planning or monitoring, then an assessment method that encompasses detailed skill profiling would be more useful. In addition, clinicians can adopt a testing strategy that maximizes the resources available to them while balancing the known impact of these strategies. Parallel and serial testing are two strategies that can be used when no single test provides enough information to assure a confident diagnosis. When a clinician is faced with two or more relatively insensitive measures, parallel testing can be initiated in which both measures are conducted independently and in concert. The net effect of this action is to provide a more sensitive diagnostic strategy, but it carries the potential of overdiagnosis and more false-positive results. The alternate strategy is serial testing in which a clinician uses an evaluation strategy that is contingent on previous test outcomes. For example a history is taken and then, based on the results, either a physical examination or an instrumental examination is performed. Although this strategy maximizes specificity, it lowers sensitivity, with the increased risk that a patient who has true dysphagia will be missed. This strategy is most often beneficial when there is significant risk attached to further testing. Last, the clinician also should consider patient preference in how testing is undertaken. Informed, patient-guided management decisions translate into improved patient compliance and outcome. This benefit also is seen with the procedures for swallowing evaluation.

Clearly, the field of diagnostic testing and screening for swallowing disorders is advancing. Methodology is improving, and data are accumulating to help researchers develop stronger, more rigorous evaluation tools. Meanwhile, practicing clinicians will benefit from a clear understanding of the goals and intended outcomes of their assessments. Moreover, appreciation of the issues and evidence surrounding test development and administration as presented in this article will help focus both practice and research in dysphagia.

References

[1] Langmore S, Logemann J. After the clinical bedside examination: what next? Am J Speech Lang Pathol 1991;9:13–20.

[2] Roeder B, Murray J, Dierkhising R. Patient localization of esophageal dysphagia. Dig Dis Sci 2004;49:697–701.

[3] Ramsey D, Smithard D, Kalra L. Early assessments of dysphagia and aspiration risk in acute stoke. Stroke 2003;34:1–6.

[4] Logemann J. Treatment efficacy summary: oropharyngeal dysphagia (difficulty in swallowing). Rockville (MD): American Speech-Language-Hearing Association; 1995.

[5] Logemann J. Evaluation and treatment of swallowing disorders. San Diego (CA): College Hill Press; 1983.

[6] Mann G. Effectiveness and efficiency: state of the art in dysphagia rehabilitation after stroke. Australian Communication Quarterly 1996;4:25–7.

[7] Smithard D, O'Neill P, England R, et al. The natural history of dysphagia following a stroke. Dysphagia 1997;12:188–93.

[8] Mann G, Hankey G, Cameron D. Swallowing disorders following acute stroke: prevalence and diagnostic accuracy. Cerebrovasc Dis 2000;10:380–6.

[9] Sorin R, Somers S, Austin W, et al. The influence of videofluoroscopy on the management of the dysphagic patient. Dysphagia 1988;2:127–35.

[10] Dodds W, Logemann J, Stewart E. Radiologic assessment of abnormal oral and pharyngeal phases of swallowing. AJR Am J Roentgenol 1990;154:965–74.

[11] McConnel F, Cerenko D, Jackson R, et al. Clinical application of the manofluorogram. Laryngoscope 1988;98:705–11.

[12] Logemann J. Manual for the video fluorographic study of swallowing. San Diego (CA): College-Hill Press; 1986.

[13] Splaingard M, Hutchins B, Sulton L, et al. Aspiration in rehabilitation patients: videofluoroscopy vs bedside clinical assessment. Arch Phys Med Rehabil 1988;69:637–40.

[14] Smithard D. Assessment of swallowing following acute stroke. Stroke Review 2002;6:7–10.

[15] Lazarus C, Logemann J. Swallowing disorders in closed head trauma patients. Arch Phys Med Rehabil 1987;68:79–84.

[16] Lof G, Robbins J. Test-retest variability in normal swallowing. Dysphagia 1990;4:236–42.

[17] Wilcox F, Liss J, Siegel G. Interjudge agreement in videofluoroscopic studies of swallowing. J Speech Hear Res 1996;39:144–52.

[18] McCullough G, Wertz T, Rosenbek J. Sensitivity and specificity of clinical/bedside examination signs for detecting aspiration in adults subsequent to stroke. J Commun Disord 2001;34: 55–72.

[19] Langmore S, Schatz K, Olsen N. Endoscopic and videofluoroscopic evaluations of swallowing and aspiration. Ann Otol Rhinol Laryngol 1991;100:678–81.

[20] Iskander E, Champion R, Mortensen L. PHAD validation and correlation with the modified barium swallow. Australian Communication Quarterly 1990:4:16–8.

[21] Gordon C, Hewer R, Wade D. Dysphagia in acute stroke. Br Med J (Clin Res Ed) 1987;295: 411–4.

[22] Garon B, Engle M, Ormiston C. Silent aspiration: results of 1000 videofluoroscopic swallow evaluations. J Neurol Rehabil 1996;10:121–6.

[23] DePippo K, Holas M, Reding M. Validation of the 3-oz water swallow test for aspiration following stroke. Arch Neurol 1992;49:1259–61.

[24] DePippo K, Holas M, Reding M. The Burke Dysphagia Screening Test: validation of its use in patients with stroke. Arch Phys Med Rehabil 1994;75:1284–6.

[25] Nathadwarawala K, Nicklin J, Wiles C. A timed test of swallowing capacity for neurological patients. J Neurol Neurosurg Psychiatry 1992;55:822–5.

[26] Hinds N, Wiles C. Assessment of swallowing and referral to speech and language therapists in acute stroke. QJM 1998;91:829–35.

[27] Wu M, Chang U, Wang T, et al. Evaluating swallowing dysfunction using a 100-mL water swallowing test. Dysphagia 2004;19:43–7.

[28] Gottlieb D, Kipnis M, Sister E, et al. Validation of the 50 mL drinking test for evaluation of post-stroke dysphagia. Disabil Rehabil 1996;18:529–32.

[29] Nathadwarawala K, Me Groary A, Wiles C. Swallowing in neurological outpatients: use of a timed test. Dysphagia 1994;9:120–9.

[30] Tohara H, Saitoh E, Mays K, et al. Three tests for predicting aspiration without videofluorography. Dysphagia 2003;18:126–34.

[31] Mari F, Matei M, Ceravolo M, et al. Predictive value of clinical indices in detecting aspiration in patients with neurological disorders. J Neurol Neurosurg Psychiatry 1997; 63:456–60.

[32] Linden P, Kuhlemeier K, Patterson C. The probability of correctly predicting subglottic penetration from clinical observations. Dysphagia 1993;8:170–9.

[33] Mann G. MASA: the Mann Assessment of Swallowing Ability. Clifton (NY): Thomson Learning, Inc; 2002.

[34] Crary M, Carnaby Mann G, Groher M. Initial psychometric assessment of a functional oral intake scale for dysphagia in stroke patients. Arch Phys Med Rehabil 2005;86:1516–20.

[35] Vanderwegen J, Guns C, Van Nuffelen G, et al. The reliability of the MASA dysphagia screening protocol compared to FEES for patients in an acute stroke unit [abstract]. Dysphagia 2006;21:327.

[36] Fleming S. Index of dysphagia: a tool for identifying deglutition problems. Dysphagia 1987; 1:206–8.

[37] Layne K, Losinski D, Zenner P, et al. Using the Fleming index of dysphagia to establish prevalence. Dysphagia 1989;4:39–42.

[38] Linden P, Siebens A. Dysphagia: predicting laryngeal penetration. Arch Phys Med Rehabil 1983;64:281–4.

[39] Mann G, Hankey G, Cameron D. Swallowing function after stroke: prognosis and prognostic factors at 6 months. Stroke 1999;30:744–8.

[40] Barer D. The natural history and functional consequences of dysphagia after hemispheric stroke. J Neurol Neurosurg Psychiatry 1989;52:236–41.

[41] Ott D, Hodge R, Pikna L, et al. Modified barium swallow: clinical and radiographic correlation and relation to feeding recommendations. Dysphagia 1996;11:187–90.

[42] Fletcher R, Fletcher S, Wagner E. Clinical epidemiology: the essentials. Baltimore (MD): Williams and Wilkins; 1998.

[43] Garcia-Romero H, Garcia-Barrios C, Ramos-Gutierrez F. Effects of uncertain results on sensitivity and specificity of diagnostic tests. Lancet 1996;348(9043):1745–6.

[44] Daniels S, McAdam C, Brailey K, et al. Clinical assessment of swallowing and prediction of dysphagia severity. Am J Speech Lang Pathol 1997;6:17–24.

[45] Horner J, Massey E, Brazer S. Aspiration in bilateral stroke patients. Neurology 1990;40: 1686–8.

[46] Martino R, Foley N, Bhogal S, et al. Dysphagia after stroke: incidence, diagnosis, and pulmonary complications. Stroke 2005;36:2756–63.

[47] World health organization. Principles and practices of screening for disease. Geneva (Switzerland): World Health Organization; 1968.

[48] Hinchey J, Shephard T, Furie K, et al. Formal dysphagia screening protocols prevent pneumonia. Stroke 2005;36:1972–6.

[49] The Joint Commission. Stroke performance measurement implementation guide. 2nd edition 2007. Available at: http://www.jointcommission.org/CertificationPrograms/PrimaryStrokeCenters/stroke_pm_edition_2.htm.

[50] Thom T, Haase N, Robamond W, et al. Heart disease and stroke statistics—2006 update. A report from the American Heart Association Statistics Committee and Stroke Statistics Subcommittee. Circulation 2006;113:e85–151.

[51] Perry L, Love C. Screening for dysphagia and aspiration in acute stroke: a systematic review. Dysphagia 2001;16:7–18.

[52] Kidd D, Lawson J, Nesbitt R, et al. The natural history and clinical consequences of aspiration in acute stroke. Q J Med 1995;88:409–13.

[53] Stanners A, Chapman A, Bamford J. Clinical predictors of aspiration soon after stroke. Age Ageing 1993;22:17–8.

ELSEVIER
SAUNDERS

Phys Med Rehabil Clin N Am
19 (2008) 769–785

PHYSICAL MEDICINE
AND REHABILITATION
CLINICS OF
NORTH AMERICA

The Videofluorographic Swallowing Study

Bonnie Martin-Harris, PhD, SLP, BRS-S[a,b,c,*],
Bronwyn Jones, MBBS, FRACP, FRCR[d]

[a]*Evelyn Trammell Institute for Voice and Swallowing,
Department of Otolaryngology, Head and Neck Surgery, Medical University
of South Carolina, Charleston, SC 29425, USA*
[b]*Department of Communication Sciences and Disorders, College of Health
and Rehabilitation Science, Medical University of South Carolina,
151 Rutledge Avenue, Building A, Charleston, SC 29425, USA*
[c]*Saint Joseph's Hospital of Atlanta, Evelyn Trammell Voice and Swallowing Center,
5665 Peachtree Dunwoody Road NE, Atlanta, GA 30342, USA*
[d]*The Russell H. Morgan Department of Radiology and Radiological Sciences,
The Johns Hopkins Hospital, 600 North Wolfe Street, Baltimore, MD 21287, USA*

The literature is dense with measurement methods used to estimate the presence and degree of oropharyngeal and esophageal swallowing dysfunction. These methods are directed toward gaining objective indexes of the timing [1–8], pressure [5,9–15], range [16–18], and strength [19–21] of structural movements, bolus flow patterns [22–26], bolus clearance and efficiency [11], airway protection [27,28], and sensation [29–32]. These studies have established a strong theoretic framework toward understanding the nature of swallowing abnormalities. Multiple assessment methods are in existence and development. Although the current health care climate demands fiscal responsibility, clinicians must choose the test that is appropriate for each patient and delivers the highest diagnostic and prognostic clinical yield. Furthermore, the test and the measurement methods used to capture oropharyngeal swallowing impairment must be practical for routine clinical application.

The videofluorographic swallowing study (VFSS), also known as a *modified barium swallowing* (MBS) examination, is often considered the

* Corresponding author. Department of Otolaryngology-Head and Neck Surgery, Medical University of South Carolina, 135 Rutledge Avenue, MSC 550, Charleston, SC 29425-5500.
E-mail address: harrisbm@musc.edu (B. Martin-Harris).

1047-9651/08/$ - see front matter © 2008 Elsevier Inc. All rights reserved.
doi:10.1016/j.pmr.2008.06.004   *pmr.theclinics.com*

preferred instrument by most practicing swallowing clinicians because it allows visualization of bolus flow in relation to structural movement throughout the upper aerodigestive tract in real time. The VFSS also permits detection of the presence and timing of aspiration (ie, entry of ingested material through the level of the true vocal folds into the trachea) [33,34] and helps identify the physiologic and often treatable causes of the aspiration [35–39]. Furthermore, clinicians are able to observe the effects of various bolus volumes, bolus textures, and compensatory strategies on swallowing physiology [37].

Clinicians evaluating and treating swallowing disorders use a videofluoroscopic radiology procedure to assess swallowing physiology in patients who have symptoms of swallowing disorders (ie, dysphagia) and to estimate the degree of swallowing impairment from observations made during the examination. The examination usually includes the collaborative expertise of a physician, most commonly a radiologist or physiatrist, and speech–language pathologist.

This MBS examination captures sequential videoradiographic images of barium contrast–impregnated food and liquid as they are transported through the oral cavity, pharyngeal cavity, and esophagus in real time. Various volumes and textures of food and liquid are administered and clinical impressions of the presence and degree of swallowing impairment are obtained from the radiographic images [35,38–43]. Judgments are also made regarding the coordination and timing of swallowing events [1,28,36,44–48]. Based on these qualitative observations, critical and sometimes life-sustaining recommendations are made regarding oral versus nonoral intake, diet type, referrals to other medical specialties, and treatment strategies that improve function or minimize the risk for aspiration [38].

Despite the clinical efficacy of the examination, clinicians must acknowledge that the patient's performance during the examination may not be entirely representative of the patient's typical eating and drinking function. Variables such as fatigue, medications, and anxiety may impact the testing results. Clinicians must observe patients during their usual eating and drinking environment to determine the external validity of the examination results and assess the patient's ability to carry-over any learned swallowing strategies. Furthermore, the VFSS is also used to monitor any changes in swallowing function over time during the course of swallowing treatment and the progression of a disease or condition.

Videofluorographic swallowing study: an indirect sensory and motor examination

Swallowing is an array of synergistic interdependent movements, initiated by a complex set of sensory inputs that generate motor responses. These motor responses create pressures and forces to propel ingested materials through the upper aerodigestive tract and simultaneously protect the upper airway. Although the VFSS does not use direct measures of sensation and muscle strength, the following evidence suggests that trained examiners can make accurate and reliable clinical judgments about the presence of sensory and motor impairment.

The following description of VFSS observations are characterized as physiologic components. Most observed components contribute to judgments of sensory and motor impairment because the initiation and integrity of the motor response partly depends on sensory input.

A prime example of this combined sensorimotor assessment is observation of the motor events that occur early in the pharyngeal swallow. If these events are delayed for several seconds, the sensory input to the pharyngeal motor response is probably decreased below the normal level required to initiate the cascade of pharyngeal motor events. Clinicians evaluate the sensorimotor relationships during the VFSS and administer various bolus consistencies, textures, and sometimes taste to assess their effect on swallowing function.

Swallowing physiology: foundation for videofluorographic swallowing study

Swallowing is a complex physiologic event comprised of simultaneous and sequential contractions of muscles of the oral–facial region, pharynx, larynx, and esophagus. Descriptions of swallowing physiology were attempted well before the development of a sophisticated modality for viewing the rapid contractions and movements of the muscles and structures associated with swallowing. In 1813, Magendie [49] was the first to separate swallowing into phases or stages representing the anatomic regions traversed by the *bolus*, or ball of material, to be swallowed. The rapid sequential and overlapping motions characterizing adult human swallowing behavior were better appreciated after radiography was introduced, especially videoradiography.

Although phase descriptions remain in current literature, evidence suggests that the physiologic components of the process overlap and are interdependent as the bolus traverses the regional phases (oral, pharyngeal, esophageal), which has led clinicians to attempt to assess the physiology of the swallowing rather than report abnormality of a given phase. Furthermore, the physiology is the target of swallowing rehabilitation, and therefore these targets must be identified before the treatment plan is developed. Swallowing clinicians attempt to evaluate components of swallowing behavior on VFSS examinations in patients presenting with clinical signs or symptoms of dysphagia (Box 1).

Clinicians also use the 15 literature-based components to estimate the severity of the impairments and make critical intake and diet texture recommendations, swallowing therapy recommendations, and predictions about functional outcomes [38,40,41].

Box 1. List of 15 physiologic components assessed during VFSS

1. Lip closure
2. Lingual elevation
3. Tongue-to-palatal seal
4. Bolus preparation/mastication
5. Bolus transport/lingual motion
6. Initiation of pharyngeal swallow
7. Soft palate elevation and retraction
8. Laryngeal elevation
9. Anterior hyoid excursion
10. Laryngeal closure
11. Pharyngeal contraction
12. Pharyngoesophageal segment opening
13. Tongue base retraction
14. Epiglottic inversion
15. Esophageal clearance

Although the late oral and early pharyngeal components of swallowing are the most critical from a safety viewpoint, the oral preparatory and early oral transport aspects of swallow are the most aesthetically and psychologically important. During the oral preparatory stage of swallow, the bolus is manipulated by lingual motion and masticated (if necessary). Although not a characteristic of natural drinking or eating behavior in most healthy individuals [50], the ability to contain a liquid bolus (component 1, Fig. 1A) in the oral cavity through an anterior lip seal and lateral and posterior tongue-to-palatal contact (Fig. 1B) is assessed. The proficiency of this task provides clinical information about a patient's ability to follow simple commands during swallowing, which is an important prognostic indicator for successful learning of compensatory swallowing strategies.

Furthermore, the ability to contain a bolus within the oral cavity provides information on oral motor control. The tongue is the major mobile element of the oral swallow and plays a complementary role in bolus preparation and mastication. The tongue also plays a major role in bolus containment and airway maintenance [51,52]. The back of the tongue assumes a slightly elevated position from contraction of various muscle groups, and opposes an actively contracted soft palate that is drawn downward and forward (component 2, see Fig. 1B). This glossopalatine mechanism (component 3, see Fig. 1B) ensures that portions of a liquid bolus do not fall prematurely over the base of the tongue [35,43]. The ingested material is mixed with saliva and tasted during rotary mandibular chewing (component 4), a motion that is integrated into the oral swallowing process and propelled through the oral cavity by way of lingual motility (component 5, Fig. 1C, D) [51–54].

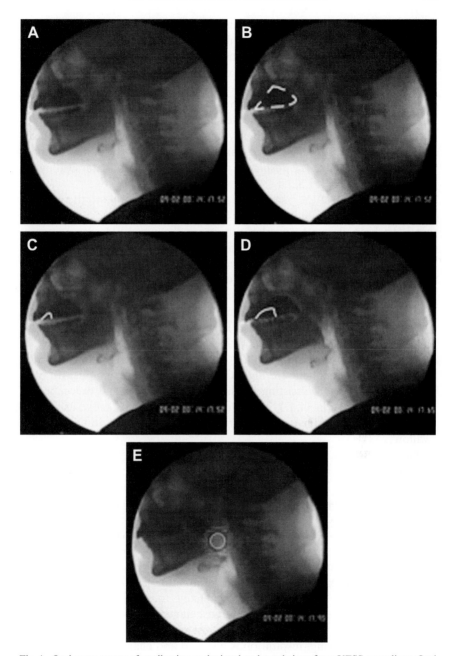

Fig. 1. Oral components of swallowing as depicted on lateral views from VFSS recordings. Oral containment through (A) anterior lip seal and (B) tongue-to-palatal contact. (C) Early and (D) mid-lingual motility during oral bolus transport. (E) Initiation of the pharyngeal swallow.

When adult humans eat natural bite sizes of solid foods, portions of the food may be propelled to and accumulate in the pharynx during mastication [54]. If the system has inefficiencies, such as muscle weakness or sensory loss, residual material may remain in the oral or pharyngeal cavity, placing the patient at risk for inadequate nutrition/hydration or airway compromise.

As the bolus is propelled through the oral cavity through upward and forward motion of the tongue, the head of the bolus reaches the region of the posterior oral cavity or oropharynx. When the sensory receptive fields in these areas are stimulated, the pharyngeal swallow is initiated (component 6, Fig. 1E) and the respiratory pause to accommodate swallowing becomes obligatory [51,52,55].

Although onset of the pharyngeal swallow varies relative to the position of the bolus [56], when initiated it is characterized by five mechanical events that have been shown to overlap during synchronized videorecordings of structural movements during swallow. These events protect the airway and clear the pharynx of ingested material, and include (1) elevation and retraction of the soft palate (component 7, Fig. 2A); (2) elevation and anterior displacement of the larynx (component 8, Fig. 2B) and hyoid bone (Fig. 2C); (3) laryngeal closure (component 10, Fig. 2D); (4) pharyngeal contraction (component 11); and (5) opening of the pharyngoesophageal region (component 12, Fig. 2E) [1,28,35,36,40,41,43–48]. Contraction of the pharyngeal constrictors (Fig. 2F) coincides with the forceful retraction of the tongue (component 13, Fig. 2G), which applies strong positive pressure on the bolus tail, assisting in pharyngeal clearance and prevention of pharyngeal residue [5,44,47]. The hyoid bone and larynx move as a functional unit in a superior and anterior trajectory during a normal, nutritive swallow.

These critical motions, observed during VFSS, are physiologically linked to effect vestibular closure (ie, through approximation of the arytenoid cartilages and the epiglottic petiole together with full inversion of the epiglottic tip) (component 14, see Fig. 2F; Fig. 2H) and to opening and distension of the pharyngoesophageal segment (PES) (see Fig. 2E). Opening of the segment permits entry of the ingested material into the cervical esophageal region [5,44,45,47,48,57]. The traction placed on the cricoid cartilage during this brisk motion pulls the cartilage anteriorly and away from the posterior pharyngeal wall, opening the compliant PES region (see Fig. 2E) [5,44,45,47,48,57]. This compliance is related to early relaxation of the cricopharyngeal muscle, the primary muscular component of the segment [55]. As the larynx descends toward its rest position in the latter stages of pharyngeal swallowing, respiration is resumed and characterized by a small expiratory airflow in most adult human swallows [58–60].

The mechanics of the esophageal body and lower esophageal sphincter are less complex and easier to study because of their slow speed relative to oropharyngeal swallow events. The bolus head enters the cervical esophageal region through the distended PES, continues through the esophagus, and is propelled and cleared (component 15, Fig. 3) through primary and secondary esophageal peristaltic muscle contractions [61,62]. These contractions continue until the bolus head and tail progress through the passively relaxed lower esophageal sphincter (LES) and advance into the stomach.

A few behavioral interventions are available to modify the contractile characteristics of the esophagus and improve esophageal clearance [41]. However, clinical evidence and preliminary research indicate that esophageal clearance in the upright position seems to have some functional impact on pharyngeal clearance and possible airway protection [63]. Therefore, clinicians observe esophageal clearance in the upright eating and drinking position during the MBS examination to gain an impression of the potential impact of incomplete or slowed esophageal clearance on oropharyngeal swallowing function; the potential for aspiration of residual esophageal contents; and the nutritional status of the patient.

The anteroposterior image projection is the optimal view for assessing the efficiency of esophageal clearance in the upright position. This viewing plane is also best suited to determine the overall symmetry of oropharyngeal swallowing function and the immediate effectiveness of compensatory postures.

Move toward standardization

By definition, a *gold standard* is a test against which all other tests are measured. The VFSS has often been described as the gold standard for the evaluation of oropharyngeal swallowing. However, a single test is unlikely to provide the best assessment of swallowing for every patient and condition. Other imaging methods, such as flexible endoscopy, may supplant or complement VFSS examination. Nonetheless, clinical use data indicate that VFSS is the preferred method by most practicing clinicians, and efforts should be taken to standardize the examination protocol, terminology used to describe swallowing behavior, and method for quantifying swallowing impairment.

Clinicians have not adopted a universally accepted terminology or tool that has been empirically based, reliable, and valid for converting clinical information into a quantifiable metric to diagnose swallowing impairment. Empiric evidence and standardization have been lacking for selecting the measured physiologic components and types of measures used, and categorizing functional swallowing components into regional domains (ie, phases). This lack of standardization in measurement methods across clinics and laboratories impedes understanding of true functional results in studies documenting rehabilitative (swallowing therapy) and restorative (surgery and medications) effects of treatment; produces ambiguous reporting of outcomes; and hinders understanding of what restorative and rehabilitative targets should be to impact the overall health and well-being of patients who have dysphagia.

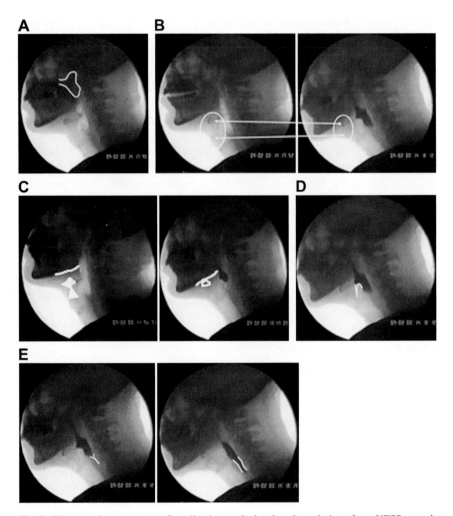

Fig. 2. Pharyngeal components of swallowing as depicted on lateral views from VFSS record-ings. (*A*) Elevation and retraction of the soft palate. Elevation and anterior displacement of the (*B*) larynx and (*C*) hyoid bone. (*D*) Laryngeal closure through apposition of arytenoid cartilages to epiglottic base. (*E*) Opening and distension of pharyngoesophageal segment. (*F*) Pharyngeal contraction and stripping wave. (*G*) Tongue base retraction and apposition with posterior pharyngeal wall. (*H*) Epiglottic inversion.

The Agency for Health Care Research and Quality (AHRQ) reports [64]:

- Standardization is critical to supporting valid comparisons and bench-marking across health care settings
- Comparability makes the information useful for quality improvement and public reporting
- Standardization assures users of the results that the validity and reliability built into the instrument by the developers are maintained

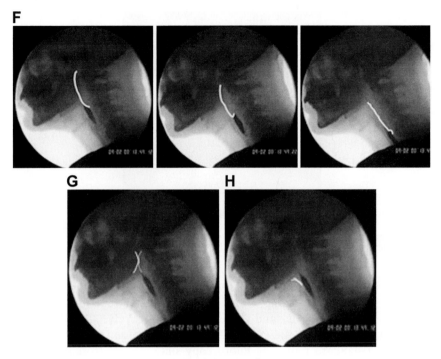

Fig. 2 (*continued*)

- Adaptation of a voluntary standards system will lead to optimization of patient care quality, safety, efficacy, and cost

AHRQ further reports that voluntary standards should be applied to the content and format of the test instrument, the data collection protocol, the analyses and interpretations, and reporting. Translating Research into Practice-II initiative focused on implementation of techniques and factors, such as those associated with successfully translating research findings into diverse applied setting. This initiative bought clinician accountability to the forefront in clinical practice. The report stated that the increased demands for accountability in health care, including reporting of clinical performance using standardized quality measures, have created a sense of urgency about improving these areas within health care organizations and clinical practices.

Standardization: videofluorographic swallowing study procedure and protocol

The descriptions if the VFSS as originally described by Logemann [40] continue to be followed in most clinical practices [42,65]. Patients are initially positioned in the lateral view, and regions of visualization include

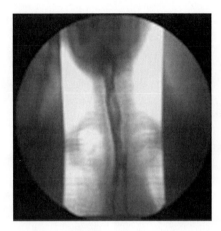

Fig. 3. Esophageal clearance in the upright position as depicted on the anteroposterior view from VFSS recording.

the oral cavity, pharyngeal cavity, larynx, and cervical esophagus. The visualization field includes the lips anteriorly, nasal cavity superiorly, cervical spinal column posteriorly, and the entire PES inferiorly [35,38,40,41,43]. The larynx should be in full view within this visualization field. The VFSS occurs in a standard radiology fluoroscopy suite. The fluoroscope is activated by the radiologist for a few seconds before and then after administration of the barium substances. The fluoroscope is deactivated shortly after the bolus tail exits the cervical esophageal region.

The lateral view is ideal for judging movements that generate pressures and open and close critical valves during swallow. Patients are then positioned in the anteroposterior (ie, frontal) viewing plane so that judgments can be made about symmetry of bolus flow, pharyngeal wall contraction, and symmetry of structure and function during bolus flow. All patients should ideally be examined in the lateral and frontal positions. An examination performed in only the lateral position can miss vital abnormalities that can be appreciated only in the frontal position. For example, examination in the frontal position is essential to detect unilateral abnormalities, such as unilateral pharyngeal paresis or paralysis and unilateral vocal fold paralysis. Total radiation exposure averages 3 to 5 minutes, an amount typically encountered in an upper gastrointestinal series. The examination may be extended depending on the nature and severity of the swallowing problem and patient condition; however, the goal of minimizing radiation exposure while maximizing clinical yield is consistently maintained.

Accurate analysis requires video freeze-frame and slow motion capability. Dynamic recording at a minimum of 30 video frames per second is essential for detecting the rapid movements and bolus flow events associated with oropharyngeal swallowing and is easily accomplished through linking a recording device to the fluoroscopic unit. A 100- or 105-mm spot-film camera with maximum frame rates of 6 to 8 frames per second is inadequate to evaluate swallowing (eg, subtle but critical laryngeal penetration or aspiration may be visible on only 1 or 2 frames of a sequence of 30 frames per second) [42,65].

The VFSS typically includes administration of various bolus volumes and textures because data have shown the potential physiologic benefits of manipulating these sensory variables. However, the consistencies of the contrast material and volumes administered have not been standardized across most clinics; one reason is that clinicians often introduce certain consistencies based on their clinical intuitions of likely patient performance. However, implementation of these practices has not been validated.

A recent study [66] has shown the need and feasibility of standardizing contrast materials. Martin and colleagues [66] determined the contribution of bolus volumes, consistencies, and textures to the overall impressions of swallowing component scores. Although the investigators identified a role for most commonly tested standardized volumes of thin liquid, nectar-thick liquid, honey-thick liquid, pudding, and cookie to one or several of the component impairment scores, 5 mL of thin and nectar-thick liquid provided sufficient information that allowed trained clinicians to make reliable assessments of the 15 physiologic swallowing components. If 5 mL of liquid (thin and nectar-thick) continues to allow judgments of impairment in subsequent studies, these two swallow trials may serve as "screening swallows" that signal the need to progress, or perhaps conclude the MBS examination. This finding certainly attests to the potentially misguided practice of foregoing the thin-liquid swallow because of the perception that patients will perform better (ie, less aspiration) with a more viscous bolus.

Standardization: videofluorographic swallowing study terminology, interpretation, and reporting

In addition to testing the role for standardizing the VFSS protocol, the study by Martin and colleagues [66] also intended to rigorously test the reliability, content, construct, and external validity of a new MBS tool (MBSImp) to quantify swallowing impairment. The tool includes an ordinal scaling methodology of each of the previously described set of physiologic components, whereby each score represents a unique observation from the VFSS. The tool shows content and construct validity and good concordance between and within clinician scoring.

Furthermore, because the VFSS represents a clinical simulation of a feeding/eating experience, any measures of impairment gained from the test should demonstrate relevance to the functional outcome of the patient. The tool was examined for this relationship, and the measures of swallowing impairment showed good external validation through statistically significant correlations with blinded outcome assessments of diet, health status, nutrition, and quality of life.

Adaptation of this voluntary standards system will lead to optimization of patient care quality, safety, efficacy, and cost. Standardized practices facilitate interinstitutional exchange of patient data using electronic data collection, aggregation, and reporting systems [64,67]. The results of this study show the achievement of a critical strategic step toward standardizing swallowing assessment. Implementation of standardized training, protocol, contrast materials, and measurements should improve the ability to compare the swallowing impairment exhibited by patients who have dysphagia during recovery or physiologic decline associated with natural histories of progressive neurologic diseases across clinics and clinical laboratories.

Videofluorographic swallowing study: a rehabilitation examination

A primary purpose of a VFSS is to determine the effect of various behavioral and sensory interventions on the physiologic function of the swallowing mechanism. Several studies have shown the ability to detect immediate effects of compensatory strategies (bolus volume, consistency and taste, postural alterations, swallowing, and respiratory maneuvers) on swallowing physiology [9,14,68–82]. The systematic application of these evidence-based strategies, if applied directly to the observed physiologic impairment, often leads to the development of eating and drinking strategies that may be immediately implemented by the patient, caregiver, and clinician. Swallowing rehabilitation strategies are described elsewhere in this edition and will not be repeated here. Although patients may not be deemed safe for immediate oral intake after examination, the importance of the VFSS for optimizing oral intake within the limits of the patient's physiologic potential cannot be understated. Proper administration and interpretation of the examination has the potential to upgrade oral intake status and diet textures and determine oral intake restrictions [38,83]. Recommendations are based not only on the patient's physiologic status but also on their cognitive status, the caregiver situation, and the nature of the underlying disease or condition.

Summary

Strong evidence has shown VFSS to be the ideally suited method for identifying and quantifying the presence and nature of oropharyngeal and cervical esophageal swallowing disorders. The ability to assess overlapping and interdependent structural movements as they relate to bolus flow in real time throughout the swallowing process has had high clinical yield. When the VFSS protocol is standardized, interpreted, and reported by trained clinicians using standardized and validated measures, treatment can be systematically applied during and after the examination according to the physiologic swallowing problem. Furthermore, change in the patient's swallowing performance and responsiveness to swallowing interventions can be consistently applied and communicated across clinics and hospitals. These standardized practices will result in seamless patient care and optimize swallowing treatment throughout the continuum of care.

Acknowledgments

We wish to thank all of the patients who have contributed to our knowledge by allowing us the opportunity to care for them and learn from them when volunteering for our clinical studies. Dr. Martin-Harris gratefully acknowledges her funding sources that include the National Institute on Deafness and Other Communication Disorders at the National Institutes of Health (NIDCD K23 DC005764) and the Mark and Evelyn Trammell Trust, Atlanta Georgia.

We wish to extend our gratitude to our colleagues at the MUSC Evelyn Trammell Institute for Voice and Swallowing and the Evelyn Trammell Voice and Swallowing Center at Saint Joseph's Hospital of Atlanta, particularly Julie Blair and Anita Cheslek for their masterful assistance in the preparation of this manuscript.

References

[1] Cook IJ, Dodds WJ, Dantas RO, et al. Timing of videofluoroscopic, manometric events, and bolus transit during the oral and pharyngeal phases of swallowing. Dysphagia 1989;4(1):8–15.

[2] Kendall K, McKenzie SW, Leonard R, et al. Timing of events in normal swallowing: a videofluoroscopic study. Dysphagia 2000;15(2):74–83.

[3] Martin-Harris B, Brodsky MB, Michel Y, et al. Breathing and swallowing dynamics across the adult lifespan. Arch Otolaryngol Head Neck Surg 2005;131(9):762–70.

[4] Martin-Harris B, Brodsky MB, Price CC, et al. Temporal coordination of pharyngeal and laryngeal dynamics with breathing during swallowing: single liquid swallows. J Appl Phys 2003;94(5):1735–43.

[5] McConnel FM, Cerenko D, Mendelsohn MS. Manofluorographic analysis of swallowing. Otolaryngol Clin North Am 1988;21(4):625–35.

[6] Perlman AL, Palmer PM, McCulloch TM, et al. Electromyographic activity from human laryngeal, pharyngeal, and submental muscles during swallowing. J Appl Phys 1999;86(5): 1663–9.

[7] Tracy JF, Logemann JA, Kahrilas PJ, et al. Preliminary observations on the effects of age on oropharyngeal deglutition. Dysphagia 1989;4(2):90–4.

[8] Van Daele DJ, McCulloch TM, Palmer PM, et al. Timing of glottic closure during swallowing: a combined electromyographic and endoscopic analysis. Ann Otol Rhinol Laryngol 2005;114(6):478–87.

[9] Castell JA, Castell DO, Schultz AR, et al. Effect of head position on the dynamics of the upper esophageal sphincter and pharynx. Dysphagia 1993;8(1):1–6.

[10] Castell JA, Dalton CB, Castell DO. Pharyngeal and esophageal sphincter manometry in humans. Am J Physiol Gastrointest Liver Physiol 1990;258(2):G173–8.

[11] Kahrilas PJ, Logemann JA, Lin S, et al. Pharyngeal clearance during swallowing: a combined manometric and videofluoroscopic study. Gastroenterology 1992;103(1):128–36.

[12] Robbins J, Hamilton JW, Lof GL, et al. Oropharyngeal swallowing in normal adults of different ages. Gastroenterology 1992;103(3):823–9.

[13] Perlman AL, Schultz JG, VanDaele DJ. Effects of age, gender, bolus volume, and bolus viscosity on oropharyngeal pressure during swallowing. J Appl Phys 1993;75(1):33–7.

[14] Shaker R, Ren J, Podvrsan B, et al. Effect of aging and bolus variables on pharyngeal and upper esophageal sphincter motor function. Am J Physiol 1993;264(3 Pt 1):G427–32.

[15] Steele CM, Huckabee ML. The influence of orolingual pressure on the timing of pharyngeal pressure events. Dysphagia 2007;22(1):30–6.

[16] Greene JR, Wang YT. Tongue-surface movement patterns during speech and swallowing. J Acoust Soc Am 2003;113(5):2820–33.

[17] Logemann JA, Pauloski BR, Rademaker AW, et al. Temporal and biomechanical characteristics of oropharyngeal swallow in younger and older men. J Speech Lang Hear Res 2000; 43(5):1264–74.

[18] Logemann JA, Pauloski BR, Rademaker AW, et al. Oropharyngeal swallow in younger and older women: videofluoroscopic analysis. Journal of Speech Language & Hearing Research 2002;45(3):434–45.

[19] Burkhead LM, Sapienza CM, Rosenbek JC. Strength-training exercise in dysphagia rehabilitation: principles, procedures, and directions for future research. Dysphagia 2007;22(3):251–65.

[20] Lazarus C, Logemann JA, Pauloski BR, et al. Effects of radiotherapy with or without chemotherapy on tongue strength and swallowing in patients with oral cancer. Head Neck 2007;29(7):632–7.

[21] Leonard RJ, Belafsky PC, Rees CJ. Relationship between fluoroscopic and manometric measures of pharyngeal constriction: the pharyngeal constriction ratio. Ann Otol Rhinol Laryngol 2006;115(12):897–901.

[22] Cerenko D, McConnel FM, Jackson RT. Quantitative assessment of pharyngeal bolus driving foces. Otolaryngol Head Neck Surg 1989;100(1):57–63.

[23] Daniels SK, Schroeder MF, DeGeorge PC, et al. Effects of verbal cue on bolus flow during swallowing. Am J Speech Lang Pathol 2007;16(2):140–7.

[24] Johnsson F, Shaw D, Gabb M, et al. Influence of gravity and body position on normal oropharyngeal swallowing. Am J Physiol 1995;269(5 Pt. 1):G653–8.

[25] McConnel FM, Guffin TNJ, Cerenko D, et al. The effects of bolus flow on vertical pharyngeal pressure measurement in the pharyngoesophageal segment: clinical significance. Otolaryngol Head Neck Surg 1992;106(2):169–74.

[26] Olsson R, Nilsson H, Ekberg O. Pharyngeal solid-state manometry catheter movement during swallowing in dysphagic and nondysphagic participants. Acad Radiol 1994;1(4): 339–44.

[27] Kahrilas PJ, Lin S, Rademaker AW, et al. Impaired deglutitive airway protection: a videofluoroscopic analysis of severity and mechanism. Gastroenterology 1997;113(5):1457–64.

[28] Logemann JA, Kahrilas PJ, Cheng J, et al. Closure mechanisms of laryngeal vestibule during swallow. Am J Physiol 1992;262(2 Pt 1):G338–44.

[29] Aviv JE, Martin JH, Keen MS, et al. Air pulse quantification of supraglottic and pharyngeal sensation: a new technique. Annals of Otology, Rhinology & Laryngology 1993;102(10): 777–80.

[30] Leow LP, Huckabee ML, Sharma S, et al. The influence of taste on swallowing apnea, oral preparation time, and duration and amplitude of submental muscle contraction. Chem Senses 2007;32(2):119–28.

[31] Logemann JA, Pauloski BR, Colangelo L, et al. Effects of a sour bolus on oropharyngeal swallowing measures in patients with neurogenic dysphagia. J Speech Hear Res 1995; 38(3):556–63.

[32] Pelletier CA, Dhanaraj GE. The effect of taste and palatability on lingual swallowing pressure. Dysphagia 2006;21(2):121–8.

[33] Robbins J, Coyle J, Rosenbek J, et al. Differentiation of normal and abnormal airway protection during swallowing using the penetration-aspiration scale [see comment]. Dysphagia 1999;14(4):228–32.

[34] Rosenbek JC, Robbins JA, Roecker EB, et al. A penetration-aspiration scale. Dysphagia 1996;11(2):93–8.

[35] Dodds WJ, Logemann JA, Stewart ET. Radiologic assessment of abnormal oral and pharyngeal phases of swallowing. Am J Roentgenol 1990;154(5):965–74.

[36] Ekberg O, Sigurjonsson SV. Movement of the epiglottis during deglutition. A cineradiographic study. Gastrointest Radiol 1982;7(2):101–7.

[37] Logemann JA. Behavioral management for oropharyngeal dysphagia. Folia Phoniatr Logop 1999;51(4–5):199–212.

[38] Martin-Harris B, Logemann JA, McMahon S, et al. Clinical utility of the modified barium swallow. Dysphagia 2000;15(3):136–41.

[39] Ramsey GH, Watson JS, Gramiak R, et al. Cinefluorographic analysis of the mechanism of swallowing. Radiology 1955;64(4):498–518.

[40] Logemann JA. Manual for the videofluorographic study of swallowing. 2nd edition. Austin (TX): ProEd; 1993.

[41] Logemann JA. Evaluation and treatment of swallowing disorders. Austin (TX): ProEd; 1998.

[42] Jones B, Donner MW. Normal and abnormal swallowing: Imaging in diagnosis and therapy. New York: Springer Verlag; 1991.

[43] Dodds WJ, Stewart ET, Logemann JA. Physiology and radiology of the normal oral and pharyngeal phases of swallowing. Am J Roentgenol 1990;154(5):953–63.

[44] Atkinson M, Kramer P, Wyman S, et al. The dynamics of swallow. I. Normal pharyngeal mechanisms. J Clin Invest 1957;36:581–98.

[45] Kahrilas PJ, Dodds WJ, Dent J, et al. Upper esophageal sphincter function during deglutition. Gastroenterology 1988;95(1):52–62.

[46] McConnel FM, Hester TR, Mendelsohn MS, et al. Manofluorography of deglutition after total laryngopharyngectomy. Plast Reconstr Surg 1988;81(3):346–51.

[47] Sokol EM, Heitmann P, Wolf BS, et al. Simultaneous cineradiographic and manometric study of the pharynx, hypopharynx, and cervical esophagus. Gastroenterology 1966;51(6): 960–74.

[48] Jacob P, Kahrilas PJ, Logemann JA, et al. Upper esophageal sphincter opening and modulation during swallowing. Gastroenterology 1989;97(6):1469–78.

[49] Magendie F. Memoire sur l'usage de l'epiglotte dans la deglutition. Paris: Meguigon-Marvis; 1813.

[50] Daniels SK, Corey DM, Hadskey LD, et al. Mechanism of sequential swallowing during straw drinking in healthy young and older adults. Journal of Speech Language & Hearing Research 2004;47(1):33–45.

[51] Storey AT. Interactions of alimentary and upper respiratory tract reflexes. In: Sessle BJ, Hannam A, editors. Mastication and swallowing: biological and clinical correlates. Toronto: University of Toronto; 1976. p. 22–36.

[52] Palmer JB, Rudin NJ, Lara G, et al. Coordination of mastication and swallowing. Dysphagia 1992;7(4):187–200.

[53] Hiiemae KM, Palmer JB. Food transport and bolus formation during complete feeding sequences on foods of different initial consistency. Dysphagia 1999;14:31–42.

[54] Hiiemae KM, Palmer JB. Cyclic motion of the soft palate in feeding. J Dent Res 2005;84: 39–42.

[55] Yoshida T. Electomyographic and x-ray investigations of normal deglutition. Otologia (Fukuoka) 1979;25:824–72.

[56] Martin-Harris B, Brodsky MB, Michel Y, et al. Delayed initiation of the pharyngeal swallow: normal variability in adult swallows. Journal of Speech Language & Hearing Research 2007;50(3):585–94.

[57] Cook IJ, Dodds WJ, Dantas RO, et al. Opening mechanisms of the human upper esophageal sphincter. Am J Physiol 1989;257(5 Pt 1):G748–59.

[58] Martin BJW. The influence of deglutition on respiration [doctoral dissertation]. Evanston (IL): Northwestern University; 1991.

[59] Martin-Harris B. Coordination of laryngeal dynamics and peripheral respiratory patterns: Isolated and sequential swallows. Presented at the Tenth Annual Meeting of the Dysphagia Research Society. Albuquerque, NM; October 11–13, 2001.

[60] Klahn MS, Perlman AL. Temporal and durational patterns associating respiration and swallowing. Dysphagia 1999;14(3):131–8.

[61] Castell DA, Diederrich LL, Castell JA. Esophageal motility and pH testing. 3rd edition. Highlands Ranch (CO): Sandhill Scientific, Inc.; 2000.

[62] Levine MS. Radiology of the esophagus. Philadelphia: Saunders Company; 1989.

[63] Mendell DA, Logemann JA. A retrospective analysis of the pharyngeal swallow in patients with a clinical diagnosis of GERD compared with normal controls: a pilot study. Dysphagia 2002;17(3):220–6.

[64] Agency for Healthcare Research and Quality. Translating research into practice (TRIP)-II. Fact Sheet. AHRQ Publication No. 01-P017, March 2001. Available at: http://www.ahrq.gov/research/trip2fac.htm. Accessed November 1, 2007.

[65] Jones B. Radiographic evaluation of motility of mouth and pharynx. GI Motility online. 2006. Available at: http://www.nature.com/gimo/index.html. Accessed December 7, 2007.

[66] Martin-Harris B, Michel Y, Brodsky MB, et al. MBS measurement tool of swallow impairment—MBSImp: establishing a standard. Presented at the 15th Annual Meeting of the Dysphagia Research Society. Vancouver, BC, Canada; March 7–10, 2007.

[67] Waters TM, Logemann JA, Pauloski BR, et al. Beyond efficacy and effectiveness: conducting economic analyses during clinical trials. Dysphagia 2004;19(2):109–19.

[68] Dodds WJ, Man KM, Cook IJ, et al. Influence of bolus volume on swallow-induced hyoid movement in normal subjects. AJR Am J Roentgenol 1988;150(6):1307–9.

[69] Ren J, Shaker R, Zamir Z, et al. Effect of age and bolus variables on the coordination of the glottis and upper esophageal sphincter during swallowing. Am J Gastroenterol 1993;88(5):665–9.

[70] Lazarus CL, Logemann JA, Rademaker AW, et al. Effects of bolus volume, viscosity, and repeated swallows in nonstroke subjects and stroke patients. Arch Phys Med Rehabil 1993;74(10):1066–70.

[71] Pouderoux P, Kahrilas PJ. Deglutitive tongue force modulation by volition, volume, and viscosity in humans. Gastroenterology 1995;108(5):1418–26.

[72] Bisch EM, Logemann JA, Rademaker AW, et al. Pharyngeal effects of bolus volume, viscosity, and temperature in patients with dysphagia resulting from neurologic impairment and in normal subjects. J Speech Hear Res 1994;37(5):1041–59.

[73] Rademaker AW, Pauloski BR, Colangelo LA, et al. Age and volume effects on liquid swallowing function in normal women. Journal of Speech Language & Hearing Research 1998;41(2):275–84.

[74] Hiss SG, Strauss M, Treole K, et al. Effects of age, gender, bolus volume, bolus viscosity, and gustation on swallowing apnea onset relative to lingual bolus propulsion onset in normal adults. J Speech Lang Hear Res 2004;47(3):572–83.

[75] Logemann JA. Noninvasive approaches to deglutitive aspiration. Dysphagia 1993;8(4):331–3.

[76] Logemann JA. Rehabilitation of oropharyngeal swallowing disorders. Acta Otorhinolaryngol Belg 1994;48(2):207–15.

[77] Robbins J. Can thickened liquids or chin down posture prevent aspiration? Ann Intern Med 2008;148(7):1–39.

[78] Welch MV, Logemann JA, Rademaker AW, et al. Changes in pharyngeal dimensions effected by chin tuck. Archives of Physical Medicine & Rehabilitation 1993;74(2):178–81.

[79] Shanahan TK, Logemann JA, Rademaker AW, et al. Chin-down posture effect on aspiration in dysphagic patients. Arch Phys Med Rehabil 1993;74(7):736–9.

[80] Shaker R, Ren J, Zamir Z, et al. Effect of aging, position, and temperature on the threshold volume triggering pharyngeal swallows. Gastroenterology 1994;107(2):396–402.

[81] Ayuse T, Ayuse T, Ishitobi S, et al. Effect of reclining and chin-tuck position on the coordination between respiration and swallowing. J Oral Rehabil 2006;33(6):402–8.

[82] Logemann JA, Rademaker AW, Pauloski BR, et al. Effects of postural change on aspiration in head and neck surgical patients. Otolaryngol Head Neck Surg 1994;110(2):222–7.

[83] Jones B. The tailored examination of the dysphagic patient. Appl Radiol 1995;24:84–9.

ELSEVIER
SAUNDERS

Phys Med Rehabil Clin N Am
19 (2008) 787–801

PHYSICAL MEDICINE
AND REHABILITATION
CLINICS OF
NORTH AMERICA

Fiberoptic Endoscopic Evaluation
of Swallowing

Steven B. Leder, PhD, CCC-SLP[a],*,
Joseph T. Murray, PhD, CCC-SLP, BRS-S[b]

[a]*Department of Surgery, Section of Otolaryngology, Yale University School
of Medicine, PO Box 208041, New Haven, CT 06520-8041, USA*
[b]*Audiology/Speech Pathology Service (126), VA Ann Arbor Healthcare System,
2215 Fuller Road, Room A-138, Ann Arbor, MI 48105, USA*

The use of flexible fiberoptic transnasal laryngoscopy to visualize swallowing function is becoming increasingly common in settings in which a practical and less resource intensive alternative is desired for the objective assessment of patients with dysphagia. The use of flexible laryngoscopy to assess swallowing was first reported by Langmore and colleagues [1] and Bastian [2]. In the 20 years since these initial reports, FEES has become a validated technique to evaluate the pharyngeal swallow [3–8]. These studies have demonstrated that FEES and the videofluoroscopic swallowing study (VFSS) (ie, modified barium swallow) have equivalent sensitivity and specificity in detecting the critical variables of delay in triggering the swallow reflex, pharyngeal residue after the swallow, as well as laryngeal penetration and tracheal aspiration of various consistencies of foods and liquids.

A comprehensive swallow evaluation has two purposes: (1) to assess dysphagia; and, (2) when appropriate, to make recommendations and implement strategies to allow for safe eating. A complete FEES examination includes surveying anatomic structures at rest and in motion, identifying the presence and management of oropharyngeal secretions, and evaluating the consequences of swallowing various consistencies of foods and liquids. If dysphagia is identified, implementation of various therapeutic interventions is performed (with the endoscope in place) to determine if postural (eg, head position), dietary (eg, bolus volume and consistency), and behavioral changes (eg, effortful swallow or two swallows per bolus) are successful in promoting safer and more efficient oral alimentation.

---

* Corresponding author.
E-mail address: steven.leder@yale.edu (S.B. Leder).

1047-9651/08/$ - see front matter © 2008 Elsevier Inc. All rights reserved.
doi:10.1016/j.pmr.2008.05.003

History of the laryngoscopic swallowing evaluation

The development of improved camera technology capable of interfacing with arrayed bundles of ever smaller flexible optical fibers has permitted visualization of anatomic areas that were previously too remote to be inspected routinely for the determination of potential medical conditions. The first of these instruments was a flexible transoral gastroscope patented in 1956. In less than 10 years, Sawashima and Hirose [9] reported the development of a smaller flexible array of optical fibers designed specifically to view the pharynx and larynx [10]. Continued improvements in camera and fiberoptic technologies have resulted in improved laryngoscopic imaging, such as the evolution from analog to digital signals and the recent development of the digital "chip tip" camera that rivals the images achieved with rigid telescopes. During the past 20 years, an ever increasing body of research has described the use of flexible laryngoscopy in patients presenting with dysphagia. The purposes of this article are to explain the use of flexible fiberoptic laryngoscopy in the assessment of swallowing, to review relevant findings, and to stimulate further research.

Purposes of dysphagia testing

The response to a consultation for the evaluation of a patient with suspected dysphagia should always include a complete medical review and clinical assessment. If the clinical evaluation does not provide sufficient information to allow for confident patient management, an instrumental assessment should be performed [11]. The goals of the two most popular instrumental assessments (ie, FEES and VFSS) are similar in construct. In the course of these examinations the clinician attempts to identify normal and abnormal anatomy relative to swallow function; to discern discrete physiologic structural movements associated with the swallow; to determine the temporal coordination of structural movements relative to bolus advancement; to assess the trajectory of the bolus through the pharynx; to ascertain bolus residue patterns; and, when indicated, to implement appropriate therapeutic interventions. Fig. 1 shows simultaneous comparisons of VFSS (on the left) and FEES (on the right) showing spillage into the vallecula and pyriform sinuses bilaterally.

The endoscopist is alert to the major salient findings of penetration of food and liquid into the laryngeal and tracheal airways as well as the retention of food and liquid in the pharynx after the initial swallow has been completed. During the examination the clinician will make adjustments to bolus volume, viscosity, and rate of delivery, as well as adjustments in positioning and implementation of maneuvers to determine if these changes have a positive effect on the safety or efficiency of the swallow. The ultimate goals are improved nutrition and hydration for the maintenance and enhancement of quality of life.

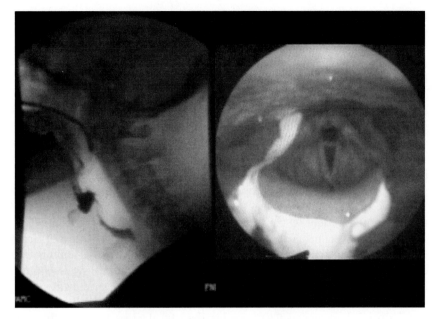

Fig. 1. Simultaneous comparison of VFSS (*left*) and FEES (*right*) showing spillage into the vallecula and right pyriform sinus.

The examination is typically tailored to meet the needs of the individual patient. The American Speech-Language-Hearing Association has developed a comprehensive triad of documents related to the performance of FEES, that is, reports on the knowledge and skills for speech-language pathologists performing endoscopic assessment of swallowing [12] and the role of the speech-language pathologist in the performance and interpretation of the endoscopic evaluation of swallowing technical report [13] and guidelines [14]. Readers are encouraged to familiarize themselves with the information provided in these reports.

Endoscopic equipment

The flexible laryngoscope is constructed to cast a "cold" light delivered from a halogen or xenon light source. The light travels along fiberoptic bundles which traverse the length of the scope. Depending on the configuration, the light is diffused through one or two lenses at the tip of the scope to illuminate the area of interest. An analog laryngoscope has a separate lens on the distal end of the scope that collects the reflected image and projects it along another bundle of light fibers to the eyepiece. The endoscopist can visualize the image by looking directly through the eyepiece or by using a chip camera, which converts the image to a video signal allowing the image to be viewed on a monitor and recorded on a video recorder. A digital chip tip scope also requires a bundled array of light fibers to illuminate the anatomy of interest but does not have an eyepiece for viewing. Instead, the image is captured on an optical chip and then projected to a video display/recorder. Ideally, when performing the laryngoscopic swallowing examination the endoscopist should be freed from viewing the image through the eyepiece. With the chip camera in place, patient positioning becomes less restrictive because close proximity of the patient and endoscopist is no longer a necessity. In addition, the image is much larger on the video monitor, allowing for better identification of potential abnormalities. It is advantageous to record the study on video tape or via digital format for archiving and later review [15].

Many fine flexible laryngoscopes on the market are suitable for the performance of FEES. The typical laryngoscope has a flexible insertion shaft that is approximately 40 cm long, with the diameters ranging from 3.2 to 4.0 mm. Smaller pediatric laryngoscopes with diameters ranging from 1.6 to 2.2 mm provide diminished but nonetheless adequate illumination capabilities for good visualization of the anatomic structures, swallow physiology, and bolus flow patterns of interest. The operation of the angulation lever on the control portion of the scope adjusts the degree of deflection. The distal tip of the scope deflects greater than 90 degrees to allow dynamic control of the image being viewed. Generally, the FEES examination rarely requires deflection beyond 90 degrees.

Laryngoscopic visualization of the pharyngeal swallow

The scope is gently inserted transnasally along the path of least resistance in the most patent naris. This path is generally along the nasal floor below the middle turbinate or between the inferior and middle turbinates. Once a passage has been determined, the scope is continuously inserted until the nasopharyngeal vault is visualized. The clinician should position the scope just anterior to the vomer bone, which demarcates the point where the hard and soft palate articulate. It is at this point that velar function should be assessed initially. The patient is then instructed to breath through the nose or hum, causing the velum to drop and opening the velopharyngeal port. At this point the angulation control lever is manipulated to angle the scope downward and allow for insertion into the nasopharynx to view the base of tongue and laryngeal inlet. After insertion, rotation of the endoscope clockwise or counter-clockwise and deflection of the endoscope tip permits the endoscopist to view the entire pharynx and larynx.

For the observation of general swallowing function, the distal end of the scope is placed superior to the epiglottis at the level of the uvula. This position allows for a view of the base of tongue, posterior pharyngeal wall, lateral pharyngeal walls, epiglottis, vallecula, larynx, and pyriform sinuses. It is important to remember that the endoscopic image is reversed, that is, the right side in the image is actually the left side anatomically and the left side in the image is actually the right side anatomically. As the scope is advanced further into the pharynx, fewer structures peripheral to the larynx are included in the field of view. The scope may be advanced to the tip of the epiglottis for optimal viewing of the pyriform sinuses, laryngeal vestibule, and subglottis, that is, the anterior tracheal wall. This location is the ideal position to observe airway closure patterns during the swallow. The typical depth of placement of the laryngoscope to view adequately swallow function and aspiration is no greater than 15 cm from the tip of the nares.

Despite concern that the presence of the flexible portion of the laryngoscope in the pharynx may have a deleterious effect on pharyngeal swallow physiology, this has been shown not to be true. Suiter and Moorhead [16] reported that the presence of a flexible fiberoptic endoscope in the pharynx during swallowing in 14 normal adults did not significantly affect pharyngeal swallow physiology in three swallow duration measures, the number of swallows necessary to clear the bolus, or Penetration-Aspiration Scale (PAS) scores.

During the examination, the laryngoscope is placed transnasally and advanced through the nasopharynx and positioned with the objective lens between the distal nasopharynx and midpharynx, with adjustments in the depth of placement to optimize the visualization of findings throughout the examination. The field of view obtainable with the laryngoscope includes only a fraction of the area that can be viewed with the fluoroscopic image; therefore, consideration should be given to the clinical signs and symptoms that the patient presents with when choosing between FEES and VFSS for the assessment of swallow. A typical fluoroscopic image will include the oral cavity, pharynx, and portions of the striated esophagus. Flexible laryngoscopy allows for the visualization of the anatomy and biomechanical movements that are immediately in front of the objective lens. The oral, upper esophageal, and esophageal stages of the swallow will not be visualized during this procedure. During the height of the pharyngeal swallow there is a brief period when the image is obliterated due to the apposition of tissue, usually the base of the tongue or velum to posterior pharyngeal wall, around the objective lens. In exchange for these disadvantages, the skilled endoscopist will be rewarded with an unequaled view of airway protective patterns and a sensitive tool for detecting laryngeal penetration and aspiration as well as an invaluable mechanism for biofeedback and patient education. Fig. 2 shows a FEES image of diffuse spillage of liquid (milk) into the vallecula and pyriform sinuses bilaterally.

Indications for the laryngoscopic evaluation of swallowing

Following a carefully conducted clinical examination (eg, a brief assessment of cognitive status and an oral-peripheral examination), the clinician should determine the field of view necessary to most completely reveal the pathophysiology of the suspected dysphagia. If questions regarding oral

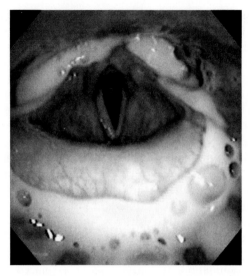

Fig. 2. FEES image of diffuse spillage of a liquid (milk) into the vallecula and pyriform sinuses bilaterally before the onset of airway closure.

stage impairments cannot be answered following the clinical examination or if there is a suspicion of an esophageal component to the dysphagia, a fluoroscopic evaluation should be performed.

Numerous clinical signs and symptoms of dysphagia can be confidently assessed by employing the flexible laryngoscope. Ideal candidates are patients with hypernasality and suspected nasal regurgitation, laryngeal penetration, or aspiration before the swallow is initiated, abnormal vocal quality, and increased swallowing difficulty over the duration of a meal secondary to fatigue. The practical reasons for employing laryngoscopy are more numerous given that a single clinician can perform the examination at bedside and on short notice. Among the practical reasons for choosing laryngoscopy are the testing of individuals who may have safety issues associated with radiation exposure (eg, women with confirmed or possible pregnancy or patients with radiation limitations) and the retesting of individuals with documented dysphagia on the endoscopic or fluoroscopic evaluation [17]. Because many patients may experience difficulty while being transported to the radiology suite, the laryngoscopic evaluation may be less taxing for bedridden or weak patients, patients with open wounds, contractures, fractures, or pain, and patients with quadriplegia or ventilator dependency. Additionally, patients who are morbidly obese, who require special positioning, or who are wheel chair dependent are challenging to assess via fluoroscopy. In the authors' experience, the greatest opportunities to apply the practicalities of the laryngoscopic evaluation are in patients who are in the intensive care unit, who are heavily monitored, or who are ventilatory dependent. Contraindications for the procedure include cases of acute facial fracture, recent refractory epistaxis, bilateral obstruction of the nasal passages, severe agitation, and possible inability to cooperate with the examination.

Risk assessment

Following placement of the tip of the laryngoscope into the pharynx but before the administration of any food and liquid, the clinician has the opportunity to survey the anatomy, elicit physiologic movements, observe the management of secretions, and monitor spontaneous swallows. Edema, postsurgical anatomic changes, and tissue changes secondary to radiation treatment can affect the configuration of the protective mechanisms of the pharynx and larynx and influence the size and shape of the valleculae and pyriform sinuses. These changes can potentially impact on the ability to contain spilled material before the swallow and retained bolus after the swallow.

The collection of persistent oropharyngeal secretions located within the laryngeal vestibule before the presentation of food and liquid is an important sign of potential poor swallowing performance (ie, increased aspiration risk) later in the examination. In a study comparing elders with neurogenic disease with age-matched controls, Murray and colleagues [18] reported that the pairing of secretions in the laryngeal vestibule with reduced frequency of swallowing was highly predictive of aspiration of food and liquid. Link and colleagues [19] in a study of pediatric patients with dysphagia found that pooled secretions in the laryngeal vestibule correlated with aspiration pneumonia. It is recommended that the endoscopist have the patient phonate and cough at the onset of the examination to get an impression of airway protection abilities before offering any food or liquid. Fig. 3 documents copious secretions indicating an increased risk of aspiration later in the examination.

Because the objective of the examination is to show ability as well as disability, the initial careful presentation of measured stimulus volumes limits the amount of penetration or aspiration early in the examination, thereby reducing the likelihood of an aborted examination due to patient distress. Small bolus volumes ranging from 3 to 5 cc are given first. As in the fluoroscopic examination, the laryngoscopic examination should not be stopped when a small amount of aspiration occurs. Discontinuing the examination prevents the implementation of adjustments to swallowing behavior that may alleviate future aspiration events. When the findings of secretions in the vestibule and reduced frequency of swallowing occur at the onset of the examination, Murray [11] recommends that the presentation of food and liquid boluses be momentarily deferred, and that the examination proceed with the more cautious offering of ice chips rather than larger spontaneous boluses of food and liquid to reduce the chance of catastrophic aspiration that may truncate the examination and reduce the degree and quality of findings.

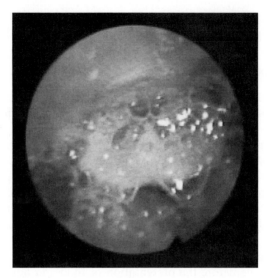

Fig. 3. FEES image of documentation of copious secretions indicating increased risk of aspiration later in the examination.

Conducting the examination

The patient can be sitting in a procedure chair or wheel chair, or can be positioned sitting upright (or as upright as possible) in bed with a hospital tray of food before them for self-feeding. The endoscopist may sit or stand during the procedure. It is recommended that the endoscopist master the performance of the examination while standing, using either hand to control the endoscope, and on either side of the patient to allow for greater mobility when the examination is performed at the bedside.

Following the insertion of the endoscope and initial risk assessment, food and liquid are presented. Ideally, the dysphagic patient can self-feed during the examination, allowing for a natural delivery of food and liquid and in a volume and rate that typifies the patient's self-feeding behaviors. Should the patient be unable to self-feed due to cognitive disability or physical limitations, an assistant may be necessary to aid in delivering the boluses to the patient's mouth. In either situation, the swallow is elicited by providing food and liquid of varying volumes and consistencies to the patient. No command to swallow is given, allowing for a more natural representation of the eating process [20].

The food and liquid should be light in color to enhance visibility [21]. Foods that are translucent (water and most juices), dark, or colored red or brown (many meats) may be more difficult to visualize because they will blend in when viewed against the pharyngeal mucosa. Milk, puddings, yoghurt, breads, and cheeses as well as many of the commercially available liquid nutrition formulas are light in color and reflect light well. Given that the direct entry of food and liquid can occur during the period when the view of the larynx and pharynx is obliterated (ie, at the height of the swallow due to tissue apposition to the objective lens, commonly called "white out"), the reflective properties of the bolus are especially important. If highly reflective food and liquid are used, it is easily observed in the pharynx and laryngeal vestibule and subglottically along the anterior tracheal wall after the brief period of visual obliteration has resolved.

Interestingly, laryngoscopy has proven to be more precise in identifying laryngeal penetration and aspiration when compared with fluoroscopy. Kelly and colleagues [7] investigated 15 simultaneous VFSS and FEES tests with 15 independent raters and reported significant differences between FEES and VFSS regarding pharyngeal residue severity scores. In a follow-up study, Kelly and colleagues [8] using the PAS [22] found that the judges ranked the PAS score significantly higher when the swallow was viewed with FEES versus VFSS. This finding may be due to the fact that the endoscopist can visualize small amounts of food particulate and mucosal coating with the laryngoscope that may not carry enough barium sulfate to cause an impression on the fluoroscopic image and are thus not perceived by the examiner when viewing the fluoroscopic study. Because both the residue and PAS scores were consistently higher with FEES than VFSS, clinicians using both instruments in their practice should make every effort to calibrate their ratings for the two examinations and not treat the results as interchangeable [7,8]. Fig. 4 is a FEES image of tracheal aspiration.

It is essential to sustain discipline in positioning the endoscope before and after the swallow to augment the visualization of findings. Because the field of view is limited, findings must be pursued actively through the dynamic placement of the scope. Before each presentation of food or liquid, the

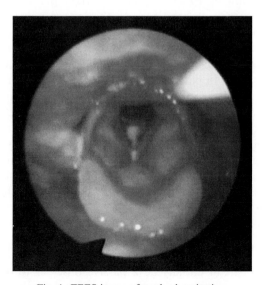

Fig. 4. FEES image of tracheal aspiration.

endoscopist must endeavor to achieve a field of view that includes the areas of interest. Following the swallow, the scope should be placed quickly deeper into the pharynx to allow for visualization of the laryngeal vestibule, pyriform sinuses, and subglottic region to determine evidence of penetration or aspiration that may have occurred during the period of obliteration.

Conventional wisdom has held that a bolus should not enter into the pharynx before the onset of hyolaryngeal elevation, and, in some cases, the endoscopist may not see the bolus enter into the pharynx in a nondysphagic subject who is holding a bolus intraorally while preparing to swallow spontaneously or waiting for a command to swallow. Nevertheless, recent research has suggested that natural feeding and swallowing without commands to swallow yields a different bolus flow pattern [20]. In a study of 15 healthy young normal subjects, 60% of liquids and 76% of solid food boluses entered into the pharynx, sometimes as deep as the pyriform sinus, before triggering the pharyngeal stage of the swallow [23].

Therapeutic interventions with the laryngoscopic swallowing evaluation

FEES is ideally suited for implementation of various diagnostic interventions before recommending oral feedings. The endoscope can be safely and atraumatically inserted via the most patent naris [24] and, if necessary, reinserted during an evaluation for optimal visualization. Scope placement can also be tolerated for relatively long periods of time (eg, 15 minutes or longer) while different food consistencies, bolus sizes, and therapeutic interventions are tried. Thickener can be added to thin liquids to assess success with nectar, honey, or custardlike consistencies using real food during the initial as well as the follow-up FEES [17]. Also, various postural changes can be assessed (ie, chin tuck or head turn to the left or right) in combination with different bolus consistencies and volumes and with different swallow strategies (eg, two swallows per bolus or a sequence of swallow–clear throat–swallow again) in an attempt to determine optimal safe and successful feeding strategies. In patients who can benefit from visual biofeedback, placing the monitor in their visual field and instructing them to swallow twice, swallow hard, or swallow–throat clear–swallow again or perform a super supraglottic swallow [25] may provide enough reinforcement for successful swallowing of at least one consistency or adequate success on which to base ongoing rehabilitation. Fig. 5 demonstrates the change in anatomy with a head turn to the left (ie, narrowing of left pyriform sinus and lateral pharyngeal area) with the goal of promoting more efficient pharyngeal clearing and a safer and more successful swallow.

Visual biofeedback with the laryngoscopic swallowing evaluation

The endoscopist can initially be a passive observer to determine if the patient will swallow on their own depending on the bolus location in the

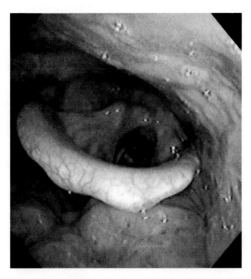

Fig. 5. FEES image of head turn to left compensatory maneuver to close off the left pyriform sinus and lateral pharyngeal area to aid in pharyngeal clearing and promote safe swallowing.

pharynx (eg, triggering of the swallow reflex when the bolus contacts the rim of the aryepiglottic folds). Once a pattern of swallowing is observed, the endoscopist can be directive and inform the patient of the most successful swallow steps or strategies. To aid in pharyngeal clearing, the patient may be instructed to swallow hard two times in rapid succession, swallow–clear throat–swallow again, or alternate a small liquid bolus after every puree bolus. These therapeutic interventions may be helpful in transitioning the patient from a nil-by-mouth status to a safe and more efficient oral diet or from a puree to a more palatable solid consistency diet.

Real-time visual feedback is a powerful intervention strategy uniquely provided by FEES. It is helpful in providing the patient objective input regarding targeted laryngeal adduction maneuvers and confirmation of attainment of successful physiology and bolus status in the pharynx [26]. The patient and relevant caregivers are positioned in front of the video monitor to be able to view the oropharyngeal swallow. This allows the patient to understand the exact nature of the swallowing impairment rather than relying only on the endoscopist's descriptions. Different bolus consistencies and bolus volumes as well as targeted therapeutic interventions (eg, head turn) can be explored. The patient and caregivers become direct participants in swallow rehabilitation and are able to see immediately successful as well as unsuccessful outcomes.

The laryngoscopic swallowing evaluation in specific populations

The applicability of FEES to both diagnose and treat pharyngeal swallowing disorders has grown as clinicians have investigated its efficacy in different patient populations. The categories are varied and include broad patient descriptors as well as specific patient diagnoses. Broad patient descriptors include trauma [27–29], pediatrics [6,30], nursing home residents [31], and patients in intensive care units [32] as well as long-term care settings [33]. More specific patient diagnoses include head and neck cancer [34,35], inhalation injuries [36], developmental disabilities [37], acute stroke [38], respiratory failure [39], amyotrophic lateral sclerosis [40], vocal fold immobility [41], and post transhiatal esophagectomy [42]. This literature attests to the generalizability of the laryngoscopic swallowing evaluation. It has gained widespread acceptability and utility for the diagnosis and treatment of pharyngeal stage swallowing disorders.

Future research

Regardless of the mechanism used to assess the swallow, precision in establishing the exact pathophysiology of the dysphagia in a patient is poor [11,43,44]. Recent research investigating pharyngeal residue [7] and laryngeal penetration and aspiration [8] using simultaneous FEES and VFSS has concluded that the examinations are not interchangeable because of the unequal judgments made by clinicians when judging pharyngeal residue, laryngeal penetration, and tracheal aspiration. Some authorities would argue that FEES and VFSS are not interchangeable but are instead complimentary [45,46] because visualization of the pharyngeal swallow is achieved from different perspectives. The mucosal surface of the pharynx is well visualized endoscopically, whereas the submucosal elements are better visualized fluoroscopically. Future research pairing the two instruments should focus on reliable and accurate identification of focal disorders of the propulsive components of the oropharyngeal swallow. Every effort should be made to link signs and symptoms from each examination so that firm inferences can be made regarding the presence of a focal swallow disorder.

Summary

FEES is a mature evaluation technique that allows for the diagnosis of pharyngeal dysphagia and the implementation of appropriate rehabilitation interventions with the goal of promoting safe and efficient swallowing. Patients of all ages, in different environmental settings, and comprising many diverse diagnoses can benefit from a laryngoscopic swallowing evaluation. The skilled endoscopist knows when to recommend additional testing methods to manage appropriately an individual who presents with dysphagia. Future research will focus on the precise reliability of FEES in comparison with other currently used objective testing procedures (eg, VFSS, scintigraphy, and functional MRI) as well as techniques not in the current diagnostic armamentarium (eg, real-time computerized axial tomography).

References

[1] Langmore SE, Schatz K, Olsen N. Fiberoptic endoscopic examination of swallowing safety: a new procedure. Dysphagia 1988;2:216–9.

[2] Bastian RW. Videoendoscopic evaluation of patients with dysphagia: an adjunct to the modified barium swallow. Otolaryngol Head Neck Surg 1991;104:339–50.

[3] Langmore SE, Schatz K, Olsen N. Endoscopic and videofluoroscopic evaluations of swallowing and aspiration. Ann Otol Rhinol Laryngol 1991;100:678–81.

[4] Wu CH, Hsiao TY, Chen JC, et al. Evaluation of swallowing safety with fiberoptic endoscope: comparison with videofluoroscopic technique. Laryngoscope 1997;107:396–401.

[5] Leder SB, Sasaki CT, Burrell MI. Fiberoptic endoscopic evaluation of dysphagia to identify silent aspiration. Dysphagia 1998;13:19–21.

[6] Leder SB, Karas DE. Fiberoptic endoscopic evaluation of swallowing in the pediatric population. Laryngoscope 2000;110:1132–6.

[7] Kelly AM, Leslie P, Beale T, et al. Fibreoptic endoscopic evaluation of swallowing and videofluoroscopy: does examination type influence perception of pharyngeal severity? Clin Otolaryngol 2006;31:425–32.

[8] Kelly AM, Drinnan MJ, Leslie P. Assessing penetration and aspiration: how do videofluoroscopy and fiberoptic endoscopic evaluation of swallowing compare? Laryngoscope 2007;117:1723–7.

[9] Sawashima M, Hirose H. New laryngoscopic technique by use of fiberoptics. J Acoust Soc Am 1968;43:168–9.

[10] Hecht J. City of light. New York: Oxford University Press; 1999. p. 67.

[11] Murray J. Manual of dysphagia assessment in adults. San Diego (CA): Singular Publishing Group; 1999.

[12] American Speech-Language-Hearing Association. Knowledge and skills for speech-language pathologists performing endoscopic assessment of swallowing functions. ASHA Position Statement 2005. Available at: www.ASHA.org. DOI:10.1044/policy.KS2002-00069.

[13] American Speech-Language-Hearing Association. Role of the speech-language pathologist in the performance and interpretation of endoscopic evaluation of swallowing. ASHA Position Statement 2005. Available at: www.ASHA.org. DOI:10.1044/policy.PS2005-00112.

[14] American Speech-Language-Hearing Association. Role of the speech-language pathologist in the performance and interpretation of endoscopic evaluation of swallowing. ASHA Technical Report 2005. Available at: www.ASHA.org. DOI:10.1044/policy.TR2005-00155.

[15] Gallivan G. FEES/FEEST and videotape recording. Chest 2002;122:1513–5.

[16] Suiter DM, Moorhead MK. Effects of flexible fiberoptic endoscopy on pharyngeal swallow physiology. Otolaryngol Head Neck Surg 2007;137:956–8.

[17] Leder SB. Serial fiberoptic endoscopic swallowing evaluations in the management of patients with dysphagia. Arch Phys Med Rehabil 1998;79:1264–9.

[18] Murray J, Langmore SE, Ginsberg S, et al. The significance of oropharyngeal secretions and swallowing frequency in predicting aspiration. Dysphagia 1996;11:99–103.

[19] Link D, Willging J, Miller C, et al. Pediatric laryngoscopic sensory testing during flexible endoscopic evaluation of swallowing: feasible and correlative. Ann Otol Rhinol Laryngol 2000;109:899–905.

[20] Daniels SK, Schroeder MF, DeGeorge PC, et al. Effects of verbal cue on bolus flow during swallowing. Am J Speech Lang Pathol 2007;16:140–7.

[21] Leder SB, Acton LA, Lisitano HL, et al. Fiberoptic endoscopic evaluation of swallowing (FEES) with and without blue dyed food. Dysphagia 2005;20:157–62.

[22] Rosenbek JC, Robbins JA, Roecker EB, et al. A penetration-aspiration scale. Dysphagia 1996;11:93–8.

[23] Dua KS, Ren J, Bardan E, et al. Coordination of deglutitive glottal function and pharyngeal bolus transit during normal eating. Gastroenterology 1997;112:73–83.

[24] Aviv JE, Kaplan S, Thomson JE, et al. The safety of flexible endoscopic evaluation of swallowing with sensory testing (FEESST): an analysis of 500 consecutive evaluations. Dysphagia 2000;15:39–44.

[25] Logemann JA, Gibbons P, Rademaker AW, et al. Mechanisms of recovery of swallow after supraglottic laryngectomy. J Speech Hear Res 1994;37:965–74.

[26] Denk DM, Kaider A. Videoendoscopic feedback: a simple method to improve the efficacy of swallowing rehabilitation of patients after head and neck surgery. ORL J Otorhinolaryngol Relat Spec 1997;59:100–5.

[27] Leder SB, Cohn SM, Moller BA. Fiberoptic endoscopic documentation of the high incidence of aspiration following extubation in critically ill trauma patients. Dysphagia 1998;13:208–12.

[28] Leder SB. Fiberoptic endoscopic evaluation of swallowing in patients with acute traumatic brain injury. J Head Trauma Rehabil 1999;14:448–53.

[29] Ajemian MS, Nirmul GB, Anderson MT, et al. Routine fiberoptic endoscopic evaluation of swallowing following prolonged intubation. Arch Surg 2001;136:434–7.

[30] Harnick CJ, Miller C, Hartley BEJ, et al. Pediatric fiberoptic endoscopic evaluation of swallowing. Ann Otol Rhinol Laryngol 2000;109:996–9.

[31] Pelletier CA. Use of FEES to assess and manage nursing home residents. In: Langmore SE, editor. Endoscopic evaluation and treatment of swallowing disorders. New York: Thieme; 2001. p. 201–12.

[32] Langmore SE. Dysphagia in neurologic patients in the intensive care unit. Semin Neurol 1996;16:329–39.

[33] Spiegel JR, Selber JC, Creed J. A functional diagnosis of dysphagia using videoendoscopy. Ear Nose Throat J 1998;77:628–32.

[34] Denk DM, Swoboda H, Schima W, et al. Prognostic factors for swallowing rehabilitation following head and neck cancer surgery. Acta Otolaryngol 1997;117:769–74.

[35] Leder SB, Sasaki CT. Use of FEES to assess and manage patients with head and cancer. In: Langmore SE, editor. Endoscopic evaluation and treatment of swallowing disorders. New York: Thieme; 2001. p. 178–87.

[36] Muehlberger T, Kunar D, Munster A, et al. Efficacy of fiberoptic laryngoscopy in the diagnosis of inhalation injuries. Arch Otolaryngol Head Neck Surg 1998;124:1003–7.

[37] Migliore LE, Scoopo FJ, Robey KL. Fiberoptic examination of swallowing in young adults with severe developmental disability. Am J Speech Lang Pathol 1999;8:303–8.

[38] Leder SB, Espinosa JF. Aspiration risk after acute stroke: comparison of clinical examination and fiberoptic endoscopic evaluation of swallowing. Dysphagia 2002;17:214–8.

[39] Leder SB. Incidence and type of aspiration in acute care patients requiring mechanical ventilation via a new tracheotomy. Chest 2002;122:1721–6.

[40] Leder SB, Novella S, Patwa H. Use of fiberoptic endoscopic evaluation of swallowing (FEES) in patients with amyotrophic lateral sclerosis. Dysphagia 2004;19:177–81.

[41] Leder SB, Ross DA. Vocal fold immobility in patients with dysphagia. Dysphagia 2005;20:163–7.

[42] Leder SB, Sasaki CT, Bayar S, et al. Fiberoptic endoscopic evaluation of swallowing in the evaluation of aspiration following transhiatal esophagectomy. J Am Coll Surg 2007;205:581–5.

[43] Ekberg O, Nylander G, Fork FT, et al. Interobserver variability in cineradiographic assessment of pharyngeal function during swallow. Dysphagia 1988;3:46–8.

[44] Kuhlemeier K, Yates P, Palmer J. Intra- and interrater variations in the evaluation of videofluorographic swallow studies. Dysphagia 1998;13:142–7.

[45] Schroter-Morasch H, Bartolome G, Troppmann N, et al. Values and limitations of pharyng-olaryngoscopy in patients with dysphagia. Folia Phoniatr Logop 1999;51:172–8.
[46] Kidder TM, Langmore SE, Martin BJW. Indications and techniques of endoscopy in eval-uation of cervical dysphagia: comparison with radiographic techniques. Dysphagia 1994;9:256–61.

ELSEVIER
SAUNDERS

Phys Med Rehabil Clin N Am
19 (2008) 803–816

PHYSICAL MEDICINE
AND REHABILITATION
CLINICS OF
NORTH AMERICA

Treatment of Oral
and Pharyngeal Dysphagia

Jeri A. Logemann, PhD, CCC-SLP, BRS-S[a,b,c,*]

[a]*Department of Communication Sciences and Disorders, Northwestern University,
2240 Campus Drive, #3-358, Evanston, IL 60208, USA*
[b]*Department of Neurology, Feinberg School of Medicine, Northwestern University,
303 East Chicago Avenue, Chicago, IL 60611, USA*
[c]*Department of Otolaryngology, Head and Neck Surgery, Feinberg School of Medicine,
Northwestern University, 303 East Chicago Avenue, Chicago, IL 60611, USA*

Over the years, treatment of swallowing disorders has been interpreted and reinterpreted by various clinicians. It is clear that many clinicians are unsure of how to manage patients who have these disorders, such that they only evaluate and follow patients regularly to see if and when their dysphagia recovers and patients become ready for oral intake or require nonoral feeding. This type of regular re-evaluation, by clinical or instrumental means, such as videofluoroscopy, is not treatment of the dysphagia. It is a watch and wait approach. Treatment of dysphagia includes active exercise and other strategies, including compensations designed to improve safety of the swallow and efficiency of surgical procedures, medications, and dental prosthetic devices. This article reviews all available options for treatment and evidence to support their effectiveness.

Treatment of dysphagia often takes two parallel courses: 1. compensations to allow patients to eat at least some foods orally without aspirating and 2. exercises to build strength and coordination so that patients no longer need the compensations and can return to full oral intake. During the diagnostic procedure for determining the nature of a patient's oropharyngeal swallow problem, treatment procedures should be introduced in an attempt to improve the swallow. Also, assessing the effectiveness of selected treatment procedures during instrumental evaluation allows clinicians to determine whether or not patients will benefit from one or another treatment procedure. If during this time a patient uses a posture, heightening of

* Northwestern University, 2240 Campus Drive, #3-358, Evanston, IL 60208.
E-mail address: j-logemann@northwestern.edu

1047-9651/08/$ - see front matter © 2008 Elsevier Inc. All rights reserved.
doi:10.1016/j.pmr.2008.06.003

sensation, or voluntary maneuver technique and it is successful, then the patient is given that procedure to use to eat or practice swallowing. In parallel, the patient may be given some types of exercises to practice, generally 10 times a day for 5 minutes each time, to improve or change the muscular control of swallow and prevent fatigue. Swallow itself does not seem to fatigue [1], but patients may tire and lose focus on exercise. Unfortunately, there are few data examining the effectiveness of various treatment paradigms in terms of optimal frequency and duration of treatment. Research on this topic is much needed for specific patient groups.

Considering the range of patients and medical etiologies for oropharyngeal dysphagia, it is important to have a range of treatment procedures, some of which require higher cognitive abilities, some of which do not, others of which require physical coordination, and others of which do not. Having these treatment variations enables clinicians to select the type of treatment that best fits a patient's abilities at the moment and diagnosis.

Postural techniques

Postural techniques often are the first line of treatment considered because they are relatively easy to do, most patients do not have trouble moving their neck or head, and most are able to use these postures with minimal direction. There are five postures and several postural combinations that can have specific effects on the oropharyngeal swallow, generally in terms of how food is flowing and where it is flowing. The effectiveness of each posture has been examined in several populations [2]. The five postures are chin down, chin elevated, head turned, head tilted, and lying down. Each posture has specific effects on the flow of food and the relationship of oropharyngeal structures.

Chin-down posture narrows the distance between the tongue base and pharyngeal wall and is helpful in patients who have a tongue base disorder. The chin-down posture widens the valleculae in some individuals, enabling the valleculae to capture the bolus during a pharyngeal delay and prevent aspiration before the swallow. The chin-down posture also is helpful when patients have reduced airway closure because the chin-down posture also narrows the airway entrance [3]. The chin-elevated posture is helpful in patients who have oral tongue problems, such as those who have amyotrophic lateral sclerosis or who have part of the tongue removed because of head and neck cancer. These patients have difficulty generating adequate lingual pressures to drive the bolus out of the mouth and into the pharynx.

The chin-up posture enables the bolus to drop by gravity into the pharynx. A requirement of use of this posture is that the patients have a timely triggering of the pharyngeal swallow and that they have good airway closure. As a protection, patients can hold their breath before lifting the head (the supraglottic swallow), such that the airway is protected before the bolus drops from the mouth.

The third posture, head rotation, is useful when there is a unilateral pharyngeal wall paresis or paralysis or unilateral laryngeal paralysis. The head should be rotated to the side of the damage [4]. This closes that side of the pharynx that the head is rotated toward and directs the bolus down the more normal side. If patients have a problem with oral transit and pharyngeal function on the same side, tilting the head toward the stronger side to direct the bolus down that side can be helpful. This can occur in patients treated for head and neck cancer at the back or base of the tongue. It also can happen to some patients who have had neurologic damage on one side of their mouth and pharynx.

The fifth posture is lying down. This is useful for patients who have bilateral pharyngeal damage or reduced laryngeal elevation causing aspiration after the swallow. Lying down changes the way gravity affects residue: it keeps residue in the pharynx from falling into the larynx and a follow-up swallow clears the residue into the esophagus.

Sensory stimuli

A second set of treatment procedures whose effectiveness can be evaluated during the radiographic study is the presentation of a heightened preliminary sensory stimulus. This includes changing the taste, volume, temperature, or carbonation to be swallowed as the bolus is the primary sensory stimulus for the swallow. Other procedures for heightening preswallow sensory stimulation include thermal tactile stimulation [5] and providing additional pressure on the tongue with a spoon as food is presented. Patients who have a swallow disorder related to reduced sensation, such as delayed oral onset, delayed pharyngeal swallow, and apraxia of swallow, may benefit from these techniques. There is a more research needed to validate these techniques and their effects on the swallow in various types of patients. It has been reported that these sensory techniques are effective in patients who have sensory disorders, but how long should the stimulation continue and for how many minutes per day? This has yet to be studied in specific types of patients.

Voluntary changes (swallow maneuvers) in the swallow

There are several voluntary changes that can be made during the pharyngeal swallow by dysphagic patients. These voluntary changes also are used spontaneously by normal patients and patients who have various disease entities [6]. Included in these voluntary changes are (1) the supraglottic swallow, (2) the super-supraglottic swallow, (3) the effortful swallow, and (4) the Mendelsohn maneuver. Each of these can be used to modify swallow physiology in specific ways.

The supraglottic swallow involves holding the breath before, during, and after the swallow and results in closure of the true vocal folds before, during, and after the swallow [7]. The super-supraglottic swallow also prolongs airway closure before, during, and after the swallow with extra effort. The effort translates to closure of the airway entrance at the false vocal folds with the arytenoid cartilages tilting forward to the base of epiglottis [8]. The effortful swallow involves contracting the muscles involved in swallowing with great effort to increase the oral and pharyngeal pressures generated during the swallow [9,10]. The Mendelsohn maneuver is designed to voluntarily increase the movement of the larynx and hyoid during the pharyngeal swallow and thereby prolong and extend the opening of the upper esophageal sphincter (UES). The Mendelsohn maneuver is useful in patients who have suffered a brainstem stroke [11]. A fifth voluntary maneuver, known as the tongue holding or Masako maneuver, involves pulling the tongue base forward, anchoring the oral tongue between the front teeth, and swallowing with the tongue in that position. This exercise involves stabilizing the oral tongue in a more forward position, thereby forcing the glossopharyngeus muscle, which connects the tongue base to the pharyngeal wall, to contract further. It may be most appropriate to use this exercise with patients who have weak pharyngeal contraction [12]. Radiographic examination of this swallow maneuver reveals greater bulging in the posterior pharyngeal wall at the level of the glossopharyngeus muscle [13].

All of these voluntary changes in the swallow result in specific changes in oropharyngeal swallow, which have been documented and measured. The length of time patients need to use these maneuvers varies with the cause of their dysphagia. There are no studies that examine the optimum number of repetitions of these voluntary maneuvers or the number of weeks needed to practice them by various types of dysphagic patients. Such studies are much needed. In some cases, patents need to use these swallow maneuvers permanently to facilitate oral feeding [2]. In other cases, frequent practice of the maneuver lead to lasting changes in swallow physiology. This also needs more study.

Exercises

There are several exercise programs needed by some types of patients to build strength and coordination of muscles in the oropharyngeal swallow and enable return to oral feeding. These exercises require pre- and postexercise assessments. Their effectiveness is not immediate. Each exercise takes time (1 to 6 weeks) to be effective. Each exercise has a specific purpose and should be used in patients who have that specific swallow disorder or cause. For example, range-of-motion exercises typically are used in patients who have had treatment of head and neck cancer or other peripheral damage, such as might occur after a motor vehicle accident. Any of these patients can sustain damage reducing range of lip, tongue, or jaw motion, which affect oropharyngeal swallow. In each range-of-motion exercise for each structure, the structure is extended as far as possible in each direction and held firmly in the extended position for at least a count of 3. Typically, patients are requested to repeat each motion 5 times for 5 to 10 times per day. Lips, tongue, and jaw movement can be improved with these range-of-motion exercises, and the improvement can be measured using a millimeter ruler and asking patients to extend the structure as far as possible in each direction [2].

Shaker exercise

The Shaker exercise is based on knowledge of the muscular mechanism controlling the opening of the UES. When doing the exercise, patients should lie down on a bed or on the floor. While leaving their shoulders lying against the bed or floor, patients lift their head just enough to see the toes while keeping the mouth closed. Patients should hold this position for 1 minute, then rest for 1 minute. Elevation should be repeated for 1 minute followed by letting the head rest for 1 minute for a total of three repetitions. Then patients should lift the head to see the toes and lower it without holding it for any length of time and repeat this 30 times. The exercise should be repeated 3 times per day for 6 weeks. Data have shown that practice of this exercise can result in improved hyolaryngeal movement and UES opening. Additional research is needed to determine which patents can benefit most from this and other exercises [14,15].

Tongue-strengthening exercises

Recently, tongue-strengthening exercises have been advocated and there is a growing body of data on the efficacy of these exercises in dysphagic patients who have suffered strokes [16] and in patients who have been treated for head and neck cancer [17]. The effect of these exercises is to improve the oral and pharyngeal transit times and improve the efficiency of the swallow. Results of studies on tongue-strengthening exercises in stroke show that the effects of these therapies generalize to all swallows, including various food consistencies and swallow maneuvers. To date, the effectiveness of the exercises has been described in small groups of subjects, but these results are encouraging.

An effect of tongue base exercises in patients who have received resection of part of the tongue base because of squamous cell cancer is the expansion in bulk of the tongue base. Clinicians from two hospitals (Northwestern University in Chicago and Royal National Throat, Nose and Ear Hospital in London) reported increasing bulk to the tongue base from doing aggressive tongue base exercises. The exercises included pulling the tongue straight back and holding it for a second or 2, gargling and holding the retracted tongue base position for a second or 2, and yawning while holding the retracted tongue base position for several seconds [18]. Repeating words starting with /k/ and /g/ even adjacent to back vowels is not a tongue base exercise. It is a back-of-tongue exercise. Repeating words with /k/ and /g/ moves the back of the tongue vertically whereas tongue base exercises move the base of the tongue horizontally toward the posterior pharyngeal wall.

Combinations of treatment approaches

During the videofluoroscopic (modified barium swallow) study of a patient, techniques can be combined and the effects observed for best results. For example, head rotation to the weak side for a patient who has unilateral pharyngeal weakness while performing the Mendelsohn maneuver can result in the best improvement in cricopharyngeal opening. In patients who have laryngeal closure problems resulting in aspiration during the swallow, best outcomes may include chin-down posture to narrow the airway entrance with the supraglottic or super-supraglottic swallow. It is critical that clinicians use a patient's instrumental diagnostic study to assess the effectiveness of procedures to improve the swallow. This constitutes an evaluation of a patient's individual treatment efficacy. The videofluoroscopic study is an excellent teaching tool for speech-language pathologists to illustrate treatment effects for the patients and families, physicians, and nurses.

Although there are few large-scale treatment studies showing the effectiveness of various treatments of oropharyngeal dysphagia, there are individual case study illustrations and several large-scale studies (described later).

Dietary change

One method to improve safety and efficiency of a patient's swallow may involve changing the food consistency in the diet. It cannot be assumed, however, that thickening liquids will solve a patient's dysphagia problem. Instead, a clinician must examine the effects of the various food viscosities on an individual patient's swallow. Unfortunately, many clinicians in nursing homes automatically thicken liquids for a patient who coughs at mealtime. Thickening liquids to various viscosities may not result in greater safety as revealed in the results from a recent clinical trial [19].

This large study, involving more than 500 patients, recently has been completed by the Communication Sciences and Disorders Clinical Trials Research Group (CSDRG). This two-part clinical trial examined the effect of two common dysphagia interventions (chin down and two viscosities of thickened liquids) on immediate prevention of aspiration during the modified barium swallow (Part I) and on the incidence of pneumonia after 3 months of use with the interventions for patients who had Parkinson's disease or dementia [19,20].

The focus of this clinical trial was pneumonia because it is "the most common cause of infectious death in the U.S. among persons over age 65 and the third leading cause of death for persons over 85 [21]. One hospital admission for pneumonia is estimated to cost $7,166 [22]. Rates of hospital discharge for Medicare beneficiaries with pneumonia as a primary diagnosis have risen by 93.5% in the last decade [23], length of stay has increased, and there has been an increase in death rates" [22,24].

Aspiration of liquids in older individuals suffering from debilitation and dementia is believed the most common type of aspiration [25]. Relative risk for aspiration leading to pneumonia is highest in demented patients followed by those who are institutionalized [26]. Research indicates that 70% to 80% of people who have Alzheimer's disease have dysphagia [25], and as many as 50% of people who have Parkinson's disease are dysphagic. An added challenge with these populations is the high incidence of silent aspiration [27].

Thickened liquid diets are a common treatment of liquid aspiration [28] even in the absence of efficacy data. This intervention is costly financially and regarding quality of life. It costs approximately $200 per month for an individual to drink thickened liquids [29,30].

A common alternative to thickened liquids is using a chin-down posture, which is believed to prevent aspiration of liquids. Welch and colleagues [31] reported that posterior shift of anterior pharyngeal structures with the chin down improved airway protection. Rasley and colleagues [32] demonstrated that many patients who have liquid aspiration can swallow safely with their chin down. Although previous reports have provided a basis for the widespread clinical use of chin-down posture, these studies do not provide long-term effects on rate of pneumonia.

The CSDRG was funded to conduct the largest randomized clinical trial ever completed in dysphagia and designed to investigate the effectiveness of two commonly used interventions for treatment of thin liquid aspiration: chin-down posture and thickened liquids (nectar thick and honey thick). The study, entitled, "Randomized Study of Two interventions for Liquid Aspiration: Short- and Long-term Effects," was funded by the National Institute on Deafness and Other Communication Disorders.

Part I of the project

The immediate effects of those methods were assessed during a videofluorographic swallow study. Long-term effects on patient health were measured by reports of the incidence of pneumonia and other health status changes during a 3-month post-assessment period (Part II).

Details of study design and methods, presented elsewhere [33], are summarized here. Between enrollment initiation on June 9, 1998, and enrollment closure on September 16, 2005, 47 acute care hospitals and 79 subacute residential facilities combined to enroll 742 participants into Part I (immediate) of the study with 515 individuals meeting criteria to continue participation in Part II (long-term). Inclusion criteria were physician-identified diagnosis of dementia (Alzheimer's type, single or multistroke type, or other nonresolving type) or Parkinson's disease, age 50 to 95 years, and suspected aspiration with liquids. Exclusion criteria were tobacco abuse in the past year, current alcohol abuse, history of head or neck cancer, greater than 20-year insulin-dependent, nasogastric tube, other progressive/infectious neurologic disease, or pneumonia within 6 weeks of enrollment.

Patients meeting these criteria were referred to acute care centers from long-term care institutions and outpatient clinics to assess swallowing function. A videofluoroscopic study was completed with patients seated and viewed in the lateral plane. Each subject was given up to six trial swallows of thin liquid: three 3-mL swallows from a spoon, followed by three self-regulated swallows selected by the patient from an 8-oz cup filled with 6 oz of liquid barium (Varibar Thin, E-Z-EM Inc., Westbury, NY). Aspiration in one or more of these trial swallows qualified the patient for part I, the immediate protocol.

Participants qualifying for Part I of the study were given boluses to perform the three interventions in random order: (1) Varibar Thin Liquid (15 centipoise) with chin-down posture, (2) Varibar Nectar (300 centipoise) swallowed in head neutral position, and (c) Varibar Honey (3000 centipoise) swallowed in head neutral position. All patients received all three interventions and randomization was stratified by age at enrollment (50–79 or 80-95 years) and by diagnosis (Parkinson's disease or dementia). Patients were given the same instructions for each of the following interventions. For chin-down posture, patients were instructed to put their chins down to touch their chests. In some cases, they were assisted with gentle pressure on their head. Patients were excluded if they could not perform a chin-down posture. Some of the patients who had dementia needed repetition of the instructions. Researchers in the central laboratory for the project carefully analyzed all videofluoroscopic data for the presence of aspiration (defined as barium below the vocal folds) and scored each swallow using the penetration-aspiration scale [34,35].

Part II of the project

Participants who did equally well on the videofluoroscopy (all interventions eliminated aspiration) or equally poorly (no interventions eliminated aspiration), but wished to continue oral intake despite being informed of the pneumonia risk, were eligible to participate in Part II of the protocol. Each participant in this subset of 515 was randomly assigned to one of the conditions as an intervention and followed for 3 months. Randomizations were assigned centrally by a telephone system controlled by the statistical and data center. Participants who aspirated when using one or two of the interventions were not randomized. This community-based trial did not include a no-treatment arm because no treatment would be unethical in the context of standard clinical care.

Performance of the interventions was supervised by on-site speech-language pathologists, nurses, and direct care and dietary staff who completed rigorous training regarding facilitation of the chin-down posture and proper techniques to thicken liquids. Clinicians were instructed to refrain from using concomitant active or compensatory interventions with participants during the study period. Site visits from research staff to monitor protocol adherence were completed monthly. The primary outcome was pneumonia diagnosed by chest radiograph or by the presence of three respiratory indicators.

Results

The primary outcome of Part I showed that overall, significantly more participants aspirated on thin liquids using the chin-down posture compared with using nectar-thick liquids (68% vs. 63%, $P < .001$) or honey-thick liquids (68% vs. 53%, $P < .0001$). Additionally, significantly more participants aspirated on nectar-thick liquids than aspirated on honey-thick liquids (63% vs. 53%, $P < .0001$). Thirty-nine percent of participants who had Parkinson's disease without dementia aspirated on all three interventions whereas more than 50% of participants who had dementia with or without Parkinson's disease aspirated on all three interventions ($P < .001$). Approximately half (49%) of the participants aspirated on all three of the interventions and 25% of participants did not aspirate on any of the three interventions. No differences were observed by race or gender.

Participants who had Parkinsons disease without dementia were given the opportunity to assess each intervention for their preference. A significantly smaller percentage of participants rated the honey-thick intervention as easy or pleasant compared with the chin-posturing intervention or the nectar-thick intervention (29% vs. 37%, $P < .05$ and $P < .01$, respectively).

More information from Part I of the study is published in detail elsewhere [19]. Further analyses of data with regard to secondary hypotheses focusing on the biomechanical mechanisms underlying swallowing are ongoing and will be the focus of future reports.

Part II: long-term outcomes

Pneumonia occurred in 52 participants (of the total 515 subjects involved in Part II) yielding an overall estimated 3-month cumulative incidence of 11%. The 3-month cumulative incidence of pneumonia was 0.098 and 0.116 in the chin-down and thickened liquids arms, respectively (hazard ratio 0.84 [95% CI, 0.49 to 1.45]; $P = .53$). The 3-month cumulative incidence of pneumonia was 0.084 in the nectar-thick arm, compared with 0.150 in the honey-thick arm (hazard ratio 0.50 [95% CI, 0.23 to 1.09]; $P = .083$). More patients assigned to thickened liquids than those assigned to the chin-down intervention experienced dehydration (6% versus 2%), urinary tract infection (6% versus 3%), and fever (4% versus 2%). Median length of hospital stay because of pneumonia for participants in the honey-thick arm was 18 days compared with 6 days for chin-down and 4 days for nectar-thick arms. More information from Part II of the study is published in detail elsewhere [20].

Results of Part I indicate that the most frequently successful intervention to eliminate thin liquid aspiration immediately was the honey-thick liquid, followed closely by the nectar-thick liquid and then the chin-down posture. This was true for all three patient diagnostic groups. Patients who had more severe dementia exhibited reduced effectiveness with all interventions compared with those who had less severe dementia, probably reflecting the importance of cognition and volitional control when using even what are considered more passive swallowing interventions (such as changes in viscosity of food). In contrast, severity of Parkinson's disease was not correlated to success with the three interventions. Clinicians caring for patients similar to those in this study must examine the effectiveness of all three interventions for each patient as this study reveals that aspiration of thin liquid could be eliminated with one or more of the three interventions in approximately half of the patients. This also means that approximately half of the patients received no benefit from any intervention, emphasizing the need to look for other interventions to eliminate aspiration.

The finding that honey-thick liquid was least successful in eliminating aspiration when it was introduced last in the order of randomized techniques may reflect the effects of fatigue. Clinicians need to be sure that older patients can sustain the increased muscle effort needed to swallow thicker liquids [36], in particularly honey thick, during an entire meal or throughout the day.

Findings reduce support for providing honey-thick fluid (3000 centipoise) as an intervention for dementia or Parkinson's disease patients who aspirate thin liquid. The common current clinical assumption that "the thicker the liquid, the safer the swallow," based largely on immediate response evaluated bedside or videofluoroscopically, is brought into question by these results. The caveat is that only participants who did not benefit preferentially from an intervention were studied. It remains to be determined whether or not participants for whom honey-thick fluid reduces aspiration preferentially in the fluoroscopy suite and then are treated with honey-thick liquids remain in better respiratory health with fewer or less severe adverse outcomes (eg, hospital length of stay if pneumonia occurred).

The outcome focuses clinicians and researchers on important issues of clinical significance. The lower than expected pneumonia incidence in this population changes the threshold at which clinicians, patients, or caregivers balance the risks and benefits of the available interventions. Chin-down posture, with the advantage of continuing to enjoy the taste and texture of thin liquids, is one option. Alternatively, choosing nectar-thick liquids, with the advantage of less need for training and oversight during the swallowing process, also is a reasonable alternative. Choices ultimately depend on the desires and judgments of the patients and their caregivers.

Future investigation of chin-down posture combined with nectar-thick liquid is warranted to determine whether or not pneumonia rates are significantly reduced when the interventions are implemented together or if the pneumonia rate is significantly influenced compared with the use of either intervention independently. The current findings should influence clinicians to question the practice of recommending very thick liquids, in this case 3000 centipoise, without first evaluating all possible intervention options, considering the relative cost burden to patients and care providers. These considerations require justification not only of the cost of thickened liquids but also their impact on quality-of-life related issues. Many more clinical trials examining treatment effects of dysphagia are needed [24].

Other studies have examined smaller groups of subjects looking at the nature of changes in swallow physiology resulting from particular treatment procedures in specific types of patients. These studies are designed to assist understanding the exact effects of specific dysphagia treatment procedures. A greater number of these studies are needed to fully understand the effectiveness of particular treatment procedures in specific patient subgroups, such as the super-supraglottic swallow in normal individuals [37] and in subjects who had received radiation treatment of head and neck cancer [38].

Questions to be answered

Although some data to support the rationale and outcomes for the swallowing therapies currently used, a great deal more data are needed on their effects on specific populations. There also are not adequate dose-response studies to tell exactly how much therapy it takes to have an effect in specific populations. Some therapies, such as postural changes, can have an immediate effect on the safety and efficiency of the oropharyngeal swallow [8,32]. The necessary duration of exercise programs in specific dysphagic populations, however, has not been clearly defined. Thus, a great deal more research is needed to allow efficient use of therapy resources to improve the oropharyngeal swallow in dysphagic patients.

Therapies with little or no evidence to support their efficacy

Some therapies, such as deep pharyngeal muscular stimulation and electrical stimulation, including VitalStim, have no or insufficient evidence to define their efficacy, especially in patients for whom recovery processes are ongoing. Deep pharyngeal muscular stimulation has no published evidence to support its efficacy. It is a noxious treatment for patients in that clinicians, wearing gloves, stimulate and press on the pharyngeal walls in the oral cavity and pharynx to stimulate various reflexes. This can be uncomfortable, as patients gag frequently.

Electrical stimulation has reportedly variable effects and success in improving swallow function [39–41]. There are two types of electrical stimulation: (1) electrodes placed externally on the neck in a vertical array, which reportedly can affect laryngeal movement by lowering it rather than elevating it as is needed for normal swallowing [42] and (2) electrodes placed internally by surgery on the muscle, such as thyrohyoid [43,44]. With surface electrodes, clinicians cannot be sure which muscles are stimulated. There is a great deal of additional research needed before electrical stimulation should be used broadly in dysphagic patients. In addition, electrical stimulation often is used in patients who have dysphagia after stroke or head injury for whom significant spontaneous recovery is anticipated. In these patients it is impossible to attribute any swallow recovery only to electrical stimulation. Most patients also receive traditional therapy in combination with electrical stimulation so that the effect of electrical stimulation itself cannot be measured.

Summary

Research on treatment of oropharyngeal dysphagia has supported several treatment approaches. Treatment can include postural changes, heightening preswallow sensory input, voluntary swallow maneuvers, and exercises. Evidence to support the efficacy of these procedures is variable. An instrumental study of a patient's oropharyngeal swallow forms the basis for treatment selection.

References

[1] Kleinjan KJ, Logemann JA. Effects of repeated wet and dry swallows in healthy adult females. Dysphagia 2002;17(1):50–6.

[2] Logemann JA. Evaluation and treatment of swallowing disorders. 2nd edition. Austin (TX): Pro-Ed; 1998.

[3] Shanahan TK, Logemann JA, Rademaker AW, et al. Chin-down posture effect on aspiration in dysphagic patients. Arch Phys Med Rehabil 1993;74(7):736–9.

[4] Logemann JA, Kahrilas PJ, Kobara M, et al. The benefit of head rotation on pharyngoesophageal dysphagia. Arch Phys Med Rehabil 1989;70(10):767–71.

[5] Lazzara G, Lazarus C, Logemann JA. Impact of thermal stimulation on the triggering of the swallowing reflex. Dysphagia 1986;1(1):73–7.

[6] Mokhlesi B, Logemann JA, Rademaker AW, et al. Oropharyngeal deglutition in stable COPD. Chest 2002;121(2):361–9.

[7] Logemann JA. Evaluation and treatment of swallowing disorders. 1st edition. Austin (TX): Pro-Ed; 1983.

[8] Logemann JA, Rademaker AW, Pauloski BR, et al. Effects of postural change on aspiration in head and neck surgical patients. Otolaryngol Head Neck Surg 1994;110(2):222–7.

[9] Kahrilas PJ, Logemann JA, Lin S, et al. Pharyngeal clearance during swallow: a combined manometric and videofluoroscopic study. Gastroenterology 1992;103(1):128–36.

[10] Kahrilas PJ, Lin S, Logemann JA, et al. Deglutitive tongue action: volume accommodation and bolus propulsion. Gastroenterology 1993;104(1):152–62.

[11] Kahrilas PJ, Logemann JA, Gibbons MS. Food intake by maneuver; an extreme compensation for impaired swallowing. Dysphagia 1992;7(3):155–9.

[12] Fujiu M, Logemann JA, Pauloski BR. Increased postoperative posterior pharyngeal wall movement in patients with anterior oral cancer: preliminary findings and possible implications for treatment. Am J Speech Lang Pathol 1995;4(1):24–30.

[13] Fujiu M, Logemann JA. Effect of a tongue holding maneuver on posterior pharyngeal wall movement during deglutition. Am J Speech Lang Pathol 1996;5(1):23–30.

[14] Shaker R, Kern M, Bardan E, et al. Effect of isotonic/isometric head lift exercise on hypopharyngeal intrabolus pressure. Dysphagia 1997;12(2):107.

[15] Shaker R, Kern M, Bardan E, et al. Augmentation of deglutitive esophageal sphincter opening in the elderly by exercise. Am J Physiol 1997;272(6 Pt 1):G1518–22.

[16] Robbins J, Kayes SA, Gangnon RE, et al. The effects of lingual exercise in stroke patients with dysphagia. Arch Phys Med Rehabil 2007;88(2):150–8.

[17] Lazarus C, Logemann JA, Pauloski BR, et al. Effects of radiotherapy with or without chemotherapy on tongue strength and swallowing in patients with oral cancer. Head Neck 2007;29(7):632–7.

[18] Veis S, Logemann JA, Colangelo L. Effects of three techniques on maximum posterior movement of the tongue base. Dysphagia 2000;15(3):142–5.

[19] Logemann JA, Gensler G, Robbins J, et al. A randomized study of three interventions for aspiration of thin liquids in patients with dementia or Parkinson's disease. J Speech Lang Hear Res 2008;51(1):173–83.

[20] Robbins J, Gensler G, Hind J, et al. Comparison of 2 interventions for liquid aspiration on pneumonia incidence: a randomized trial. Ann Intern Med 2008;148(7):509–18.

[21] LaCroix AZ, Lipson S, Miles TP, et al. Prospective study of pneumonia hospitalizations and mortality of U.S. older people: the role of chronic conditions, health behaviors, and nutritional status. Public Health Rep 1989;104:350–60.

[22] Niederman MS, McCombs JS, Unger AN, et al. The cost of treating community-acquired pneumonia. Clin Ther 1998;20:820–37.

[23] Baine WB, Yu W, Summe JP. Epidemiologic trends in hospitalization of elderly medicare patients for pneumonia, 1991–1998. Am J Public Health 2001;91:1121–3.

[24] Robbins JA, Hind J. Overview of results from the largest clinical trial for dysphagia treatment efficacy. Perspectives on Swallowing and Swallowing Disorders 2008;17(2):59–66.

[25] Feinberg MJ, Knebl J, Tully J, et al. Aspiration and the elderly. Dysphagia 1990;5:61–71.

[26] Lipsky BA, Boyko EJ, Inui TS, et al. Risk factors for acquiring pneumococcal infections. Arch Intern Med 1986;146:2179–85.

[27] Fonda D, Schwarz J. Parkinsonian medication one hour before mealtime improves symptomatic swallowing: a case study. Dysphagia 1995;10:165–6.

[28] Groher ME, McKaig N. Dysphagia and dietary levels in skilled nursing facilities. J Am Geriatr Soc 1995;43:1–5.

[29] Chernoff R. Nutritional requirements and physiological changes in aging. Nutr Rev 1994;52:3–5.

[30] Chidester JC, Spangler AA. Fluid intake in the institutionalized elderly. J Am Diet Assoc 1997;97:23–8.

[31] Welch M, Logemann JA, Rademaker AW, et al. Changes in pharyngeal dimensions affected by chin tuck. Arch Phys Med Rehabil 1993;74:178–81.

[32] Rasley A, Logemann JA, Kahrilas PJ, et al. Prevention of barium aspiration during videofluoroscopic swallowing studies: value of change in posture. AJR Am J Roentgenol 1993;160(5):1005–9.

[33] Brandt DK, Hind JA, Robbins J, et al, Communication Sciences and Disorders Clinical Trials Research Group. Challenges in the design and conduct of a randomized study of two interventions for liquid aspiration. Clin Trials 2006;3(5):457–68.

[34] Rosenbek JC, Robbins JA, Roecker EB, et al. A penetration-aspiration scale. Dysphagia 1996;11:93–8.

[35] Robbins J, Coyle J, Rosenbek J, et al. Differentiation of normal and abnormal airway protection during swallowing using the penetration-aspiration scale. Dysphagia 1999;14(4): 228–32.

[36] Reimers-Neils L, Logemann J, Larson C. Viscosity effects on EMG activity in normal swallow. Dysphagia 1994;9:101–6.

[37] Ohmae Y, Logemann JA, Kaiser P, et al. Effects of two breath-holding maneuvers on oropharyngeal swallow. Ann Otol Rhinol Laryngol 1996;105(2):123–31.

[38] Logemann JA, Pauloski BR, Rademaker AW, et al. Super-supraglottic swallow in irradiated head and neck cancer patients. Head Neck 1997;19(6):535–40.

[39] Freed ML, Freed L, Chatburn RL, et al. Electrical stimulation for swallowing disorders caused by stroke. Respir Care 2001;46(5):466–74.

[40] Kiger M, Brown CS, Watkins L, et al. Dysphagia management: an analysis of patient outcomes using VitalStim therapy compared to traditional swallow therapy. Dysphagia 2006; 21(4):243–53.

[41] Suiter DM, Leder SB, Ruark JL. Effects of neuromuscular electrical stimulation on submental muscle activity. Dysphagia 2006;21(1):56–60.

[42] Ludlow CL, Humbert I, Saxon K, et al. Effects of surface electrical stimulation both at rest and during swallowing in chronic pharyngeal Dysphagia. Dysphagia 2007;22(1):1–10.

[43] Burnett TA, Mann EA, Stoklosa JB, et al. Self-triggered functional electrical stimulation during swallowing. J Neurophysiol 2005;94(6):4011–8.

[44] Burnett TA, Mann EA, Cornell SA, et al. Laryngeal elevation achieved by neuromuscular stimulation at rest. J Appl Physiol 2003;94(1):128–34.

ELSEVIER
SAUNDERS

Phys Med Rehabil Clin N Am
19 (2008) 817–835

PHYSICAL MEDICINE
AND REHABILITATION
CLINICS OF
NORTH AMERICA

Surgical Treatment of Dysphagia

Liat Shama, MD, Nadine P. Connor, PhD,
Michelle R. Ciucci, PhD,
Timothy M. McCulloch, MD*

Division of Otolaryngology-Head & Neck Surgery, Department of Surgery,
University of Wisconsin School of Medicine and Public Health, 600 Highland Avenue,
Madison, WI 53792-7373, USA

Dysphagia encompasses a wide range of etiologies. Its proper evaluation and treatment uses tools and expertise from a variety of specialties working toward the common goals of safety and satisfactory quality of life. Most causes of dysphagia do not require surgical intervention to accomplish these goals; however, several entities warrant surgery to treat a specific problem or to augment medical/therapeutic management. As medicine has made amazing technological and pharmacologic advances, it also has sought a more holistic approach to patients, including quality of life as an integral part of care. Certain surgical therapies for dysphagia address this perspective.

The head and neck surgeon can be an important member of the dysphagia rehabilitation team. This role maybe underemphasized in the current era of percutaneous gastrostomy tubes and accelerated medical care. The role of surgery is well defined for some causes of dysphagia and is less well defined for others. For example, the management of glottic insufficiency, Zenker's diverticulum, cricopharyngeal dysfunction, pharyngoesophageal stricture, and sialorrhea, as related to dysphagia, routinely includes surgery (Table 1). In contrast, the role of surgery for dysphagia in patients who have progressive neuromuscular disease, stroke, or polyneuropathy is less well defined and controversial. This article includes a general overview of the causes of dysphagia that can be addressed successfully with surgery as well as a discussion of why surgery may be less appropriate for other conditions associated with dysphagia.

---

* Corresponding author.
E-mail address: mccull@surgery.wisc.edu (T.M. McCulloch).

1047-9651/08/$ - see front matter © 2008 Elsevier Inc. All rights reserved.
doi:10.1016/j.pmr.2008.05.009

Table 1
Surgical intervention for dysphagia

Indication	Intervention
Cricopharyngeal dysfunction	Botox injection
	Cricopharyngeal myotomy
Zenker's diverticulum	Cricopharyngeal myotomy with diverticulum resection, endoscopic or external approach
Glottic insufficiency	Temporary: injection laryngoplasty
	Permanent: repeated injection laryngoplasty, medialization thyroplasty with or without arytenoid adduction
Intractable aspiration	Laryngotracheal separation
	Total laryngectomy
Sialorrhea	Relocation of salivary ducts
	Excision of submandibular salivary glands

Cricopharyngeal dysfunction

The cricopharyngeus muscle is situated at the junction of the hypopharynx and the esophagus and is integral to the complex swallowing action. This muscle maintains a static contraction with momentary relaxation during the pharyngeal swallow to allow passage of the bolus into the esophagus. The cricopharyngeus muscle then contracts actively, initiating the primary peristaltic wave of the esophagus [1]. Accordingly, temporal parameters of muscle relaxation and contraction are critical to the initiation of the esophageal phase of the swallow.

Nearly all cases of cricopharyngeal dysfunction produce signs and symptoms of dysphagia, including reported choking or difficulty swallowing, multiple attempts at swallowing a bolus, nasopharyngeal reflux, globus, aspiration, and regurgitation. Cricopharyngeal dysfunction generally manifests as a cricopharyngeal bar (Fig. 1A, B), cricopharyngeal spasm, or a sluggish, incoordinated cricopharyngeus muscle visualized on lateral-view barium-contrast video swallow studies [2,3]. The mechanisms of dysfunction include isolated or esophageal reflux-induced spasm and hypertonicity; neuropathy with poor coordination, muscular contractions, and incomplete cricopharyngeus muscle relaxation; muscular stiffening secondary to inflammation from internal (myositis) and external (radiation) sources; and combined causes as seen with aging [4]. Disorders such as myasthenia gravis, muscular dystrophy, and stroke may be associated with incoordination of the pharyngeal constrictors and the cricopharyngeal muscle, which may lead to dysphagia [1]. Other conditions that may cause cricopharyngeal dysfunction resulting in dysphagia include amyotrophic lateral sclerosis, multiple sclerosis, and injuries to the vagus nerve, pharyngeal nerve plexus, and recurrent laryngeal or superior laryngeal nerves [5,6]. Additionally, cricopharyngeal opening is related to hyolaryngeal elevation and forward traction as well to pharyngeal bolus-propulsive forces; therefore any weakness

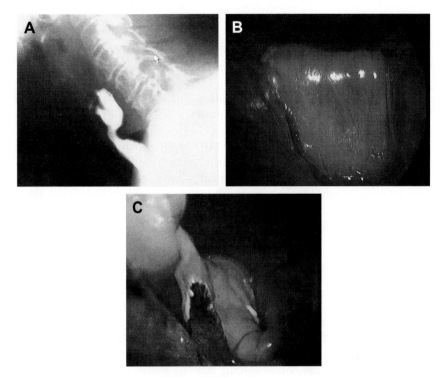

Fig. 1. The cricopharyngeal bar and the endoscopic surgical approach. (*A*) Lateral videofluorographic view of the cricopharyngeal bar. (*B*) Endoscopic view of cricopharyngeal bar. (*C*) Endoscopic view of completed carbon dioxide laser myotomy.

of the lingual or pharyngeal muscle can decrease cricopharyngeal opening, resulting in abnormally high hypopharyngeal pressures during swallowing.

Cricopharyngeal dysfunction should be considered in any patient who presents with dysphagia [1]. Factors indicating potential cricopharyngeal dysfunction include diet modification, weight loss, globus sensation, aspiration, cough, and regurgitation [2]. Patients who have symptomatic cricopharyngeal dysfunction should be referred to the dysphagia team for assessment and management to prevent malnutrition, dehydration, and aspiration pneumonia [3]. Therapeutic modalities for cricopharyngeal dysfunction include mechanical dilatation and chemical denervation with botulinum toxin injections as well as surgical weakening with cricopharyngeal myotomy.

Management of cricopharyngeal dysfunction: botulinum toxin injection

Botulinum toxin injection of the cricopharyngeus muscle leads to relaxation of the upper esophageal sphincter. It is useful for cricopharyngeal achalasia and spasm. It often is done under general anesthesia for direct

visualization of the cricopharyngeus muscle to ensure accurate drug placement, but it can be done in an awake patient in the office aided by electromyography [7–11]. The effect of botulinum toxin is temporary, and repeat
injections may be required. Because botulinum toxin may spread to adjacent
tissues, the accuracy of the injection and the use of the lowest effective dose
are essential for success. Inadvertent diffusion to the adjacent muscles of the
larynx can lead to voice and airway problems.

Botulinum toxin injection for cricopharyngeal muscle dysfunction has
been shown to improve swallowing ability in approximately 75% of patients
[9]. Improvement was assessed via patient report and by objective measures
of esophageal manometry, videofluoroscopy, and laryngeal electromyography. In patients who did not have a positive response to botulinum toxin
injection, cricopharyngeal myotomy was shown to improve dysphagia
70% of the time [12].

Management of cricopharyngeal dysfunction: cricopharyngeal myotomy

Cricopharyngeal myotomy is a surgical procedure that involves cutting
the cricopharyngeus muscle, using either an external or an endoscopic approach. The endoscopic approach may be performed with the use of a laser
such as a carbon dioxide or neodymium-doped yttrium aluminum garnet
laser. The former is favored because it has less collateral thermal tissue
interaction (Fig. 1C) [4,13]. Myotomy has the advantage of affecting both
the muscular and connective tissue components of the cricopharyngeus.
It can be effective in the treatment of inflammatory and fibrotic disorders
where botulinum toxin may fail. It is the recommended surgical treatment
for hypertonicity of the cricopharyngeus muscle as determined by esophageal manometry and is part of the surgical therapy for Zenker's diverticula
[2]. Cricopharyngeal myotomy generally is indicated if patients have moderate to severe dysphagia and sequelae such as weight loss and pneumonia, if
there are obvious physical findings on radiographic studies, and if the
patient can tolerate surgery [4]. Cricopharyngeal myotomy has been shown
to normalize the upper esophageal sphincter relaxation pattern, allowing
a more normal swallow and thereby decreasing dysphagia [2]. Generally,
the endoscopic approach is preferred because it is shorter in duration and
is less invasive than the external approach. The endoscopic approach has
fewer associated risks but may have a slightly higher a risk of mediastinitis
and is not possible in all patients because of the limitations of rigid endoscopy [4]. Possible complications of the external approach include hemorrhage, hematoma, damage to the recurrent laryngeal nerve, wound
infection, and pharyngocutaneous fistula.

The role and timing of surgery for patients who have mild or intermittent
symptoms and less obvious cricopharyngeal pathology on swallowing studies is controversial. These patients maybe taught swallowing strategies such
as the Mendelsohn maneuver (ie, lifting or elevating the larynx with the

muscles of the neck for a few seconds during the swallow to encourage the upper esophageal sphincter to open) or effortful swallowing (ie, bearing down or "squeezing" the neck muscles during the swallow) with the goal of compensating for the poor cricopharyngeus function. The addition of simple procedures such as transoral myotomy, cricopharyngeal dilatation, and/or botulinum toxin injections could augment the swallowing therapy and, in many cases, could guarantee its success.

Zenker's diverticulum

Zenker's diverticulum (Fig. 2) is within the spectrum of cricopharyngeal dysfunction. Although the pathophysiology of the diverticulum is not completely clear, it is apparent that incomplete or poorly timed cricopharyngeal relaxation plays a central role in its development and expansion. It is suggested that intrapharyngeal pressure with inadequate relaxation of the cricopharyngeus muscle leads to fibrosis of the muscle fibers over the area of increased pressure [14]. Surgical treatment for Zenker's diverticulum should be considered in patients who are symptomatic, because the sequelae may be life threatening: patients may have significant weight loss and be at risk of aspiration of the diverticulum contents. Additionally, dietary limitations may require lifestyle modifications and alter the patient's quality of life,

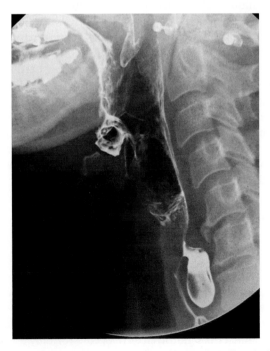

Fig. 2. Lateral videofluorographic view of a Zenker's diverticulum.

which may be improved with surgical treatment. If patients are asymptomatic, or if the diverticulum causes minimal symptoms, long-term monitoring may be considered in lieu of immediate surgical management.

Most of these patients have intact hypopharyngeal contraction forces, and in most cases the surgical intervention of cricopharyngeal myotomy, with or without removal of the diverticulum pouch, alleviates symptoms. Most patients who have Zenker's diverticulum have a relatively obvious problem with severe symptoms. Because the surgery is simple and has a high probability of a positive outcome, the choice to proceed is straightforward. The trend in the United States has been toward using transoral approaches and to complete the myotomies with either laser techniques or endoscopic stapling. The outcomes are equally good with either approach, and the risks are the same, so either approach is justified [15]. Open cricopharyngeal myotomy now is used primarily when neck anatomy and/or cervical spine stiffness prevent the placement of a necessary pharyngoscope.

The external approach to resection of a Zenker's diverticulum involves a cervical neck incision with dissection to identify the diverticulum, which then is freed from the surrounding tissues. A cricopharyngeal myotomy is performed next, followed by excision, inversion, or suspension of the pouch using a suture or staple technique [4]. This approach has a higher rate of complications, including fistulas, recurrent laryngeal nerve palsy, pneumomediastinum, and mediastinitis, and has been passed over for newer, safer endoscopic techniques. Compared with open surgery, endoscopic methods lead to a shorter postoperative course with very low rates of serious complications such as mediastinitis [15,16]. Additionally, most patients report relief of symptoms after endoscopic surgery [13]. Endoscopic techniques include an endoscopic staple diverticulostomy and a laser-assisted technique. This technique uses a modified bivalved laryngoscope to visualize the diverticulum. Division of the common wall between the diverticulum and the esophagus is performed with electrocautery, carbon dioxide laser, or staples, thereby performing an internal cricopharyngeal myotomy and creating a single lumen [13]. Some controversy remains as to which endoscopic approach is best. Each has merits and limitations, but the published data show little or no significant difference in outcomes and risk (Table 2).

Glottic insufficiency

The larynx contains the glottis, which is the space between the true vocal folds and which has three primary functions: airway protection, respiration, and phonation [17–20]. Glottal insufficiency is defined as the inability of the vocal folds to adduct fully and thus protect the lower airway during swallowing or voice production (Fig. 3A).

The laryngopharyngeal events that allow a safe swallow are highly orchestrated. Sphincterlike glottic closure occurs for only a brief time at the point of bolus transfer from the pharynx to the esophagus [21]. Although

Table 2
Risks and outcomes of cricopharyngeal myotomy for Zenker's diverticulum

Type of cricopharyngeal myotomy	Advantages	Risks and disadvantages	Outcomes
External approach	Access to large diverticula	Fistula, recurrent laryngeal nerve palsy, mediastinitis	Effective, with a higher complication rate than endoscopic approaches
Endoscopic staple-assisted	Least operative time	Esophageal perforation, pneumomediastinum	2.6% complication rate
	Fastest return to oral diet	Cannot always be placed through scope or used for smaller diverticula	0.3% mortality rate
	Shortest hospital stay	Produces an incomplete myotomy at the tip	6% recurrence rate
Endoscopic laser-assisted	Intermediate return to oral diet	Thermal tissue injury	3%–8.1% complication rate 0.2% mortality rate
		Postoperative fever, pneumomediastinum, hemorrhage	3 to 11.5% recurrence rate
Endoscopic cautery	Longest operative time	Thermal tissue injury, fistula, mediastinitis, hemorrhage	7.4% complication rate
	Longest return to oral diet		0% mortality rate 3.4% recurrence rate

From: Chang CY, Payyapilli RJ, Scher RL. Endoscopic staple diverticulostomy for Zenker's diverticulum: review of literature and experience in 159 consecutive cases. Laryngoscope 2003;113:962; with permission.

the glottic closure is only one of the mechanisms of airway protection during the swallow, its importance is shown by the fact that the maximal glottic (thyroarytenoid and interarytenoid) muscle contraction occurs during the swallow and by the high incidence of aspiration and penetration identified in patients who have vocal fold paralysis [22–24]. The simple mechanical benefit of complete glottic closure is confirmed by the immediate benefits in swallowing associated with static vocal fold medialization procedures [25,26].

Glottic insufficiency secondary to vocal fold paralysis may be coupled with sensory and motor defects, depending on the site of neural injury (high vagal trunk or isolated recurrent laryngeal nerve). These conditions may be temporary or permanent. Temporary causes may include stroke, postintubation trauma, and stretching of the nerves during surgeries of the neck such as thyroidectomy, anterior-approach cervical spine surgery, and thoracic surgery. These medical conditions and surgeries also may

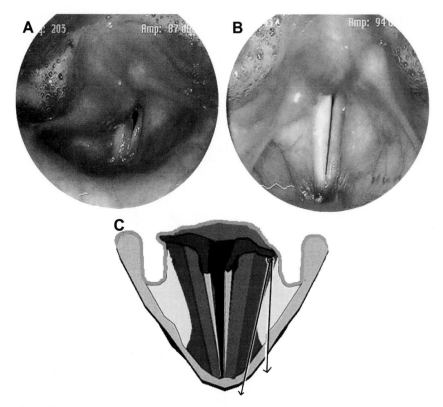

Fig. 3. Glottic insufficiency and arytenoid adduction. (*A*) Endoscopic view of a paralyzed vocal fold (*left*). (*B*) Endoscopic view after medialization laryngoplasty and arytenoid adduction (*left*). (*C*) Diagram of suture traction vectors (*arrows*) on the arytenoid muscular process and vocal process rotation to midline.

lead to permanent nerve deficits. It is not always immediately apparent whether the damage will be temporary or permanent, and establishing a prognosis can be problematic. The role of laryngeal electromyography in determining the status of laryngeal innervation and the prognosis of functional recovery is controversial [27,28]. Fortunately, because of the multiple therapeutic choices available, a successful rehabilitation strategy can be implemented even with imperfect information regarding recovery prognosis.

Clinical signs of glottic insufficiency include a hoarse and breathy vocal quality, coughing in response to secretions or oral intake (primarily with thin liquids), and the inability to produce an adequate clearing cough [29]. When glottic insufficiency is suspected, the patient should be evaluated by both an otolaryngologist and a speech-language pathologist who specializes in the evaluation and treatment of voice and swallowing. Evaluation may include a bedside swallow evaluation to determine the risk of aspiration with continued oral feeding and probably will continue with imaging studies to define better the extent of dysfunction. The common studies include videofluoroscopic swallowing study or an endoscopic examination of swallowing, during which the speech-language pathologist examines the patient's ability to swallow liquids, purees, and solids and determines the usefulness of various compensatory maneuvers and behavioral strategies to prevent aspiration and identify evidence of silent aspiration. Although these behavioral and compensatory strategies are effective in many patients, those who have severe swallowing deficits or cognitive impairments may not be good candidates for behavioral treatment and may require surgery to avoid aspiration pneumonia. Vocal fold injection with temporary agents could be offered to any symptomatic patient as an adjunct to swallow therapy, because these injections aid in voice stability and cough respiratory function and improves the mechanics of swallowing.

The spectrum of surgical therapy for glottic insufficiency is quite large when all the subtle modifications are considered, but the two basic groups are injection procedures and open laryngeal procedures. Injection procedures use both temporary and permanent injection materials. The choice of surgical therapy for glottic insufficiency depends on a multitude of factors including the likelihood of spontaneous normal recovery, the anticipated time until recovery, the degree of impairment in voice, swallowing, and coughing, the position of the paretic vocal fold, the patient's relative tolerance of aspiration and the risk of pneumonia, the patient's cognitive status, the patient's willingness to modify diet and eating habits, and the expected length of overall survival because of medical conditions. In this article the authors emphasize the advantages of the currently available procedures (Table 3) and provide an example of a decision tree to assist in appropriate treatment triage (Fig. 4).

Management of glottal insufficiency: injection laryngoplasty

Injection laryngoplasty involves the placement of a filler substance into the paraglottic space occupied by the connective tissues and muscles primarily responsible for glottic closure. The filler material simply occupies space and displaces the mobile edge of the vocal fold toward the midline, thus positioning it as close as possible to its phonatory location; this placement allows vocal fold contact and glottic closure during swallowing, voicing, and coughing. The injections can be done transcutaneously or transorally and with flexible or rigid endoscopy. Nearly all patients can be treated in a clinic setting, but if the patient prefers or if injection precision is essential, as with polytetrafluoroethylene (a permanent material), a brief general anesthetic can be used. Most injection materials used today would be considered temporary, but the ease of the technique lends itself to repeat procedures (see Table 3) [24]. In most cases of injection laryngoplasty, an attempt is made to over-augment slightly, because bulk loss is anticipated when the injection swelling resolves and injection carrier materials are resorbed (Fig. 5).

Table 3
Common vocal fold injection materials

Material	Active component	Duration of effect	Advantages	Disadvantages
Fat	Human adipose tissue	4 months–permanent	Low antigenicity, similar to native vocal fold tissue	Unpredictable resorption and long-term results
Cymetra (Life Cell, Branchburg, NJ)	Micronized acellular dermis	2–12 months	Low antigenicity	Preparation time, unpredictable duration
Voice Gel (Bioform Medical, San Mateo, CA)	Carboxymethylcellulose	2–3 months	Low antigenicity	Intermediate duration
Polytetrafluoroethylene	Synthetic	Permanent	Long-lasting	Irreversible, foreign body reaction, unpredictable
Hyaluronic acid gels	Glycosaminoglycan from human extracellular matrix	4–6 months	Low antigenicity	Limited history, not effective with vocal fold scars
Gel foam	Bovine gelatin	4–6 weeks	Long track record	Short duration

Data from Kwon TK, Buckmore R. Injection laryngoplasty for management of unilateral vocal fold paralysis. Curr Opin Otolaryngol Head Neck Surg 2004;12(6):538–42; King JM, Simpson CB. Modern injection augmentation for glottic insufficiency. Curr Opin Otolaryngol Head Neck Surg 2007;15(3):153–8; Courey MS. Injection laryngoplasty. Otolaryngol Clin North Am 2004;37:121–38.

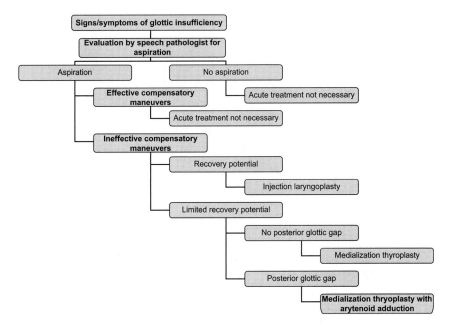

Fig. 4. Algorithm for treatment of glottic insufficiency.

Management of glottal insufficiency: medialization thyroplasty

Open laryngoplasty and medialization thyroplasty are reserved to treat permanent conditions of glottic insufficiency and to treat patients in whom recovery is impossible because of nerve or tissue resection. The available techniques all require the placement of an implant into the same

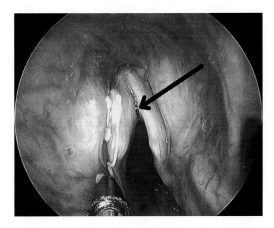

Fig. 5. Endoscopic view of injection laryngoplasty. The arrow indicates the site of the initial midcord injection. The needle is at the site of the second injection lateral to the vocal process.

paraglottic space exploited with injections; however these techniques rely on the framework of the thyroid cartilage to retain stability. These implants are intended to be permanent and are incrementally sized and positioned to procure optimum glottic closure. In most cases the procedures are done with local anesthesia and intravenous sedation to allow an awake, cooperative patient to assist with phonation during the positioning of the implant. Several types of implants have been described, all requiring slight modifications in surgical technique but with the same ultimate goal. The quality of the outcome depends more on the experience of the surgeon than on the material implanted.

Management of glottal insufficiency: arytenoid adduction

It can be difficult, at times, using either injection techniques or open aryngoplasty, to close a wide posterior glottic gap completely. This recognized deficiency led to the development of suture arytenoid adduction (see Fig. 3B, C). Arytenoid adduction first was described as a stand-alone procedure, but now it almost always is combined with open implant laryngoplasty [30,31]. Arytenoid adduction leads to better and more durable voice outcomes secondary to more complete glottic closure. This benefit is manifested in measures such as improved maximum phonation times and presumably also leads to better swallowing function [31]. Arytenoid adduction, however, is a much more complicated surgical procedure with higher risks and longer operating times, so its use is limited primarily to patients who have a wide posterior glottic gap.

Other management techniques: hyoid suspension, epiglottoplasty, and laryngeal stents

The use of hyoid suspension to improve swallowing is limited currently to augmentation of glottic closure after supraglottic laryngectomy. In this setting, it temporarily improves glottic protection during swallowing by positioning the exposed glottis under the tongue base and may supplement cricopharyngeal opening with static anterior traction. It has been reported as a method of dysphagia control, but its role other than in laryngeal cancer therapy has not been defined.

A variety of other supraglottic surgical procedures have been described to close the larynx completely or partially. These procedures have not been adopted widely, however, because they are difficult to perform, have high failure rates, limit or eliminate voicing, and require the placement of a tracheotomy. One simple technique that has a place in treating recoverable severe dysphagia is the placement of a laryngeal stent combined with tracheotomy [32]. In this simple technique the silicone elastomer stent is placed in the glottis and subglottis and is secured with a suture through the laryngeal cartilages. The stent sits above the tracheotomy tube and acts as a physiologic cork, preventing aspiration. Once the patient has recovered swallowing function, the stent can be removed, leaving the normal larynx intact.

Total laryngectomy and laryngotracheal separation

Although adult patients develop and acquire medical problems throughout life, their difficulties with swallowing often stem from a single cause that may lead to various difficulties. Children, on the other hand, may sustain a single insult in utero, perinatally, or while young that results in numerous medical problems leading to dysphagia of multifactorial causes. As in adults, the impairment of laryngeal and pharyngeal function leads to repeated pulmonary insults such as aspiration pneumonia and to microaspiration leading to chronic lung damage. This problem is prevalent in patients who have cerebral palsy, anoxic encephalopathy, and traumatic brain injuries and has a cumulative effect [33]. Pharmacologic treatment and surgical interventions such as the placement of a tracheotomy may lessen but do not eliminate the morbidity from chronic aspiration [33]. Aspiration can be prevented in the pediatric population by the complete surgical separation of the airway from the alimentary tract [20,33]. The pediatric population with permanent injuries such as cerebral palsy will have lifelong and cumulative difficulties with swallowing. These children merit special consideration when evaluated and should be followed on a long-term basis by the dysphagia team.

Many dysphagia-associated disease states cannot be managed by simple surgical treatments, swallowing therapies, or diet modifications and lead to repeated and intractable aspiration, with a risk of malnutrition and life-threatening pneumonia. These entities often are neuromuscular disorders or neurologic diseases, such as amyotrophic lateral sclerosis, stroke, and severe cerebral palsy. They also can occur in patients treated for head and neck cancer with partial laryngectomy or high-dose radiation therapy, leading to anatomic and/or functional laryngeal defects. In many of these patients multiple interventions to control aspiration may have been unsuccessful, or the patients may not be suitable candidates for these interventions. These patients have complex medical, social, and quality-of-life issues that require consideration, but if prevention of aspiration and its side effects coincides with the therapy goals, the two best operative options are laryngotracheal separation and laryngectomy.

Laryngotracheal separation (Fig. 6), which involves complete separation of the alimentary and respiratory pathways, completely eliminates aspiration [34]. It involves separation of the lower respiratory tract from the upper aerodigestive tract at the level of the second and third tracheal rings. It leaves a blind pouch at the proximal end of the trachea and generally is considered reversible [20]. Although the surgery requires general anesthesia, it is not considered complex. It is important to realize that this surgery eliminates the ability to phonate, but not the potential to phonate in the future, should the surgery be reversed. Laryngotracheal separation generally is used

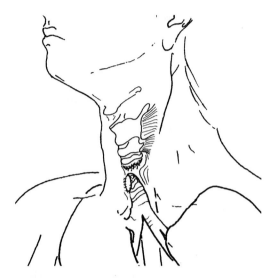

Fig. 6. Diagram of laryngotracheal separation.

to treat patients who have severe neurologic disease and patients who have chronic aspiration after major head and neck surgery for cancer. It is well tolerated but does require a tracheostoma for respiration. Because most patients undergoing this procedure already have lost the ability to communicate with the voice, the loss of usable speech is not considered a deterrent for the procedure [34]. The laryngotracheal separation procedure retains an intact anatomic larynx, which may be valuable in vocal rehabilitation when the procedure is reversed. Otherwise neurologically intact patients can improve communication by using an electrolarynx or can be coupled with tracheoesophageal puncture and voicing valve placement. The retention of a body part such as the larynx also may have psychologic benefits in some patients.

A total laryngectomy involves the removal of the larynx, completely and permanently separating the upper aerodigestive tract from the respiratory system and eliminating aspiration. It is the best choice for nonverbal patients and for patients without hope of recovery of laryngeal function.

Tracheotomy tubes and their effect on dysphagia and aspiration

Tracheotomy tubes are a common part of the management of patients who have complex medical issues. Their primary role is an adjunct to pulmonary support and ventilation, but they frequently are placed in an attempt to control respiratory secretions and, in some cases, to manage aspiration. There is no doubt that a tracheotomy tube eases the access to the lower airway for frequent suctioning and certainly aids in the visualization of the aspiration. A tracheotomy, however, does not prevent aspiration and may be associated with an increased risk of aspiration. Nasogastric and percutaneous gastrostomy tubes are used commonly in dysphagic patients for the delivery of nutrition, but aspiration is not totally prevented by the use of these tubes because refluxate from the stomach into the hypopharynx can be aspirated.

The population of patients predisposed to combined respiratory failure and dysphagia include those who have brain injuries from trauma or stroke, acute or progressive neurologic disease, neuromuscular diseases, or multisystem failure caused by infection or other illness [35]. These patients are more likely to require placement of a tracheotomy because of their underlying disease process. Debate continues around the impact of tracheotomy on dysphagia and aspiration. Some argue that tracheotomies are associated with an increased risk of aspiration, because there is an alteration in laryngeal elevation and swallow reflex [35–39]. Some studies of trauma patients and of patients who have head and neck cancer in the early postsurgical period, however, have shown that tracheotomy tubes neither increase nor decrease aspiration [35,40,41]. The impact of tracheal occlusion also has been controversial. Tracheotomy tube occlusion status was not shown to influence the presence of aspiration in the early postsurgical period in patients who had head and neck cancer [42]. Examination of aspiration status with occluded and unoccluded tracheotomy tubes in patients 6 to 8 months after surgery for head and neck cancer, however, demonstrated increased aspiration with unoccluded tracheotomy tubes [42–44]. The reason for the discrepancy with respect to tracheotomy tube occlusion status and aspiration between the early and late postsurgical periods in patients who have cancer is not clear. Numerous theories have been postulated, including differences in study designs, differences in dysphagia patterns over time, and the timeline for physiologic impairment of adductor laryngeal reflexes [42–46]. Generally, the tracheotomy should be considered a tool for respiratory management and not a treatment for dysphagia.

Sialorrhea

Sialorrhea is defined as excess or poor control of salivary flow. Sialorrhea can overlap with the broader definition of dysphagia and often is coupled with posterior salivary overflow and recurrent cough and eating impairment. This condition differs from drooling, which implies normal salivary volume but difficulty managing the saliva [47]. The causes of sialorrhea include neurologic and/or muscular dysfunction as well as hypersecretion. It is common in children who have cerebral palsy and in adults who have neurologic diseases such as Parkinson's disease and stroke [48].

The treatment modalities for sialorrhea are similar to those for drooling, because the presence of sialorrhea also has physical, social, and quality-of-life implications. Physical complications include chapping and maceration of the lips and perioral skin and possible secondary infection. The social implications include isolation, barriers to education, increased dependency on caregivers, and decreased quality of life from possible stigmatization [48].

Generally, patients who do not have severe disease processes are able to compensate for increased salivation by swallowing, but most patients who have neuromuscular disorders are not able to compensate and have difficulty managing their secretions. Patients who have surgical defects after major head and neck surgery and reconstruction may present with drooling. These patients may benefit from therapy for the sialorrhea and/or drooling to prevent physical and psychosocial sequelae and to improve quality of life.

The treatment modalities for sialorrhea include both medical and surgical therapies. Orthodontic appliances can aid in lip closure and tongue movement to improve management of saliva [48,49]. Biofeedback and cueing have worked for patients who have mild neurologic dysfunction. Unfortunately, these techniques lose effectiveness over time [50,51]. Medications such as anticholinergics block the parasympathetic innervation of the salivary glands, thereby decreasing saliva production. Glycopyrrolate and scopolamine are effective but are limited by their side-effect profiles, which include constipation, urinary retention, blurry vision, and irritability [52–56]. Botulinum toxin improved sialorrhea in a small study with 10 patients [56]. The main drawback to therapy with botulinum toxin injection is that it is temporary and therefore requires repeated injections. Radiation therapy is effective for patients who do not respond to or cannot tolerate other modalities for control of sialorrhea, but the xerostomia related to this treatment can be permanent or last for months to years. The main risk with radiation therapy for sialorrhea is the development of radiation-induced malignancies [57,58].

Surgical therapy for sialorrhea usually is performed for constant, profuse drooling when other modalities have failed, secondary to either the patient or the caregiver [59]. Surgical therapy for sialorrhea includes denervation procedures, relocating the salivary gland ducts, and excision of the major salivary glands. Denervation procedures are performed through the middle ear and are relatively simple, but the nerve fibers regenerate as early as 6 months after surgery, and salivary function returns [58]. Relocation of the submandibular duct has been studied in patients who have cerebral palsy and drooling. The procedure was found to be effective and safe [47]. Different combinations of duct relocation and salivary gland excision have been investigated. The addition of sublingual gland excision to submandibular duct relocation was found to have a higher morbidity than relocation alone [60]. Submandibular gland excision was found to be superior to submandibular and parotid duct relocation in children with drooling [61]. The definitive surgical treatment for sialorrhea is excision of the major salivary glands. It is completely effective and may be the best treatment for severe sialorrhea [62].

Summary

The role of surgery in the management of dysphagia is clear in some areas and controversial in others. Evaluation for the causes of dysphagia elucidates conditions that have been shown to benefit from surgery for safety, for improved quality of life, or both. Surgical therapy, when indicated, is safe and effective for many causes of dysphagia.

References

[1] Calcaterra T, Kadell BM, Ward PH. Dysphagia secondary to cricopharyngeal muscle dysfunction, surgical management. Arch Otolaryngol 1975;101:726–9.

[2] Yip HT, Leonard R, Kendall KA. Cricopharyngeal myotomy normalizes the opening size of the upper esophageal sphincter in cricopharyngeal dysfunction. Laryngoscope 2006;116: 93–6.

[3] Parameswaran MS, Soliman AM. Endoscopic botulinum toxin injection for cricopharyngeal dysphagia. Ann Otol Rhinol Laryngol 2002;111:871–4.

[4] Lawson G, Remacle M. Endoscopic cricopharyngeal myotomy: indications and technique. Curr Opin Otolaryngol Head Neck Surg 2006;14:437–41.

[5] McKenna JA, Dedo HH. Cricopharyngeal myotomy: indications and technique. Ann Otol Rhinol Laryngol 1992;101:216–21.

[6] Ahsan SF, Meleca RJ, Dworkin JP. Botulinum toxin injection of the cricopharyngeus muscle for the treatment of dysphagia. Otolaryngol Head Neck Surg 2000;122: 691–5.

[7] Schneider I, Thumfart WF, Pototschnig C, et al. Treatment of dysfunction of the cricopharyngeal muscle with botulinum A toxin: introduction of a new, noninvasive method. Ann Otol Rhinol Laryngol 1994;103:31–5.

[8] Haapaniemi JJ, Laurikainen EA, Pulkkinen J, et al. Botulinum toxin in the treatment of cricopharyngeal dysphagia. Dysphagia 2001;16:171–5.

[9] Moerman MB. Cricopharyngeal Botox injection: indications and technique. Curr Opin Otolaryngol Head Neck Surg 2006;14:431–6.

[10] Atkinson SI, Rees J. Botulinum toxin for cricopharyngeal dysphagia: case reports of CT-guided injection. J Otolaryngol 1997;26:273–6.

[11] Crary MA, Glowasky AL. Using botulinum toxin A to improve speech and swallowing function following total laryngectomy. Arch Otolaryngol Head Neck Surg 1996;122:760–3.

[12] Zaninotto G, Marchese Ragona R, Briani C, et al. The role of botulinum toxin injection and upper esophageal sphincter myotomy in treating oropharyngeal dysphagia. J Gastrointest Surg 2004;8:997–1006.

[13] Lim RY. Endoscopic CO2 laser cricopharyngeal myotomy. J Clin Laser Med Surg 1995;13: 241–7.

[14] Ferreira LE, Simmons DT, Baron TH. Zenker's diverticula: pathophysiology, clinical presentation, and flexible endoscopic management. Dis Esophagus 2008;21:1–8.

[15] Chang CY, Payyapilli RJ, Scher RL. Endoscopic staple diverticulostomy for Zenker's diverticulum: review of literature and experience in 159 consecutive cases. Laryngoscope 2003; 113:957–65.

[16] Cook RD, Huang PC, Richstmeier WJ, et al. Endoscopic staple-assisted esophagodiverticulostomy: an excellent treatment of choice for Zenker's diverticulum. Laryngoscope 2000;110: 2020–5.

[17] Flint PW, Purcell LL, Cummings CW. Pathophysiology and indications for medialization thyroplasty in patients with dysphagia and aspiration. Otolaryngol Head Neck Surg 1997; 116:349–54.

[18] Courey MS. Injection laryngoplasty. Otolaryngol Clin North Am 2004;37:121–38.

[19] Eisele DW, Yarington CT Jr, Lindeman RC. Indications for the tracheoesophageal diversion procedure and the laryngotracheal separation procedure. Ann Otol Rhinol Laryngol 1988;97:471–5.

[20] Eisele DW, Yarington CT Jr, Lindeman RC, et al. The tracheoesophageal diversion and laryngotracheal separation procedures for treatment of intractable aspiration. Am J Surg 1989;157:230–6.

[21] Van Daele DJ, McCulloch TM, Palmer PM, et al. Timing of glottic closure during swallowing: a combined electromyographic and endoscopic analysis. Ann Otol Rhinol Laryngol 2005;114:478–87.

[22] Perlman AL, Palmer PM, McCulloch TM, et al. Electromyographic activity from human laryngeal, pharyngeal, and submental muscles during swallowing. J Appl Physiol 1999;86: 1663–9.

[23] McCulloch TM, Perlman AL, Palmer PM, et al. Laryngeal activity during swallow, phonation, and the valsalva maneuver: an electromyographic analysis. Laryngoscope 1996;106:1351–8.

[24] McCulloch TM, Andrews BT, Hoffman HT, et al. Long-term follow-up of fat injection laryngoplasty for unilateral vocal cord paralysis. Laryngoscope 2002;112:1235–8.

[25] Bhattacharyya N, Kotz T, Shapiro J. Dysphagia and aspiration with unilateral vocal cord immobility: incidence, characterization, and response to surgical treatment. Ann Otol Rhinol Laryngol 2002;111:672–9.

[26] Nayak VK, Bhattacharyya N, Kotz T, et al. Patterns of swallowing failure following medialization in unilateral vocal fold immobility. Laryngoscope 2002;112:1840–4.

[27] Sataloff RT, Mandel S, Mann EA, et al. Practice parameter: laryngeal electromyography (an evidence-based review). Otolaryngol Head Neck Surg 2004;130:770–9.

[28] Sulica L, Blitzer A. Electromyography and the immobile vocal fold. Otolaryngol Clin North Am 2004;37:59–74.

[29] Lewy RB. Experience with vocal cord injection. Ann Otol Rhinol Laryngol 1976;85:440–50.

[30] Sato K, Kurita S, Hirano M, et al. Distribution of elastic cartilage in the arytenoids and its physiologic significance. Ann Otol Rhinol Laryngol 1990;99:363–8.

[31] McCulloch TM, Hoffman HT, Andrews BT, et al. Arytenoid adduction combined with GoreTex medialization thyroplasty. Laryngoscope 2000;110:1306–11.

[32] Weisberger EC. Treatment of intractable aspiration using a laryngeal stent or obturator. Ann Otol Rhinol Laryngol 1991;100:101–7.

[33] Lawless ST, Cook S, Luft J, et al. The use of a laryngotracheal separation procedure in pediatric patients. Laryngoscope 1995;105:198–202.

[34] Eibling DE, Snyderman CH, Eibling C. Laryngotracheal separation for intractable aspiration: a retrospective review of 34 patients. Laryngoscope 1995;105:83–5.

[35] Sharma OP, Oswanski MF, Singer D, et al. Swallowing disorders in trauma patients: impact of tracheostomy. Am Surg 2007;73:1117–21.

[36] Smith Hammond CA, Goldstein LB. Cough and aspiration of food and liquids due to oral-pharyngeal dysphagia: ACCP evidence-based clinical practice guidelines. Chest 2006;129: 154S–68S.

[37] Cameron JL, Reynolds J, Zuidema GD. Aspiration in patients with tracheostomies. Surg Gynecol Obstet 1973;136:68–70.

[38] Bone DK, Davis JL, Zuidema GD, et al. Aspiration pneumonia. Prevention of aspiration in patients with tracheostomies. Ann Thorac Surg 1974;18:30–7.

[39] Nash M. Swallowing problems in the tracheotomized patient. Otolaryngol Clin North Am 1988;21:701–9.

[40] Leder SB, Joe JK, Ross DA, et al. Presence of a tracheotomy tube and aspiration status in early, postsurgical head and neck cancer patients. Head Neck 2005;27:757–61.

[41] Leder SB, Ross DA. Investigation of the causal relationship between tracheotomy and aspiration in the acute care setting. Laryngoscope 2000;110:641–4.

[42] Leder SB, Ross DA, Burrell MI, et al. Tracheotomy tube occlusion status and aspiration in early postsurgical head and neck cancer patients. Dysphagia 1998;13:167–71.

[43] Muz J, Mathog RH, Nelson R, et al. Aspiration in patients with head and neck cancer and tracheostomy. Am J Otolaryngol 1989;10:282–6.

[44] Muz J, Hamlet S, Mathog R, et al. Scintigraphic assessment of aspiration in head and neck cancer patients with tracheostomy. Head Neck 1994;16:17–20.

[45] Buckwalter JA, Sasaki CT. Effect of tracheotomy on laryngeal function. Otolaryngol Clin North Am 1984;17:41–8.

[46] Sasaki CT, Suzuki M, Horiuchi M, et al. The effect of tracheostomy on the laryngeal closure reflex. Laryngoscope 1977;87:1428–33.

[47] Puraviappan P, Dass DB, Narayanan P. Efficacy of relocation of submandibular duct in cerebral palsy patients with drooling. Asian J Surg 2007;30:209–15.

[48] Hockstein NG, Samadi DS, Gendron K, et al. Sialorrhea: a management challenge. Am Fam Physician 2004;69:2628–34.

[49] Asher RS, Winquist H. Appliance therapy for chronic drooling in a patient with mental retardation. Spec Care Dentist 1994;14:30–2.

[50] Domaracki LS, Sisson LA. Decreasing drooling with oral motor stimulation in children with multiple disabilities. Am J Occup Ther 1990;44:680–4.

[51] Lancioni GE, Brouwer JA, Coninx F. Automatic cueing to reduce drooling: a long-term follow-up with two mentally handicapped persons. J Behav Ther Exp Psychiatry 1994;25: 149–52.

[52] Blasco PA, Stansbury JC. Glycopyrrolate treatment of chronic drooling. Arch Pediatr Adolesc Med 1996;150:932–5.

[53] Mier RJ, Bachrach SJ, Lakin RC, et al. Treatment of sialorrhea with glycopyrrolate: a double-blind, dose-ranging study. Arch Pediatr Adolesc Med 2000;154:1214–8.

[54] Talmi YP, Finkelstein Y, Zohar Y. Reduction of salivary flow with transdermal scopolamine: a four-year experience. Otolaryngol Head Neck Surg 1990;103:615–8.

[55] Lewis DW, Fontana C, Mehallick LK, et al. Transdermal scopolamine for reduction of drooling in developmentally delayed children. Dev Med Child Neurol 1994;36:484–6.

[56] Porta M, Gamba M, Bertacchi G, et al. Treatment of sialorrhoea with ultrasound guided botulinum toxin type A injection in patients with neurological disorders. J Neurol Neurosurg Psychiatry 2001;70:538–40.

[57] Borg M, Hirst F. The role of radiation therapy in the management of sialorrhea. Int J Radiat Oncol Biol Phys 1998;41:1113–9.

[58] Frederick FJ, Stewart IF. Effectiveness of transtympanic neurectomy in management of sialorrhea occurring in mentally retarded patients. J Otolaryngol 1982;11:289–92.

[59] Martin TJ, Conley SF. Long-term efficacy of intra-oral surgery for sialorrhea. Otolaryngol Head Neck Surg. 2007;137:54–8.

[60] Glynn F, O'Dwyer TP. Does the addition of sublingual gland excision to submandibular duct relocation give better overall results in drooling control? Clin Otolaryngol 2007;32: 103–7.

[61] Greensmith AL, Johnstone BR, Reid SM, et al. Prospective analysis of the outcome of surgical management of drooling in the pediatric population: a 10-year experience. Plast Reconstr Surg 2005;116:1233–42.

[62] Shott SR, Myer CM III, Cotton RT. Surgical management of sialorrhea. Otolaryngol Head Neck Surg 1989;101:47–50.

**ELSEVIER
SAUNDERS**

Phys Med Rehabil Clin N Am
19 (2008) 837–851

PHYSICAL MEDICINE
AND REHABILITATION
CLINICS OF
NORTH AMERICA

Pediatric Dysphagia

Maureen A. Lefton-Greif, PhD, CCC-SLP

*Department of Pediatrics, Eudowood Division of Pediatric Respiratory Sciences, The Johns
Hopkins University School of Medicine, The David M. Rubenstein Child Health Building,
200 N. Wolfe Street, Baltimore, MD 21287, USA*

Feeding and swallowing disorders during childhood are on the increase [1–5] and typically occur in conjunction with multiple and complex medical, health, and developmental conditions. A multidisciplinary approach is essential for the evaluation of these disorders and the prompt initiation of appropriate treatment. Following a brief description of the terms "feeding" and "swallowing," this article provides an overview of the available epidemiologic data on dysphagia and its common diagnostic conditions, impact, evaluation, and management in the pediatric population.

Feeding and swallowing processes are linked inextricably during infancy and early childhood. Feeding provides children and their caregivers with communication and social experiences that form the basis for many future interactions. "Swallowing" refers to process of deglutition that occurs after liquids or foods enter the mouth. Mealtime disruptions that occur early in life may result in long-term feeding problems or exacerbate pre-existing dysphagia. Consequently, unless distinguishing between feeding and swallowing is relevant to the discussion, the generic term "feeding/swallowing" is used henceforth in this article.

Epidemiologic data

The prevalence of feeding disorders in the pediatric population is estimated to range from 25% to 45% in typically developing children and from 33% to 80% in children who have developmental disorders [4,6–12]. The incidence of pediatric dysphagia is increasing [1–5]. A partial explanation for this increase is the improved survival rates of children who have histories of prematurity (<37 weeks' gestation), low birth weights, and

E-mail address: mlefton1@jhmi.edu

1047-9651/08/$ - see front matter © 2008 Elsevier Inc. All rights reserved.
doi:10.1016/j.pmr.2008.05.007   *pmr.theclinics.com*

complex medical conditions [13,14]. The percentage of infants delivered pre-term has increased 20% since 1990 [14], and the proportion of infants born with low birth weight (<2500 g or 5 lb, 8 oz) is at the highest level reported in the past 50 years [14]. Early gestational age, low birth weight, and espe-cially very low birth weight (<500 g or 1 lb, 2 oz) are strong predictors of infant mortality, morbidity, and cerebral palsy (CP) [3,15].

Approximately 37% to 40% of infants and children assessed for feeding/ swallowing problems were born prematurely [1,4,5,11,16] and are at increased risk for respiratory, neurologic, and developmental problems. Immaturity of organ systems and the presence of concurrent disease pro-cesses contribute to morbidities associated with prematurity [17]. For exam-ple, preterm infants are at risk for poorly coordinated feeding, and those who have bronchopulmonary dysplasia (BPD, chronic lung disease associ-ated with prematurity) have poorer feeding endurance and performance than those who do not have bronchopulmonary dysplasia [18].

Another potential reason for the rising incidence of pediatric feeding/ swallowing disorders during the last 20 years is the increased life expectancy of children who have CP and developmental disabilities [19]. CP has been reported in 20% of infants born between 24 and 26 weeks' gestation and in 4% of infants born at 32 weeks' gestation [3]. In one survey, approxi-mately 30% of children who had CP and were referred to a feeding program had histories of preterm births [20]. Additionally more children with other developmental disorders are surviving [21]. Finally, swallowing dysfunction is being identified in children who previously had not been recognized as having impairments in deglutition [22–25].

Despite the presentation of this information, data on the prevalence and incidence feeding problems in the pediatric population are limited. Possible reasons for this paucity are that disabling or disease conditions are more likely to be counted than are symptoms of diseases (eg, dysphagia) [26–28], terminology for the coding of feeding-related behaviors may be reflected by multiple underlying diagnostic conditions [16], standardized diagnostic protocols are lacking, and differences exist in methods of ascer-tainment [3,21]. Additionally, it may be challenging to distinguish between feeding patterns associated with variability during normal development and those associated with impairment. For example, identifying children who have delays in the acquisition of specific feeding behaviors (eg, drink-ing from an open cup or with a straw) requires an appreciation of the wide age range in which typically developing children first acquire the same be-haviors [29].

Diagnostic conditions associated with pediatric dysphagia

Causes of dysphagia may evolve from five broad diagnostic categories: neurologic disorders (eg, immaturity, delays, or defects), anatomic abnor-malities involving the aerodigestive tract, genetic conditions, conditions affecting suck/swallow/breathing coordination, and other comorbidities influencing deglutition (Table 1). Regardless of age, similar diagnostic conditions and comorbidities probably would present with comparable impairments in deglutition. Nonetheless, specific diagnostic conditions are likely to differ across the age spectrum. Neurologic conditions are the etiologies most frequently associated with dysphagia. Although CP is the most common neurogenic condition associated with dysphagia in children, stroke is the most common neurologic condition in adults. Similarly, airway and craniofacial anomalies may be associated with dysphagia regardless of age; however, congenital conditions are more common in children, and acquired conditions occur more often in adults.

Table 1
Common diagnostic conditions and comorbidities associated with pediatric dysphagia

Site or process	Examples of diagnostic conditions
Neurologic disorders (immaturity, delays, or defects)	Prematurity
	Central nervous system conditions (cerebral palsy, Arnold-Chiari malformation, brain stem tumor, traumatic brain injury, cerebral vascular accidents)
	Neuromuscular junction disease (myasthenia gravis)
	Muscle disease (spinal muscular atrophy, muscular dystrophy, Guillain-Barré syndrome)
Anatomic abnormalities of the aerodigestive tract	Congenital or acquired anomalies (cleft lip/palate, vocal-fold paralysis or paresis, laryngeal cleft, tracheoesophageal fistula, laryngomalacia[a], tracheomalacia)
	Iatrogenic (tracheostomy)
Genetic conditions	Syndromes (eg, Down syndrome, velocardiofacial syndrome)
	Craniofacial anomalies (Pierre Robin sequence; CHARGE syndrome [coloboma, heart anomalies, choanal atresia, retardation of growth and development, and genital abnormalities]; Treacher-Collins syndrome)
	Degenerative systemic diseases
Conditions affecting suck-swallowing/ breathing coordination	Choanal atresia
	Laryngomalacia[a]
	Bronchopulmonary dysplasia
	Cardiac disease
	Respiratory syncytial virus
Other comorbidities	Gastroesophageal reflux disease
	Pervasive developmental delay

[a] Laryngomalacia appears twice in this table because it is a common anatomic abnormality associated with pediatric dysphagia and it may compromise suck/swallow/breathing coordination.

Adapted from Lefton-Greif MA, McGrath-Morrow SA. Deglutition and respiration: development, coordination, and practical implications. Semin Speech Lang 2007;28(3):173; with permission.

Approximately 50% of children who have feeding disorders have multiple causes contributing to their feeding difficulties [16,30], and 90% have at last one medical diagnosis [11]. Swallowing problems are prevalent in infants and young children who have histories of preterm births, BPD, congenital heart disease, anatomic abnormalities, and various syndromes and neurologic abnormalities [31]. Gastroesophageal reflux disease (GERD) has been identified as a common underlying medical condition associated with feeding problems [9,16].

For some children, dysphagic symptoms may be the first sign of other underlying conditions. Feeding problems during infancy have been predictive of severe illness [32]. Despite the increased risk of dysphagia associated with varying medical or developmental conditions, isolated swallowing dysfunction has been documented in otherwise neurologically normal children without identifiable causes at the time of presentation [23,25,33]. Dysphagia also may occur after the acute states of respiratory infections in previously healthy children [22,34].

Manifestations of feeding/swallowing disorders in infants and young children

Presentations of pediatric feeding/swallowing disorders are variable and may include poor sucking coordination [18], pharyngeal phase dysfunction [1,8,9,24,35,36], respiratory distress [24,37], GERD [9], nutrition compromise [12], oral motor delays [7–9], food refusal or selectivity [8], delayed transition or refusal to consume developmentally appropriate textures or foods [5,8,9], or some combination of these presentations. Differing patterns of clinical presentation may be associated with specific underlying diagnostic conditions. Oral motor dysfunction or delays are common in children who have developmental delays and occur in up to 90% of children diagnosed as having CP [7] and in 80% of children who have Down syndrome [8]. In contrast, children diagnosed as having specific developmental delays (eg, the autistic spectrum) are more likely to exhibit selectivity of type and texture of food than oropharyngeal dysphagia [8].

Infants who have unexplained causes of dysphagia at the time of presentation are likely to represent a heterogeneous cohort of patients with varying degrees of dysphagia [37]. Presentations of "unexplained" dysphagia have ranged from profound problems characterized by "very weak or absent pharyngeal contraction" or "incomplete pharyngeal palsy" [23,38], to moderate pharyngeal dyscoordination [23,33], to suck/swallow/breathing incoordination [18,23]. Investigations are needed to provide careful details regarding the types of presentation of dysphagia and their relationship to feeding/swallowing development and general well being.

Impact of pediatric dysphagia

Influential factors

Infants and young children who have dysphagia are at increased risk for the development of aspiration-induced chronic lung disease, malnutrition, neurodevelopmental problems, and stressful interactions with their caregivers [4,39–42]. Unfortunately, little is known about the impact of pediatric dysphagia and the efficacy of interventions on the long-term health and quality-of-life outcomes for affected children [43]. With sparse evidence to guide clinical decision making, clinicians have made decisions by using information extrapolated from studies of adults who have dysphagia or from anecdotal reports or by adhering to institutional routines. Given the current state of knowledge, Lefton-Greif and McGrath [44] proposed adapting a pediatric asthma model as a framework to view the impact of pediatric dysphagia as an interaction among host characteristics, environmental/social factors, and age or timing of dysphagic exposure (Fig. 1).

Although comparable factors modify the impact of dysphagia across the lifespan, the impact of specific factors is likely to differ with age. For example, when considering host characteristics, infants and young children may be especially sensitive to the effects of dysphagia at certain ages or developmental periods. The respiratory and nutritional sequelae associated with dysphagia may exert a profound influence on overall growth and on the growth and development of specific organs [45–47]. Likewise, environmental/social factors (eg, access to appropriate health and rehabilitation services and adherence to management recommendations) influence the impact of dysphagia in all affected persons, but the patient's age and neurodevelopmental status alter the specific features of these factors. Age or timing of exposure to the swallowing dysfunction probably is the most critical factor

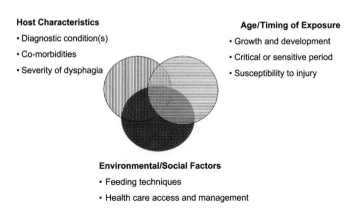

Fig. 1. Factors that can modify the impact of dysphagia. (*Adapted from* Lefton-Greif MA, McGrath-Morrow SA. Deglutition and respiration: development, coordination, and practical implications. Semin Speech Lang 2007; 28(3):170; with permission).

that distinguishes between impact of the dysphagia in pediatric and adult populations. Interruptions at critical stages may interfere with the development of optimal function or may compromise the functioning of current systems.

Critical or sensitive periods

Critical or sensitive periods seem to emerge soon after the relevant sensory information first becomes available to the specific organism [48]. When swallowing dysfunction is present, it may interrupt normal development at critical or sensitive periods of time, delay or interfere with typical development or established patterns of feeding/swallowing, and facilitate the development of feeding aversions. Case studies suggest that children who are not given the opportunity to eat solid foods shortly after they learn to chew may have difficulty taking solids or may refuse to chew [49]. Recently, the introduction of tastes during the first 5 months of life has been shown to influence later food preferences [50].

Successful feeding requires sufficient experience in addition to neurologic maturity [51,52]. Further research is needed to define the critical stages of development in children who have dysphagia and identify necessary stimuli and appropriate dose–response relationships when oral feedings are interrupted or modified. Additionally, investigations are needed to determine whether swallowing disruptions that occur in early childhood have consequences later in life, particularly in the setting of adult-onset dysphagia.

Long-term outcomes

Unfortunately, outcome data for the resolution of dysphagia are limited. The prognosis for the recovery from dysphagia is dictated by the underlying diagnostic condition, by whether the condition is an acute or chronic condition, and, if the condition is chronic, by whether it is static or progressive (see [53] for a detailed description of the progression of disease conditions).

For some children, dysphagic symptoms may be one of the first indications of an underlying condition [23,54]. That said, children may present with severe feeding problems even if they were without difficulty with early sucking behaviors. One study reported feeding problems in 55% of adults who had CP [55].

Another way to view outcomes is to consider the long-term sequelae associated with the respiratory and nutritional consequences associated with pediatric dysphagia. Although the influence of recurrent aspiration on the developing airways is not well understood, many lung diseases in adults are thought to begin during childhood [56,57]. Recurrent aspiration during the first decade of life may interfere with normal or compensatory lung growth [45].

Malnutrition is another complication associated with pediatric dysphagia and is linked with adverse cognitive and developmental outcomes [58].

Additionally, specific micronutrient deficiencies during the childhood periods critical to brain development may interfere with brain development, behavior, and cognition [46,47].

Evaluation of infants and young children suspected of having dysphagia

Clinical or bedside evaluation

Input from multiple medical, health, and developmental disciplines is essential for establishing a diagnosis and developing an appropriate treatment plan for pediatric patients who have feeding/swallowing problems. Moreover, early evaluation of the swallowing dysfunction and prompt initiation of appropriate therapies are critical to lessen the impact of the morbidities associated with dysphagia.

Evaluation of all children who have feeding/swallowing difficulties begins with taking a thorough history and completing a physical examination. Foci of the clinical examination are organ and symptom specific and are directed toward identifying the appropriate diagnostic tests to determine the nature and extent of the swallowing impairment. The clinical examination process is complicated by the variability in the presentations of feeding/swallowing disorders.

Regardless of patient age, dysphagia may present as respiratory distress, nutritional compromise, and stressful mealtimes. Critical issues to consider when evaluating all children for feeding/swallowing concerns include the presence of episodic or chronic signs of respiratory distress and patterns of weight gain. Respiratory presentations differ with age and neurodevelopmental status (Table 2) [44,59–65]. Unlike adults, children are expected to gain weight. Consequently, either weight loss or failure to gain weight is concerning [65], particularly during the first 2 years of life when appropriate nutrition is critical for brain and lung development. The duration of meals and reports of stressful meals may provide some clues about the extent of the feeding/swallowing problems. Mealtimes in excess of 30 minutes on a regular basis are too long [66] and may compromise the balance between the nutritional value and the energy expended with the feeding.

Instrumental evaluation

When the clinical evaluation identifies problems that may be caused by or reflect conditions that are not visible, an instrumental evaluation typically is recommended. The rationale and goals for completing instrumental evaluations are similar for all patients who have dysphagia, regardless of age. Instrumental evaluations are conducted to understand the nature and pathophysiology of the dysphagia and to obtain the information needed to develop appropriate management plans. Videofluoroscopic swallow studies (VFSSs) and flexible endoscopic evaluations of swallowing (FEESs) are the

Table 2
Common respiratory presentations associated with oropharyngeal dysphagia in infants and
young children

Common respiratory presentation	Age	
	Infants (0–6 months)	Young children (6 months or older)
Acute or episodic presentations		
Apnea/bradycardia [41]	+ [60–63]	—
Apparent life-threatening episode	+	—
Coughing or choking during/after oral feeding	+	+
Cyanosis during oral feeding	+	+
Wheezing or stridor	+	+
Chronic presentations (>4 weeks in duration) [59,64]		
[a]Congestion (upper ± lower airway) [41]	+	+
Coughing [41]	+	+
Frequent or persistent respiratory illnesses	+	+
[a]Intractable wheezing or reactive airway disease [41]	+	+
Unexpected need for supplemental oxygen	+	+
Recurrent pneumonia or bronchitis	+	+ [59]

[a] Also may be episodic and occur in association with oral feeding.

Adapted from Lefton-Greif MA, McGrath-Morrow SA. Deglutition and respiration: development, coordination, and practical implications. Semin Speech Lang 2007;28(3):174; with permission.

most common instrumental evaluations recommended for assessment of oropharyngeal dysphagia in infants and children.

Videofluoroscopic swallow study

Radiologic evaluations are directed at determining whether anatomic or structural abnormalities are present, determining whether appropriate coordination exists during bolus passage, and identifying strategies that enhance the safety and efficiency of feeding while minimizing the dysphagic patterns. (See [67,68] and for extensive reviews of VFSS procedures.) Considerations for completing VFSSs in infants and young children include the use of developmentally appropriate protocols and utensils and efforts to minimize radiation exposure. The latter precaution is particularly important because even low-dose radiation from repeated routine procedures may increase the risk of cancer for some children [69]. Additionally, children must be able to participate in evaluation protocols. Some children who have feeding refusal may not be willing or able to participate in VFSS procedures.

Specific radiologic findings in infants and young children

Interpretation of radiologic findings requires that clinicians distinguish between radiologic findings that represent normal variability and those that are indications of swallowing dysfunction. Unfortunately, the paucity of radiologic data from nondysphagic persons and the lack of standardized evaluation approaches are challenges across the life span and particularly in the pediatric population. (See the article by Martin-Harris in this issue.) Common radiologic findings in pediatric patients that are worthy of mention include onset of the pharyngeal swallow and the presence of supraglottic penetration, nasopharyngeal reflux, and silent aspiration.

Onset of pharyngeal phase of swallowing

Although there has been debate about the location of bolus aggregation at the time of pharyngeal swallow onset in adults [70,71], cine-radiologic frame tracings of infants during suckle feeding demonstrate that bolus accumulation in the valleculae precedes swallow initiation, particularly when one or more suckles occur before swallowing [72]. Nonetheless, on VFSSs, the lingering or accumulation of boluses in pyriform sinuses before swallow onset is likely to increase the risk of aspiration [1,24,67].

Nasopharyngeal reflux

Radiologic evidence of nasopharyngeal reflux may indicate velopharyngeal insufficiency or incoordination; however, trace amounts of nasopharyngeal reflux during the first few weeks of life may not be atypical, particularly when infants are asymptomatic or the findings are incidental. Although trace nasopharyngeal reflux in the neonate typically resolves with age or maturation, it has been associated with apnea in preterm infants [62].

Supraglottic penetration

Although the incidence of supraglottic penetration in typically developing children is unknown, isolated penetration on upper gastrointestinal examinations in children younger than 2 years of age who are without history or clinical suspicion of dysphagia may reflect immaturity of the swallowing mechanism [73]. In children at risk for oropharyngeal dysphagia, however, VFSS findings of supraglottic penetration to the lower portion of the laryngeal vestibule are predictive of aspiration [1,74].

Silent aspiration

Silent aspiration is frequent among infants and young children who have dysphagia and concomitant aspiration [1,24,33,35,75]. As reviewed by Thach [76], laryngeal chemoreflexes are the primary defense against aspiration of fluids throughout the life span, and the cough component of the laryngeal chemoreflexes becomes increasingly prominent with age and maturation [77]. Whether the absence of a cough in response to aspiration represents incomplete maturation of the vagal response [76,78], blunting of the cough response secondary to recurrent aspiration [41], or some interaction between the two manifestations remains unclear. Regardless of the reason for the lack of a cough response, findings of silent aspiration are particularly concerning in children younger than 2 years of age, given that the primary airway clearance response to aspiration is absent during the greatest period of postnatal lung development [79].

Flexible endoscopic evaluation of swallowing

FEES and FEES plus sensory testing (FEES-ST) are used in the pediatric population for all the same reasons that they are used with adults. (See the article by Leder in this issue.) Recently, the usefulness of FEES and FEES-ST was demonstrated during the evaluation and treatment of children who had specific diagnostic conditions (ie, type I laryngeal clefts [supraglottic interarytenoid defect]) [80] and during preoperative evaluations for pediatric airway reconstruction [81]. FEES-ST has demonstrated elevated laryngopharyngeal sensory thresholds with clinical diagnoses of recurrent pneumonia, neurologic disorders, and GERD [82].

Other diagnostic evaluations

Other diagnostic tests may be needed to determine the cause of the swallowing dysfunction. For example, imaging of the brain stem may be needed to diagnose abnormalities of the skull base or spine as potential underlying conditions. Specialized evaluations may be needed for children who have refractory respiratory conditions. Chest radiographs, pulmonary function tests, high-resolution CT, and bronchoscopy provide information regarding the extent of lung injury. Endoscopy may be beneficial for patients who have histories or presentations suggestive of gastrointestinal conditions.

Treatment of infants and young children who have dysphagia

The primary goals of dysphagia interventions are to fix or control treatable causes and to avoid or minimize the impact of the swallowing dysfunction. Medical or surgical interventions may be appropriate for anatomic conditions (eg, laryngeal cleft or tracheoesophageal fistula), GERD, and some inflammatory conditions (eg, esophagitis). Even after underlying conditions have been corrected, some children may require behaviorally based interventions to treat feeding refusal secondary to learned aversions [83].

Outcome data for treatment of pediatric feeding/swallowing disorders are limited. Although there are no tools or algorithms that predict the best treatment modalities for children who have dysphagia, treatment that is diagnosis specific improves nutritional status and decreases morbidities, as shown by a reduction in acute hospitalization rates [9]. The impact of the dysphagia may be lessened by the implementation of interventions that facilitate the development of oral motor skills, lessen the swallowing dysfunction, or provide supplemental nutrition. Additionally, given that swallowing is the best exercise for swallowing [84] and that interruptions in oral feeding carry social, learning, and emotional burdens [4], clinicians first should consider the implementation of the safest, least invasive, and most functional management options.

Common oral motor and swallowing therapies that address the pathophysiology of the swallowing dysfunction in infants and young children include modifications in the texture of foods or liquids [34], the use of utensils [85], the position or scheduling of feeding [86], tactile simulation [87,88], and activities that focus on swallowing musculature or the integration of developmentally appropriate movement patterns. In one study, behavioral therapy was successful in approximately two thirds of former preterm children treated for severe feeding problems; however, the presence of tube feedings and swallowing dysfunction were the best predictors of failure to respond to interventions [89]. Compensatory swallowing maneuvers (eg, supraglottic and effortful swallows) may be appropriate for older children, depending on the pathophysiology as defined by instrumental examination and the ability of children to follow directions. Oral hygiene is a reasonable component of all intervention programs, because poor oral hygiene is a risk factor for lung infections in adults who have dysphagia [90].

Further research is needed to determine the appropriateness of treating pediatric patients with techniques that have been validated in adults. It is not clear that techniques aimed at treating impairments in a neurologically mature system are appropriate for the developing system. Moreover, treatments used with adult patients may be dangerous when applied to children. For example, neck flexion, as used during a chin tuck, predisposes some infants to obstructive apnea [91].

Short- or long-term supplemental tube feedings may be considered for children who have oropharyngeal dysphagia associated with respiratory compromise or the inability to meet nutrition needs safely. Some factors that influence decisions about feeding tube placement include the anticipated duration of the dysphagia, the presence of comorbidities, and the presence of vomiting or extra-esophageal reflux leading to potential aspiration of gastric contents. Again, whenever possible, efforts should be made to offer tastes to children for swallowing practice and to optimize child and caregiver interactions during mealtimes.

Summary

Feeding/swallowing problems commonly occur in the setting of complex medical, health, and developmental conditions. These problems are increasing in frequency and may be associated with long-term respiratory, nutritional, and developmental sequelae. Evidence-based practices in pediatric dysphagia have not kept pace with the recognition of these problems. Rigorous investigations are needed to identify the best clinical practices for optimal outcomes of affected children. Evaluation and treatment of pediatric feeding/swallowing problems require input from multiple disciplines.

References

[1] Newman LA, Keckley C, Petersen MC, et al. Swallowing function and medical diagnoses in infants suspected of dysphagia. Pediatrics 2001;108:E106.

[2] Marlow N. Neurocognitive outcome after very preterm birth. Arch Dis Child Fetal Neonatal Ed 2004;89:F224–8.

[3] Ancel PY, Livinec F, Larroque B, et al. Cerebral palsy among very preterm children in relation to gestational age and neonatal ultrasound abnormalities: the EPIPAGE cohort study. Pediatrics 2006;117:828–35.

[4] Burklow KA, Phelps AN, Schultz JR, et al. Classifying complex pediatric feeding disorders. J Pediatr Gastroenterol Nutr 1998;27:143–7.

[5] Hawdon JM, Beauregard N, Slattery J, et al. Identification of neonates at risk of developing feeding problems in infancy. Dev Med Child Neurol 2000;42:235–9.

[6] Linscheid TR. Behavioral treatments for pediatric feeding disorders. Behav Modif 2006;30: 6–23.

[7] Reilly S, Skuse D, Poblete X. Prevalence of feeding problems and oral motor dysfunction in children with cerebral palsy: a community survey. J Pediatr 1996;129:877–82.

[8] Field D, Garland M, Williams K. Correlates of specific childhood feeding problems. J Paediatr Child Health 2003;39:299–304.

[9] Schwarz SM, Corredor J, Fisher-Medina J, et al. Diagnosis and treatment of feeding disorders in children with developmental disabilities. Pediatrics 2001;108:671–6.

[10] Palmer S, Horn S. Feeding problems in children. In: Palmer S, Ekvall E, editors. Pediatric nutrition in developmental disorders. Springfield (IL): Charles Thomas; 1978. p. 107–29.

[11] Burklow KA, McGrath AM, Valerius KS, et al. Relationship between feeding difficulties, medical complexity, and gestational age. Nutr Clin Pract 2002;17:373–8.

[12] Dahl M, Thommessen M, Rasmussen M, et al. Feeding and nutritional characteristics in children with moderate or severe cerebral palsy. Acta Paediatr 1996;85:697–701.

[13] Martin JA, Hamilton BE, Sutton PD, et al. Births: final data for 2003. Natl Vital Stat Rep 2005;54:1–116.

[14] Hamilton BE, Minino AM, Martin JA, et al. Annual summary of vital statistics: 2005. Pediatrics 2007;119:345–60.

[15] Mathews TJ, MacDorman MF. Infant mortality statistics from the 2003 period linked birth/ infant death data set. Natl Vital Stat Rep 2006;54:1–29.

[16] Rommel N, De Meyer AM, Feenstra L, et al. The complexity of feeding problems in 700 infants and young children presenting to a tertiary care institution. J Pediatr Gastroenterol Nutr 2003;37:75–84.

[17] Symington A, Pinelli J. Developmental care for promoting development and preventing morbidity in preterm infants. Cochrane Database Syst Rev 2006:CD001814.

[18] Mizuno K, Nishida Y, Taki M, et al. Infants with bronchopulmonary dysplasia suckle with weak pressures to maintain breathing during feeding. Pediatrics 2007;120:e1035–42.

[19] Strauss D, Shavelle R, Reynolds R, et al. Survival in cerebral palsy in the last 20 years: signs of improvement? Dev Med Child Neurol 2007;49:86–92.

[20] Selley WG, Parrott LC, Lethbridge PC, et al. Objective measures of dysphagia complexity in children related to suckle feeding histories, gestational ages, and classification of their cerebral palsy. Dysphagia 2001;16:200–7.

[21] Hirtz D, Thurman DJ, Gwinn-Hardy K, et al. How common are the "common" neurologic disorders? Neurology 2007;68:326–37.

[22] Khoshoo V, Edell D. Previously healthy infants may have increased risk of aspiration during respiratory syncytial viral bronchiolitis. Pediatrics 1999;104:1389–90.

[23] Heuschkel RB, Fletcher K, Hill A, et al. Isolated neonatal swallowing dysfunction: a case series and review of the literature. Dig Dis Sci 2003;48:30–5.

[24] Lefton-Greif MA, Carroll JL, Loughlin GM. Long-term follow-up of oropharyngeal dysphagia in children without apparent risk factors. Pediatr Pulmonol 2006;41:1040–8.

[25] Lefton-Greif MA, Crawford TO, Winkelstein JA, et al. Oropharyngeal dysphagia and aspi-
     ration in patients with ataxia-telangiectasia. J Pediatr 2000;136:225–31.
[26] Donner MW. Editorial. Dysphagia 1986;1:1–2.
[27] Threats TT. Dysphagia as a disability: World Health Organization framework. Presented at
     the 14th Annual Meeting of the Dysphagia Research Society. Scottsdale (AZ), March 24,
     2006.
[28] Threats TT. Towards an international framework for communication disorders: use of the
     ICF. J Commun Disord 2006;39:251–65.
[29] Carruth BR, Skinner JD. Feeding behaviors and other motor development in healthy chil-
     dren (2–24 months). J Am Coll Nutr 2002;21:88–96.
[30] Lifschitz CH. Feeding problems in infants and children. Curr Treat Options Gastroenterol
     2001;4:451–7.
[31] Mercado-Deane MG, Burton EM, Harlow SA, et al. Swallowing dysfunction in infants less
     than 1 year of age. Pediatr Radiol 2001;31:423–8.
[32] The Young Infants Clinical Signs Study Group. Clinical signs that predict severe illness in
     children under age 2 months: a multicentre study. Lancet 2008;371:135–42.
[33] Sheikh S, Allen E, Shell R, et al. Chronic aspiration without gastroesophageal reflux as
     a cause of chronic respiratory symptoms in neurologically normal infants. Chest 2001;120:
     1190–5.
[34] Khoshoo V, Ross G, Kelly B, et al. Benefits of thickened feeds in previously healthy infants
     with respiratory syncytial viral bronchiolitis. Pediatr Pulmonol 2001;31:301–2.
[35] Arvedson J, Rogers B, Buck G, et al. Silent aspiration prominent in children with dysphagia.
     Int J Pediatr Otorhinolaryngol 1994;28:173–81.
[36] Kirby M, Noel RJ. Nutrition and gastrointestinal tract assessment and management of chil-
     dren with dysphagia. SemIn Speech Lang 2007;28:180–9.
[37] Inder TE, Volpe JJ. Recovery of congenital isolated pharyngeal dysfunction: implications
     for early management. Pediatr Neurol 1998;19:222–4.
[38] Mbonda E, Claus D, Bonnier C, et al. Prolonged dysphagia caused by congenital pharyngeal
     dysfunction. J Pediatr 1995;126:923–7.
[39] Tawfik R, Dickson A, Clarke M, et al. Caregivers' perceptions following gastrostomy
     in severely disabled children with feeding problems. Dev Med Child Neurol 1997;39:
     746–51.
[40] Nair RH, Kesavachandran C, Shashidhar S. Spirometric impairments in undernourished
     children. Indian J Physiol Pharmacol 1999;43:467–73.
[41] Loughlin GM. Respiratory consequences of dysfunctional swallowing and aspiration. Dys-
     phagia 1989;3:126–30.
[42] Abrams SA. Chronic pulmonary insufficiency in children and its effects on growth and
     development. J Nutr 2001;131:938S–41S.
[43] Cass H, Wallis C, Ryan M, et al. Assessing pulmonary consequences of dysphagia in
     children with neurological disabilities: when to intervene? Dev Med Child Neurol
     2005;47:347–52.
[44] Lefton-Greif MA, McGrath-Morrow SA. Deglutition and respiration: development, coor-
     dination, and practical implications. Semin Speech Lang 2007;28:166–79.
[45] Jobe AJ. The new BPD: an arrest of lung development. Pediatr Res 1999;46:641–3.
[46] Yehuda S, Rabinovitz S, Mostofsky DI. Nutritional deficiencies in learning and cognition.
     J Pediatr Gastroenterol Nutr 2006;43(Suppl 3):S22–5.
[47] Fanjiang G, Kleinman RE. Nutrition and performance in children. Curr Opin Clin Nutr
     Metab Care 2007;10:342–7.
[48] Sengpiel F. The critical period. Curr Biol 2007;17:R742–3.
[49] Illingworth RS, Lister J. The critical or sensitive period, with special reference to certain feed-
     ing problems in infants and children. J Pediatr 1964;65:839–48.
[50] Mennella JA, Griffin CE, Beauchamp GK. Flavor programming during infancy. Pediatrics
     2004;113:840–5.

[51] Pickler RH, Best AM, Reyna BA, et al. Prediction of feeding performance in preterm infants. Newborn Infant Nurs Rev 2005;5:116–23.

[52] Mizuno K, Ueda A. Development of sucking behavior in infants who have not been fed for 2 months after birth. Pediatr Int 2001;43:251–5.

[53] Rogers B. Neurodevelopmental presentation of dysphagia. SemIn Speech Lang 1996;17: 269–80.

[54] Kohda E, Hisazumi H, Hiramatsu K. Swallowing dysfunction and aspiration in neonates and infants. Acta Otolaryngol Suppl (Stockholm) 1994;517:11–6.

[55] Ferrang TM, Johnson RK, Ferrara MS. Dietary and anthropometric assessment of adults with cerebral palsy. J Am Diet Assoc 1992;92:1083–6.

[56] Jeffrey PK. The development of large and small airways. Am J Respir Crit Care Med 1998; 157:S174–80.

[57] Von Mutius E. Paediatric origins of adult lung disease. Thorax 2001;56:153–7.

[58] Sigman M, Neumann C, Baksh M, et al. Relationship between nutrition and development in Kenyan toddlers. J Pediatr 1989;115:357–64.

[59] Matsuse T, Teramoto S, Matsui H, et al. Widespread occurrence of diffuse aspiration bronchiolitis in patients with dysphagia, irrespective of age. Chest 1998;114:350–1.

[60] Guilleminault C, Coons S. Apnea and bradycardia during feeding in infants weighing > 2000 gm. J Pediatr 1984;104:932–5.

[61] Thach BT. Can we breathe and swallow at the same time? J Appl Physiol 2005;99:1633.

[62] Plaxico DT, Loughlin GM. Nasopharyngeal reflux and neonatal apnea. Am J Dis Child 1981;135:793–4.

[63] Steinschneider A, Weinstein SL, Diamond E. The sudden infant death syndrome and apnea/obstruction during neonatal sleep and feeding. Pediatrics 1982;70:858–63.

[64] Hay AD, Wilson A, Fahey T, et al. The duration of acute cough in pre-school children presenting to primary care: a prospective cohort study. Fam Pract 2003;20:696–705.

[65] Hamill PV, Drizd TA, Johnson CL, et al. Physical growth: national center for health statistics percentiles. Am J Clin Nutr 1979;32:607–29.

[66] Reau NR, Senturia YD, Lebailly SA, et al. Infant and toddler feeding patterns and problems: normative data and a new direction. J Dev Behav Pediatr 1996;17:149–53.

[67] Arvedson JC, Lefton-Greif MA. Pediatric videofluoroscopic swallow studies: a professional manual with caregiver handouts. San Antonio (TX): Communication Skill Builders; 1998.

[68] Logemann JA. Manual for the videofluorographic study of swallowing. 2nd edition. Austin (TX): Pro-Ed; 1993.

[69] de Jong PA, Mayo JR, Golmohammadi K, et al. Estimation of cancer mortality associated with repetitive computed tomography scanning. Am J Respir Crit Care Med 2006;173: 199–203.

[70] Matsuo K, Hiiemae KM, Gonzalez-Fernandez M, et al. Respiration during feeding on solid food: alterations in breathing during mastication, pharyngeal bolus aggregation and swallowing. J Appl Physiol 2007;104:674–81.

[71] Palmer JB, Hiiemae KM. Eating and breathing: interactions between respiration and feeding on solid food. Dysphagia 2003;18:169–78.

[72] Bosma JF. Development of feeding. Clin Nutr 1986;5:210–8.

[73] Delzell PB, Kraus RA, Gaisie G, et al. Laryngeal penetration: a predictor of aspiration in infants? Pediatr Radiol 1999;29:762–5.

[74] Friedman B, Frazier JB. Deep laryngeal penetration as a predictor of aspiration. Dysphagia 2000;15:153–8.

[75] Smith CH, Logemann JA, Colangelo LA, et al. Incidence and patient characteristics associated with silent aspiration in the acute care setting. Dysphagia 1999;14:1–7.

[76] Thach BT. Maturation and transformation of reflexes that protect the laryngeal airway from liquid aspiration from fetal to adult life. Am J Med 2001;111(Suppl 8A): 69S–77S.

[77] Thach BT. Maturation of cough and other reflexes that protect the fetal and neonatal airway. Pulm Pharmacol Ther 2007;20:365–70.

[78] Miller HC, Proud GO, Behrle FC. Variations in the gag, cough and swallow reflexes and tone of the vocal cords as determined by direct laryngoscopy in newborn infants. Yale J Biol Med 1952;24:284–91.

[79] Thurlbeck WM. Postnatal human lung growth. Thorax 1982;37:564–71.

[80] Chien W, Ashland J, Haver K, et al. Type 1 laryngeal cleft: establishing a functional diagnostic and management algorithm. Int J Pediatr Otorhinolaryngol 2006;70:2073–9.

[81] Willging JP. Benefit of feeding assessment before pediatric airway reconstruction. Laryngoscope 2000;110:825–34.

[82] Link DT, Willging JP, Miller CK, et al. Pediatric laryngopharyngeal sensory testing during flexible endoscopic evaluation of swallowing: feasible and correlative. Ann Otol Rhinol Laryngol 2000;109:899–905.

[83] Di Scipio WJ, Kaslon K. Conditioned dysphagia in cleft palate children after pharyngeal flap surgery. Psychosom Med 1982;44:247–57.

[84] Perlman AL, Luschei ES, DuMond CE. Electrical activity from the superior pharyngeal constrictor during reflexive and nonreflexive tasks. J Speech Hear Res 1989;32:749–54.

[85] Mathew OP, Belan M, Thoppil CK. Sucking patterns of neonates during bottle feeding: comparison of different nipple units. Am J Perinatol 1992;9:265–9.

[86] McCain GC. An evidence-based guideline for introducing oral feeding to healthy preterm infants. Neonatal Netw 2003;22:45–50.

[87] Fucile S, Gisel EG, Lau C. Effect of an oral stimulation program on sucking skill maturation of preterm infants. Dev Med Child Neurol 2005;47:158–62.

[88] Gaebler CP, Hanzlik JR. The effects of a prefeeding stimulation program on preterm infants. Am J Occup Ther 1996;50:184–92.

[89] Schadler G, Suss-Burghart H, Toschke AM, et al. Feeding disorders in ex-prematures: causes—response to therapy—long term outcome. Eur J Pediatr 2007;166:803–8.

[90] Langmore SE, Terpenning MS, Schork A, et al. Predictors of aspiration pneumonia: how important is dysphagia? Dysphagia 1998;13:69–81.

[91] Thach BT, Stark AR. Spontaneous neck flexion and airway obstruction during apneic spells in preterm infants. J Pediatr 1979;94:275–81.

ELSEVIER
SAUNDERS

Phys Med Rehabil Clin N Am
19 (2008) 853–866

PHYSICAL MEDICINE
AND REHABILITATION
CLINICS OF
NORTH AMERICA

Dysphagia in the Elderly

Ianessa A. Humbert, PhD[a], JoAnne Robbins, PhD[b,c],*

[a]Department of Physical Medicine and Rehabilitation, Johns Hopkins University School
of Medicine, 98 North Broadway, Suite 413, Baltimore, MD 21231, USA
[b]University of Wisconsin School of Medicine and Public Health, Department of Medicine,
Madison, WI, USA
[c]William S. Middleton Memorial Veterans Hospital, Geriatric Research,
Education and Clinical Center (11G), 2500 Overlook Terrace GRECC 11G, Madison,
WI 53705, USA

The capacity to swallow effectively and safely or eat is one of the most basic human needs and can be a great pleasure. Sustaining oneself nutritionally and maintaining adequate hydration while enjoying the process has become intertwined with the activities of society. Older adults look forward to more opportunities to share mealtimes and participate in social interactions, including holidays, family occasions, and traditions centered on meals and specific foods. Therefore, the loss of the capacity to swallow safely and dine enjoyably can have far-reaching implications from sustaining life to quality of life. An ultimate irony is that as we grow older, the ability to swallow, a function taken for granted, undergoes changes that increase the risk for disordered swallowing. This occurs with increasing age and exposure to age-related diseases and conditions. The loss of the capacity to swallow can have devastating health implications, including nutrition and hydration deficits, especially for older adults.

According to the United States Census Bureau, as of July 1, 2005, there were an estimated 78.2 million American baby boomers (those born between 1946 and 1964). In 2006, baby boomers began turning 60 at a rate of approximately 330 every hour. With the rapid and dramatic growth in the United States aging population, dysphagia is becoming a national health care burden and concern.

Dysphagia prevalence depends on the specific population sampled, with community-dwelling and more independent individuals having rates near

* Corresponding author. William S. Middleton Memorial Veterans Hospital, Geriatric Research, Education and Clinical Center (11G), 2500 Overlook Terrace GRECC 11G, Madison, WI 53705.
E-mail address: jrobbin2@wisc.edu (J. Robbins).

1047-9651/08/$ - see front matter. Published by Elsevier Inc.
doi:10.1016/j.pmr.2008.06.002

15%. Upward of 40% of people living in institutionalized settings, such as assisted living facilities and nursing homes, are dysphagic [1]. With the projected growth of individuals living in nursing homes, there is a compelling need to address dysphagia not only in ambulatory and acute care settings but also in long-term care settings.

Presbyphagia versus dysphagia

Although the anatomic, physiologic, psychologic, and functional changes that occur in the dynamic process referred to as "aging" place older adults at risk for dysphagia; a healthy older adult's swallow is not inherently impaired. Presbyphagia refers to characteristic changes in the swallowing mechanism of otherwise healthy older adults [2]. Clinicians are becoming more aware of the need to distinguish among dysphagia, presbyphagia (an old yet healthy swallow), and other related diagnoses to avoid overdiagnosing and overtreating dysphagia. With the increased threat of acute illness, multiple medications, and several age-related conditions, older adults are more vulnerable and can cross the line from having a healthy older swallow to having dysphagia in association with certain perturbations, including acute illness, surgery, chemoradiation, and other factors. Previous work has focused primarily on the anatomy and physiology of the oropharyngeal swallowing mechanism. Age effects on the temporal evolution of isometric and swallowing pressure [2–8] indicate a progression of change that, when combined with naturally diminished functional reserve (the resilient ability of the body to adapt to physiologic stress [9], make the older population more susceptible to dysphagia. This article reviews age-related changes in peripheral and central nervous system control of head and neck structures for swallowing. In addition, promising strategies for neurorehabilitation of dysphagia are discussed that are based on the recognition that swallowing disruption may, in part, be a manifestation of sarcopenia (the age-related loss of skeletal muscle mass, organization, and strength) [10] and age-related changes in sensorimotor acuity and efficiency.

Healthy swallowing overview

Normal oropharyngeal swallowing involves closely integrated sensory and motor events that begin with the sight and smell of approaching food until material has safely entered the esophagus. The tongue propels the bolus posteriorly into the pharynx and numerous and varied sensory receptors are stimulated along the way, triggering the pharyngeal swallow [11]. The oral cavity and pharynx contain some of the richest and most diverse sensory receptors of the body, represented by dense intricate nerve supply to the oral cavity, pharynx, and larynx. Thus, exact timing of the onset of the pharyngeal swallow is imperative and highly sensory reliant, such that even a 1-second delay, or less, in initiation can result in airway invasion of ingested material [12]. Dysphagia and subsequent aspiration often are the manifestation of a breakdown in one or more of the many sensory-motor events that comprise normal swallowing.

Peripheral sensory-motor swallowing

Age-related changes in specific physiologic parameters

Sensory-motor function becomes increasingly dampened with senescence throughout the body [13–17], and rate and extent depend on personal habits (eg, smoking and alcohol may increase physiologic change). Structures of the head and neck that are important for normal swallowing also are prone to age-related changes in the peripheral nervous system. These changes have been defined by measures of specific physiologic parameters, such as muscle activity, motor-unit density, or assessments of somatosensory perception. Physiologic parameters (ie, reduced pharyngeal pressure) are the basis of age-related differences in swallowing function and behavior (ie, slow swallow) between young and elderly adults. Anatomic differences in the old include a smaller cross-sectional area of masticatory muscles (masseter and medial pterygoid), increased lingual atrophy and fatty infiltration, decreased lingual muscle fiber diameter [18,19], and atrophied type 1 (slow twitch) fibers in the thyroarytenoid muscle [20]. Beyond anatomic measures, functional changes in muscle activity between young and old include longer muscle activity (twitch prolongation) of the masseter [21], obicularis oris, supra- and infrahyoid muscles [22], and thyroarytenoid muscle [23]; slower waveforms of the pharyngeal constrictors; and lower resting tone of the upper esophageal sphincter [24,25]. Age-related diminishment in strength, mobility, and endurance also is evident in the tongue [3,5,26,27] and lips [28,29]. Sensory function, which is understudied in the swallowing literature, despite its influence on the pharyngeal swallow response, also changes with age and is influenced by declining perception of spatial tactile recognition on the lip and tongue [30–32], diminished perception of viscosity in the oral cavity [33], poorer oral stereognosis [34,35], and reductions in taste perception [36,37] with increasing age. Although physiologic parameters typically are measured at rest, post mortem, or during nonswallowing tasks and may not show immediate or direct clinical relevance to general swallowing function, they can be extrapolated or inferred to age-related changes in swallowing behavior and enhance the global understanding of swallowing abnormalities.

Age-related changes in general sensory-motor swallowing function

It is generally accepted in published studies that swallowing, as in sensory-motor physiology throughout the body, becomes slower with increasing age [2,38–40] beginning in middle age [2]. Also, the pharyngeal swallow response often initiates later in older adults [2,8,41].

In normal swallowing, the properties of a bolus (ie, volume, viscosity, and temperature) are detected by oropharyneal sensory receptors and are used to guide motor function for swallowing. Increasing bolus volume and viscosity minimizes the delay in pharyngeal swallow initiation [42–44] and increases laryngeal closure durations [2,43] in healthy adults. Taste stimuli also have modified swallowing timing [45,46], contraction of muscles in the submental region (laryngeal movement) [47–49], and lingual pressure [50] compared with a neutral stimulus. To date, much of swallowing research has examined sensory or motor components with little consideration for the complementary dynamic, despite the intimate synchrony of sensation and movement. Furthermore, given the known multimodal deficiencies in oral-pharyngeal sensation, it is no surprise that the swallowing motor response in older adults is less responsive to taste and somatosensory stimuli [51] compared with a younger cohort. A recent study found that combining sensory stimuli (consistency and taste) minimizes the age differences in motor responses to sensation [47], likely because older adults benefit from increased exogenous sensory input to drive motor responses.

Central swallowing control

Dysphagia prevalence increases in advancing age resulting from more frequent neurologic damage or disorders, such as stroke [52], Alzheimer 's disease [53], and Parkinson's disease [54]. Therefore, it has become important that peripheral differences be investigated alongside central nervous system control. Recent advances in medical technology have facilitated functional brain imaging studies of swallowing, incorporating techniques that include positron emission tomography [55–58], magnetoencephalography [59–63], transcranial magnetic stimulation [55,64–66], electroencephalography [67–69], and functional MRI (fMRI) [65,70–81]. fMRI is among the fastest growing brain-imaging technologies because it is minimally invasive compared with some other brain imaging systems and is becoming increasingly accessible for research purposes.

In a systematic review of fMRI studies of healthy swallowing [82], the primary motor cortex was the most prevalent region of activation, followed by the primary sensory cortex. Activation also was common in the insula and the anterior cingulate gyrus, but fewer studies found activation in the prefrontal, parietal, or temporal lobes consistently or across subjects. Other areas of activation included motor planning areas (supplementary motor area and premotor area), other subcortical regions (internal capsule, thalamus, basal ganglia, putamen, and globus palidus), and the cerebellum. All but one of the studies included in this review involved young adults (mean age 35 years). These pioneering fMRI studies of normal swallowing included primarily younger individuals likely because of increased procedure tolerance, task compliance, and reduced head movement.

Only one known neuroimaging study (fMRI) examined swallowing in healthy older women and reported similar patterns of activity as in younger individuals in the bilateral sensory-motor cortices, insula/operculum, and cingulate cortex for saliva and water swallows [75]. Although Martin and colleagues [76] did not include young adults for a prospective comparison, two separate studies of young women and old healthy adults have shown strong left-hemisphere lateralization for swallowing [75]. A difference was that the older women recruited far more activity for water swallows [75], primarily in motor planning areas (bilateral middle frontal gyrus and right superior frontal gyrus), whereas younger women showed more activation for saliva swallows [76].

When a bolus is manipulated in the oral cavity, afferent signals enter the brainstem and their representative cranial nerve nuclei, synapsing in the thalamus, and then projecting to sensory specific areas of the cortex [83]. Before the primary motor area can execute movement, the primary sensory cortex sends information to higher-order association areas for a single sensory modality (ie, temperature or pressure) and for multimodal processing for attention, motor planning, and memory [84]. These data suggest that the older women required more motor planning for safe swallowing than the young women did. Increased activity in motor planning areas might be the result of reduced peripheral sensory abilities in the oral cavity, requiring motor planning areas to become more active (or work harder) in the absence of adequate stimulation to guide motor movements. Overall, Martin and colleagues [75,76] has provided the first look into the central control of swallowing in older adults. Future neuroimaging studies should focus on normal aging and swallowing to enhance what is known about peripheral sensory-motor swallowing across the age span. Furthermore, the effects of increased oropharyngeal sensory stimuli on central control remain uninvestigated. So far, there is only one known experiment where sensation was manipulated (anesthesia) to determine how the brain responds during swallowing (decreased cortical activation in primary sensory-motor regions) [85].

Changes in skeletal muscle in limbs are similar to head and neck

Age-related sensory-motor changes have been more extensively studied in the limbs, with findings similar to those described previously in the head and neck. Muscle loss in the limbs, reviewed elsewhere [86–88], begins in middle age and may be the result of loss of muscle fibers [89–92], fewer motor units [14,93–95], and progressive denervation and changes in nerve conduction [17,96]. Sensory losses in the extremities with age involve declining ability to detect vibratory stimulation [97] and spatial tactile discrimination (particularly in the hands and feet). These sensory-motor losses translate into gross functional deficiencies in manual dexterity [13,98], limb strength [15,99,100], and walking speed [16,101,102].

Peripheral changes to limb anatomy and function occur alongside increased neural activation during limb movement in old compared with young within certain brain regions [103–107]. Heuninckx and colleagues [104] recently investigated whether or not the elaborate cortical responses in the old is related to compensation for increased task effort or dedifferentiation (age-related inability to activate specialized neural mechanisms unrelated to task performance) using a complex interlimb coordination task. Results showed that additional cortical recruitment (primary sensory-motor cortices and motor planning areas) was positively correlated with increased motor success within older adults but not in younger adults. Therefore, the overactivation in the old for motor tasks compared with young is consistent with the compensation hypothesis, where task-related changes are positively correlated with neural activation.

Although some investigators discourage extrapolating limb muscle function to head and neck musculature [108], over-activation in the brain relative to limb motor function may be useful leads toward hypotheses for swallowing studies of neurophysiology in healthy aging. Future studies of the effects of age on swallowing neurophysiology should determine whether or not age-related differences in peripheral movement (ie, slower swallows in older individuals) [2] seem to occur along side differences in neural control of swallowing. Furthermore, incorporating effortful swallowing might convey information about increased neural activation with increased effort with a swallowing task in elders. Overall, knowledge of swallowing neurophysiology in healthy aging is becoming more important as the possibility approaches of using neuroimaging techniques for clinical purposes to understand dysphagia. Without age-matched controls, dysphagic patients who have decreased brain activation for swallowing might show "normal" activation compared with young healthy adults, who normally have less activation than their older counterparts.

Therapy

With advancing age, lean protein tissue diminishes, contributing to the loss of muscle protein mass, whereas adipose tissue increases in skeletal muscle of the limbs [109]. Many studies are showing increased rates of muscle protein synthesis with acute resistance exercise and resistance exercise training programs in middle aged and frail older adults [110–112]. Functional gains with exercise include upper- and lower-body strength and balance, agility, and endurance [113–117].

In traditional swallowing, compensatory treatment strategies are used to alter the flow of material in the pharynx. Chin tuck and head rotation decreased choking during swallowing immediately [118], reduced aspiration in 81% of patients [119], and reduced aspiration in 25% of patients who used it for all volumes swallowed [120]. Head rotation was 20% to 75% effective in reducing aspiration [120–122] and increasing the duration of laryngeal elevation [122]. A large multisite randomized clinical trial recently indicated the need to better understand the relationship between material properties of thickened fluids often provided to elders who aspirate thin fluids relative to changes in health status. The investigators conclude that the future need is to examine efficacy of a combination of physiologically sound interventions relative to solely modifying diet (based on a cohort of 512 research participants) [123,124], particularly in the older populations who had dysphagia secondary to dementia or Parkinson's disease. Despite some success with compensatory maneuvers and modifying food consistencies, these techniques offer patients little in the way of rehabilitation for functional swallowing. Research to date primarily has focused on nonswallow and enhanced swallowing (ie, effortful swallowing) [125] motor exercises to increase muscle strength and range of motion in oropharyngeal structures. Exercise has shown to be effective in increasing strength of the tongue and improving functional swallowing in the healthy old [3,5,126,127] and in dysphagic individuals [128,129].

Sensory modalities have garnered little attention for long-term swallowing treatment, despite many reports of positive effects of increased intra-oral stimulation (ie, taste, texture, temperature, and viscosity) on swallowing biomechanics and bolus flow kinematics [45,47–49,130]. In addition to intraoral stimulation, electrical stimulation to the submental and neck regions at low sensory threshold levels reduced aspiration frequency and residue amounts in individuals who have chronic pharyngeal dysphagia [131]. Each of these sensory modalities is exogenous or externally cued forms of stimulation to improve a motor response. Endogenous or internally cued stimulation involves increased attention to a task, resulting in top-down initiation and increased neural activation of motor planning and execution areas of the cortex during a motor task in healthy adults [132]. All forms of increased sensory stimulation or attention to a task should be incorporated into swallowing therapy, especially given known diminishment in oropharyngeal sensation, attention, and memory in the old.

Sensory-based swallowing therapies that aim to increase a motor response (ie, sour or cold bolus), rather than modify bolus flow (ie, thickened liquids), might receive little attention because they are not routinely included in assessments of swallowing function. Also, their usefulness has not been researched over the long term, despite the likelihood that adaptation to a sensory stimulus might gradually decrease the effect of stimulus on the motor response. Some studies have reported oral and tongue sensory assessments [133,134]; these could be included in swallowing assessments. Also, older participants demonstrated more difficulty with taste components of the sensory assessments compared with oral somatosensory measures [135]. Sensory assessments of the oropharynx for swallowing to understand healthy aging might be limited by the use of psychophysical measures (relationship between physical stimuli and their subjective percepts), where a clinician relies heavily on subjective reports of intensity for stimuli.

Thus, cognitive differences may affect the accuracy of responses. In addition, assessing sensory ability requires knowledge and expertise to create, conduct, and interpret valid and reliable measures of oropharyngeal sensation. Therefore, as in many clinical and research foci of swallowing, multidisciplinary collaborations are necessary to derive useful sensory assessments for swallowing.

As medical technology for neuroimaging becomes more useful and available, more neurorehabilitation treatments will be examined for peripheral and central changes in disordered populations as a means of determining effectiveness [136]. With impending changes, it is imperative that sensory-motor abilities in healthy older adults are researched thoroughly so that correlations between the brain and swallowing biomechanics can be interpreted accurately for comparison to the dysphagic population.

References

[1] Barczi SR, Sullivan SP, Robbins J. How should dysphagia care of older adults differ? Establishing optimal practice patterns. Semin Speech Lang 2000;21(4):347–61.
[2] Robbins J, Hamilton JW, Lof GL, et al. Oropharyngeal swallowing in normal adults of different ages. Gastroenterology 1992;103(3):823–9.
[3] Nicosia MA, Hind JA, Roecker EB, et al. Age effects on the temporal evolution of isometric and swallowing pressure. J Gerontol A Biol Sci Med Sci 2000;55(11):M634–40.
[4] Robbins J, Coyle J, Rosenbek J, et al. Differentiation of normal and abnormal airway protection during swallowing using the penetration-aspiration scale. Dysphagia Fall 1999;14(4):228–32.
[5] Robbins J, Levine R, Wood J, et al. Age effects on lingual pressure generation as a risk factor for dysphagia. J Gerontol A Biol Sci Med Sci 1995;50(5):M257–62.
[6] Shaw DW, Cook CI, Dent J, et al. Age influence oropharyngeal and upper esophageal sphincter function during swallowing. Gastroenterology 1990;98:73–8.
[7] Shaw DW, Cook CI, Gabb M, et al. Influence of normal aging on oropharyngeal and upper esophageal sphincter function during swallow. Am J Physiol 1995;L68:G389–90.
[8] Tracy JF, Logemann JA, Kahrilas PJ, et al. Preliminary observations on the effects of age on oropharyngeal deglutition. Dysphagia 1989;4(2):90–4.
[9] Pendergast DR, Fisher NM, Calkins E. Cardiovascular, neuromuscular, and metabolic alterations with age leading to frailty Spec No. J Gerontol 1993;48:61–7.
[10] Rosenberg IH. Sarcopenia: origins and clinical relevance. J Nutr 1997;127(5 Suppl):990S–1S.
[11] Miller AJ. Oral and pharyngeal reflexes in the mammalian nervous system: their diverse range in complexity and the pivotal role of the tongue. Crit Rev Oral Biol Med 2002;13(5):409–25.
[12] Perlman AL, Booth BM, Grayhack JP. Videofluoroscopic predictors of aspiration in patients with oropharyngeal dysphagia Spring. Dysphagia 1994;9(2):90–5.
[13] Aniansson A, Rundgren A, Sperling L. Evaluation of functional capacity in activities of daily living in 70-year-old men and women. Scand J Rehabil Med 1980;12(4):145–54.
[14] Brown WF. A method for estimating the number of motor units in thenar muscles and the changes in motor unit count with ageing. J Neurol Neurosurg Psychiatry 1972;35(6):845–52.
[15] Danneskiold-Samsoe B, Kofod V, Munter J, et al. Muscle strength and functional capacity in 78-81-year-old men and women. Eur J Appl Physiol Occup Physiol 1984;52(3):310–4.
[16] Himann JE, Cunningham DA, Rechnitzer PA, et al. Age-related changes in speed of walking. Med Sci Sports Exerc 1988;20(2):161–6.

[17] LaFratta CW, Canestrari R. A comparison of sensory and motor nerve conduction velocities as related to age. Arch Phys Med Rehabil 1966;47(5):286–90.

[18] Bassler R. Histopathology of different types of atrophy of the human tongue. Pathol Res Pract 1987;182(1):87–97.

[19] Nakayama M. [Histological study on aging changes in the human tongue]. Nippon Jibiinkoka Gakkai Kaiho 1991;94(4):541–55.

[20] Malmgren LT, Fisher PJ, Bookman LM, et al. Age-related changes in muscle fiber types in the human thyroarytenoid muscle: an immunohistochemical and stereological study using confocal laser scanning microscopy. Otolaryngol Head Neck Surg 1999;121(4):441–51.

[21] Newton J, Yemm R. Age changes in contractile properties of masseter muscle in man. J Oral Rehabil 1990;17:204–5.

[22] Vaiman M, Eviatar E, Segal S. Surface electromyographic studies of swallowing in normal subjects: a review of 440 adults. Report 1. Quantitative data: timing measures. Otolaryngol Head Neck Surg 2004;131(4):548–55.

[23] Takeda N, Thomas GR, Ludlow CL. Aging effects on motor units in the human thyroarytenoid muscle. Laryngoscope 2000;110(6):1018–25.

[24] Bardan E, Xie P, Brasseur J, et al. Effect of ageing on the upper and lower oesophageal sphincters. Eur J Gastroenterol Hepatol 2000;12(11):1221–5.

[25] McKee GJ, Johnston BT, McBride GB, et al. Does age or sex affect pharyngeal swallowing? Clin Otolaryngol Allied Sci 1998;23(2):100–6.

[26] Crow HC, Ship JA. Tongue strength and endurance in different aged individuals. J Gerontol A Biol Sci Med Sci 1996;51(5):M247–50.

[27] Price PA, Darvell BW. Force and mobility in the ageing human tongue. Med J Aust 1981; 1(2):75–8.

[28] Wohlert AB. Reflex responses of lip muscles in young and older women. J Speech Hear Res 1996;39(3):578–89.

[29] Wohlert AB. Perioral muscle activity in young and older adults during speech and non-speech tasks. J Speech Hear Res 1996;39(4):761–70.

[30] Johnson KO, Phillips JR. Tactile spatial resolution. I. Two-point discrimination, gap detection, grating resolution, and letter recognition. J Neurophysiol 1981;46(6):1177–92.

[31] Stevens JC, Choo KK. Spatial acuity of the body surface over the life span. Somatosens Mot Res 1996;13(2):153–66.

[32] Wohlert AB. Tactile perception of spatial stimuli on the lip surface by young and older adults. J Speech Hear Res 1996;39(6):1191–8.

[33] Smith CH, Logemann JA, Burghardt WR, et al. Oral and oropharyngeal perceptions of fluid viscosity across the age span. Dysphagia 2006;21(4):209–17.

[34] Calhoun KH, Gibson B, Hartley L, et al. Age-related changes in oral sensation. Laryngoscope 1992;102(2):109–16.

[35] Williams WN, La Pointe LL. Intra-oral recognition of geometric forms by normal subjects. Percept Mot Skills 1971;32(2):419–26.

[36] Bartoshuk LM. Taste. Robust across the age span? Ann N Y Acad Sci 1989;561:65–75.

[37] Chauhan J, Hawrysh ZJ. Suprathreshold sour taste intensity and pleasantness perception with age. Physiol Behav 1988;43(5):601–7.

[38] Cook IJ, Weltman MD, Wallace K, et al. Influence of aging on oral-pharyngeal bolus transit and clearance during swallowing: scintigraphic study. Am J Physiol 1994; 266(6 Pt 1):G972–7.

[39] Dejaeger E, Pelemans W. Swallowing and the duration of the hyoid movement in normal adults of different ages. Aging (Milano) 1996;8(2):130–4.

[40] Logemann JA, Pauloski BR, Rademaker AW, et al. Oropharyngeal swallow in younger and older women: videofluoroscopic analysis. J Speech Lang Hear Res 2002;45(3):434–45.

[41] Logemann JA, Pauloski BR, Rademaker AW, et al. Temporal and biomechanical characteristics of oropharyngeal swallow in younger and older men. J Speech Lang Hear Res 2000; 43(5):1264–74.

[42] Bisch EM, Logemann JA, Rademaker AW, et al. Pharyngeal effects of bolus volume, viscosity, and temperature in patients with dysphagia resulting from neurologic impairment and in normal subjects. J Speech Hear Res 1994;37(5):1041–59.

[43] Lazarus CL, Logemann JA, Rademaker AW, et al. Effects of bolus volume, viscosity, and repeated swallows in nonstroke subjects and stroke patients. Arch Phys Med Rehabil 1993; 74(10):1066–70.

[44] Logemann JA, Kahrilas PJ, Cheng J, et al. Closure mechanisms of laryngeal vestibule during swallow. Am J Physiol 1992;262(2 Pt 1):G338–44.

[45] Chee C, Arshad S, Singh S, et al. The influence of chemical gustatory stimuli and oral anaesthesia on healthy human pharyngeal swallowing. Chem Senses 2005;30(5):393–400.

[46] Hamdy S, Jilani S, Price V, et al. Modulation of human swallowing behaviour by thermal and chemical stimulation in health and after brain injury. Neurogastroenterol Motil 2003; 15(1):69–77.

[47] Ding R, Logemann JA, Larson CR, et al. The effects of taste and consistency on swallow physiology in younger and older healthy individuals: a surface electromyographic study. J Speech Lang Hear Res 2003;46(4):977–89.

[48] Leow LP, Huckabee ML, Sharma S, et al. The influence of taste on swallowing apnea, oral preparation time, and duration and amplitude of submental muscle contraction. Chem Senses 2007;32(2):119–28.

[49] Palmer PM, McCulloch TM, Jaffe D, et al. Effects of a sour bolus on the intramuscular electromyographic (EMG) activity of muscles in the submental region Summer. Dysphagia 2005;20(3):210–7.

[50] Pelletier CA, Dhanaraj GE. The effect of taste and palatability on lingual swallowing pressure. Dysphagia 2006;21(2):121–8.

[51] Shaker R, Ren J, Bardan E, et al. Pharyngoglottal closure reflex: characterization in healthy young, elderly and dysphagic patients with predeglutitive aspiration. Gerontology 2003; 49(1):12–20.

[52] Robbins J, Levine RL, Maser A, et al. Swallowing after unilateral stroke of the cerebral cortex. Arch Phys Med Rehabil 1993;74(12):1295–300.

[53] Priefer BA, Robbins J. Eating changes in mild-stage Alzheimer's disease: a pilot study. Dysphagia. Fall 1997;12(4):212–21.

[54] Robbins JA, Logemann JA, Kirshner HS. Swallowing and speech production in Parkinson's disease. Ann Neurol 1986;19(3):283–7.

[55] Hamdy S, Rothwell JC, Brooks DJ, et al. Identification of the cerebral loci processing human swallowing with H2(15)O PET activation. J Neurophysiol 1999;81(4):1917–26.

[56] Harris ML, Julyan P, Kulkarni B, et al. Mapping metabolic brain activation during human volitional swallowing: a positron emission tomography study using [18F]fluorodeoxyglucose. J Cereb Blood Flow Metab 2005;25(4):520–6.

[57] Raichle ME, Fiez JA, Videen TO, et al. Practice-related changes in human brain functional anatomy during nonmotor learning. Cereb Cortex 1994;4(1):8–26.

[58] Zald DH, Pardo JV. The functional neuroanatomy of voluntary swallowing. Ann Neurol 1999;46(3):281–6.

[59] Abe S, Wantanabe Y, Shintani M, et al. Magnetoencephalographic study of the starting point of voluntary swallowing. Cranio 2003;21(1):46–9.

[60] Dziewas R, Soros P, Ishii R, et al. Neuroimaging evidence for cortical involvement in the preparation and in the act of swallowing. Neuroimage 2003;20(1):135–44.

[61] Furlong PL, Hobson AR, Aziz Q, et al. Dissociating the spatio-temporal characteristics of cortical neuronal activity associated with human volitional swallowing in the healthy adult brain. Neuroimage 2004;22(4):1447–55.

[62] Loose R, Hamdy S, Enck P. Magnetoencephalographic response characteristics associated with tongue movement Summer. Dysphagia 2001;16(3):183–5.

[63] Watanabe Y, Abe S, Ishikawa T, et al. Cortical regulation during the early stage of initiation of voluntary swallowing in humans Spring. Dysphagia 2004;19(2):100–8.

[64] Ertekin C, Turman B, Tarlaci S, et al. Cricopharyngeal sphincter muscle responses to transcranial magnetic stimulation in normal subjects and in patients with dysphagia. Clin Neurophysiol 2001;112(1):86–94.

[65] Fraser C, Power M, Hamdy S, et al. Driving plasticity in human adult motor cortex is associated with improved motor function after brain injury. Neuron 2002;34(5):831–40.

[66] Rodel RM, Laskawi R, Markus H. Tongue representation in the lateral cortical motor region of the human brain as assessed by transcranial magnetic stimulation. Ann Otol Rhinol Laryngol 2003;112(1):71–6.

[67] Hiraoka K. Movement-related cortical potentials associated with saliva and water bolus swallowing Summer. Dysphagia 2004;19(3):155–9.

[68] Huckabee ML, Deecke L, Cannito MP, et al. Cortical control mechanisms in volitional swallowing: the Bereitschaftspotential Fall. Brain Topogr 2003;16(1):3–17.

[69] Satow T, Ikeda A, Yamamoto J, et al. Role of primary sensorimotor cortex and supplementary motor area in volitional swallowing: a movement-related cortical potential study. Am J Physiol Gastrointest Liver Physiol 2004;287(2):G459–70.

[70] Birn RM, Bandettini PA, Cox RW, et al. Event-related fMRI of tasks involving brief motion. Hum Brain Mapp 1999;7(2):106–14.

[71] Hamdy S, Mikulis DJ, Crawley A, et al. Cortical activation during human volitional swallowing: an event-related fMRI study. Am J Physiol 1999;277(1 Pt 1):G219–25.

[72] Kern M, Birn R, Jaradeh S, et al. Swallow-related cerebral cortical activity maps are not specific to deglutition. Am J Physiol Gastrointest Liver Physiol 2001;280(4):G531–8.

[73] Kern MK, Jaradeh S, Arndorfer RC, et al. Cerebral cortical representation of reflexive and volitional swallowing in humans. Am J Physiol Gastrointest Liver Physiol 2001;280(3): G354–60.

[74] Komisaruk BR, Mosier KM, Liu WC, et al. Functional localization of brainstem and cervical spinal cord nuclei in humans with fMRI. AJNR Am J Neuroradiol 2002;23(4): 609–17.

[75] Martin R, Barr A, Macintosh B, et al. Cerebral cortical processing of swallowing in older adults. Exp Brain Res 2007;176(1):12–22.

[76] Martin RE, MacIntosh BJ, Smith RC, et al. Cerebral areas processing swallowing and tongue movement are overlapping but distinct: a functional magnetic resonance imaging study. J Neurophysiol 2004;92(4):2428–43.

[77] Mosier K, Bereznaya I. Parallel cortical networks for volitional control of swallowing in humans. Exp Brain Res 2001;140(3):280–9.

[78] Mosier K, Patel R, Liu WC, et al. Cortical representation of swallowing in normal adults: functional implications. Laryngoscope 1999;109(9):1417–23.

[79] Mosier KM, Liu WC, Maldjian JA, et al. Lateralization of cortical function in swallowing: a functional MR imaging study. AJNR Am J Neuroradiol 1999;20(8):1520–6.

[80] Suzuki M, Asada Y, Ito J, et al. Activation of cerebellum and basal ganglia on volitional swallowing detected by functional magnetic resonance imaging Spring. Dysphagia 2003; 18(2):71–7.

[81] Toogood JA, Barr AM, Stevens TK, et al. Discrete functional contributions of cerebral cortical foci in voluntary swallowing: a functional magnetic resonance imaging (fMRI) "Go, No-Go" study. Exp Brain Res 2005;161(1):81–90.

[82] Humbert IA, Robbins J. Normal swallowing and functional magnetic resonance imaging: a systematic review. Dysphagia 2007;22(3):266–75.

[83] Kandel ER, Schwartz JH, Jessell TM. Principles of neural science. 4th edition. Health Professions Division. New York: McGraw-Hill; 2000.

[84] Kandel E, Schwartz J. Principles of neuroscience. New York: McGraw Hill; 2000.

[85] Teismann IK, Steinstraeter O, Stoeckigt K, et al. Functional oropharyngeal sensory disruption interferes with the cortical control of swallowing. BMC Neurosci 2007;8:62.

[86] Doherty TJ, Vandervoort AA, Brown WF. Effects of ageing on the motor unit: a brief review. Can J Appl Physiol 1993;18(4):331–58.

[87] Grimby G. Muscle performance and structure in the elderly as studied cross-sectionally and longitudinally. J Gerontol A Biol Sci Med Sci 1995;50, Spec No:17–22.

[88] Young A. Ageing and physiological functions. Philos Trans R Soc Lond B Biol Sci 1997; 352(1363):1837–43.

[89] Faulkner JA, Brooks SV, Zerba E. Skeletal muscle weakness and fatigue in old age: underlying mechanisms. Annu Rev Gerontol Geriatr 1990;10:147–66.

[90] Klitgaard H, Mantoni M, Schiaffino S, et al. Function, morphology and protein expression of ageing skeletal muscle: a cross-sectional study of elderly men with different training backgrounds. Acta Physiol Scand 1990;140(1):41–54.

[91] Lexell J, Henriksson-Larsen K, Winblad B, et al. Distribution of different fiber types in human skeletal muscles: effects of aging studied in whole muscle cross sections. Muscle Nerve 1983;6(8):588–95.

[92] Lexell J, Taylor CC, Sjostrom M. What is the cause of the ageing atrophy? Total number, size and proportion of different fiber types studied in whole vastus lateralis muscle from 15- to 83-year-old men. J Neurol Sci 1988;84(2-3):275–94.

[93] Campbell MJ, McComas AJ, Petito F. Physiological changes in ageing muscles. J Neurol Neurosurg Psychiatry 1973;36(2):174–82.

[94] Doherty TJ, Brown WF. The estimated numbers and relative sizes of thenar motor units as selected by multiple point stimulation in young and older adults. Muscle Nerve 1993;16(4): 355–66.

[95] Doherty TJ, Vandervoort AA, Taylor AW, et al. Effects of motor unit losses on strength in older men and women. J Appl Physiol 1993;74(2):868–74.

[96] Lexell J, Downham DY. The occurrence of fibre-type grouping in healthy human muscle: a quantitative study of cross-sections of whole vastus lateralis from men between 15 and 83 years. Acta Neuropathol 1991;81(4):377–81.

[97] de Neeling JN, Beks PJ, Bertelsmann FW, et al. Sensory thresholds in older adults: reproducibility and reference values. Muscle Nerve 1994;17(4):454–61.

[98] Lundgren-Lindquist B, Sperling L. Functional studies in 79-year-olds. II. Upper extremity function. Scand J Rehabil Med 1983;15(3):117–23.

[99] Frontera WR, Hughes VA, Lutz KJ, et al. A cross-sectional study of muscle strength and mass in 45- to 78-yr-old men and women. J Appl Physiol 1991;71(2):644–50.

[100] Johnson T. Age-related differences in isometric and dynamic strength and endurance. Phys Ther 1982;62(7):985–9.

[101] Bendall MJ, Bassey EJ, Pearson MB. Factors affecting walking speed of elderly people. Age Ageing 1989;18(5):327–32.

[102] Samson MM, Crowe A, de Vreede PL, et al. Differences in gait parameters at a preferred walking speed in healthy subjects due to age, height and body weight. Aging (Milano) 2001;13(1):16–21.

[103] Calautti C, Serrati C, Baron JC. Effects of age on brain activation during auditory-cued thumb-to-index opposition: a positron emission tomography study. Stroke 2001;32(1): 139–46.

[104] Heuninckx S, Wenderoth N, Debaere F, et al. Neural basis of aging: the penetration of cognition into action control. J Neurosci 2005;25(29):6787–96.

[105] Hutchinson S, Kobayashi M, Horkan CM, et al. Age-related differences in movement representation. Neuroimage 2002;17(4):1720–8.

[106] Mattay VS, Fera F, Tessitore A, et al. Neurophysiological correlates of age-related changes in human motor function. Neurology 2002;58(4):630–5.

[107] Ward NS, Frackowiak RS. Age-related changes in the neural correlates of motor performance. Brain 2003;126(Pt 4):873–88.

[108] McComas AJ. Oro-facial muscles: internal structure, function and ageing. Gerodontology 1998;15(1):3–14.

[109] Cohn SH, Vartsky D, Yasumura S, et al. Compartmental body composition based on total-body nitrogen, potassium, and calcium. Am J Physiol 1980;239(6):E524–30.

[110] Hasten DL, Pak-Loduca J, Obert KA, et al. Resistance exercise acutely increases MHC and mixed muscle protein synthesis rates in 78–84 and 23–32 yr olds. Am J Physiol Endocrinol Metab 2000;278(4):E620–6.

[111] Schulte JN, Yarasheski KE. Effects of resistance training on the rate of muscle protein synthesis in frail elderly people. Int J Sport Nutr Exerc Metab 2001;11(Suppl):S111–8.

[112] Yarasheski KE, Pak-Loduca J, Hasten DL, et al. Resistance exercise training increases mixed muscle protein synthesis rate in frail women and men >/=76 yr old. Am J Physiol 1999;277(1 Pt 1):E118–25.

[113] Helbostad JL, Sletvold O, Moe-Nilssen R. Effects of home exercises and group training on functional abilities in home-dwelling older persons with mobility and balance problems. A randomized study. Aging Clin Exp Res 2004;16(2):113–21.

[114] Judge JO, Lindsey C, Underwood M, et al. Balance improvements in older women: effects of exercise training. Phys Ther 1993;73(4):254–62.

[115] Takeshima N, Rogers NL, Rogers ME, et al. Functional fitness gain varies in older adults depending on exercise mode. Med Sci Sports Exerc 2007;39(11):2036–43.

[116] Taylor-Piliae RE, Haskell WL, Stotts NA, et al. Improvement in balance, strength, and flexibility after 12 weeks of Tai chi exercise in ethnic Chinese adults with cardiovascular disease risk factors. Altern Ther Health Med 2006;12(2):50–8.

[117] Toraman NF, Erman A, Agyar E. Effects of multicomponent training on functional fitness in older adults. J Aging Phys Act 2004;12(4):538–53.

[118] Bryant M. Biofeedback in the treatment of a selected dysphagic patient. Dysphagia 1991;6(3):140–4.

[119] Lewin JS, Hebert TM, Putnam JB Jr, et al. Experience with the chin tuck maneuver in post-esophagectomy aspirators Summer. Dysphagia 2001;16(3):216–9.

[120] Rasley A, Logemann JA, Kahrilas PJ, et al. Prevention of barium aspiration during video-fluoroscopic swallowing studies: value of change in posture. AJR Am J Roentgenol 1993;160(5):1005–9.

[121] Logemann JA, Rademaker AW, Pauloski BR, et al. Effects of postural change on aspiration in head and neck surgical patients. Otolaryngol Head Neck Surg 1994;110(2):222–7.

[122] Logemann JA, Kahrilas PJ. Relearning to swallow after stroke–application of maneuvers and indirect biofeedback: a case study. Neurology 1990;40(7):1136–8.

[123] Logemann JA, Gensler G, Robbins J, et al. A randomized study of three interventions for aspiration of thin liquids in patients with dementia or Parkinson's disease. J Speech Lang Hear Res 2008;51(1):173–83.

[124] Robbins JA, Gensler G, Hind JA, et al. Comparison of two interventions for liquid aspiration on pneumonia incidence: a randomized controlled trial. Annals of Internal Medicine 2008;148(7):509–18.

[125] Hind JA, Nicosia MA, Roecker EB, et al. Comparison of effortful and noneffortful swallows in healthy middle-aged and older adults. Arch Phys Med Rehabil 2001;82(12):1661–5.

[126] Easterling C, Grande B, Kern M, et al. Attaining and maintaining isometric and isokinetic goals of the Shaker exercise Spring. Dysphagia 2005;20(2):133–8.

[127] Robbins J, Gangnon RE, Theis SM, et al. The effects of lingual exercise on swallowing in older adults. J Am Geriatr Soc 2005;53(9):1483–9.

[128] Robbins J, Kays SA, Gangnon RE, et al. The effects of lingual exercise in stroke patients with dysphagia. Arch Phys Med Rehabil 2007;88(2):150–8.

[129] Shaker R, Easterling C, Kern M, et al. Rehabilitation of swallowing by exercise in tube-fed patients with pharyngeal dysphagia secondary to abnormal UES opening. Gastroenterology 2002;122(5):1314–21.

[130] Logemann JA, Pauloski BR, Colangelo L, et al. Effects of a sour bolus on oropharyngeal swallowing measures in patients with neurogenic dysphagia. J Speech Hear Res 1995;38(3):556–63.

[131] Ludlow CL, Humbert I, Saxon K, et al. Effects of surface electrical stimulation both at rest and during swallowing in chronic pharyngeal Dysphagia. Dysphagia 2007;22(1):1–10.

[132] Jenkins IH, Jahanshahi M, Jueptner M, et al. Self-initiated versus externally triggered movements. II. The effect of movement predictability on regional cerebral blood flow. Brain 2000;123(Pt 6):1216–28.

[133] Boliek CA, Rieger JM, Li SY, et al. Establishing a reliable protocol to measure tongue sensation. J Oral Rehabil 2007;34(6):433–41.

[134] Jacobs R, Wu CH, Van Loven K, et al. Methodology of oral sensory tests. J Oral Rehabil 2002;29(8):720–30.

[135] Fukunaga A, Uematsu H, Sugimoto K. Influences of aging on taste perception and oral somatic sensation. J Gerontol A Biol Sci Med Sci 2005;60(1):109–13.

[136] Kononen M, Kuikka JT, Husso-Saastamoinen M, et al. Increased perfusion in motor areas after constraint-induced movement therapy in chronic stroke: a single-photon emission computerized tomography study. J Cereb Blood Flow Metab 2005;25(12):1668–74.

ELSEVIER
SAUNDERS

Phys Med Rehabil Clin N Am
19 (2008) 867–888

PHYSICAL MEDICINE
AND REHABILITATION
CLINICS OF
NORTH AMERICA

Dysphagia in Stroke and Neurologic Disease

Marlís González-Fernández, MD, PhD[a],*, Stephanie K. Daniels, PhD[b]

[a]Department of Physical Medicine and Rehabilitation, Johns Hopkins University,
School of Medicine, 600 North Wolfe Street, Phipps 174, Baltimore, MD 21287, USA
[b]Research Service, Rehabilitation Research (153), Michael E. Debakey VA Medical Center,
Department of Physical Medicine and Rehabilitation, Baylor College of Medicine,
2002 Holcombe Boulevard, Houston, TX 77030, USA

Epidemiology

Dysphagia is common in multiple neurologic diseases (Table 1), particularly in Parkinson's disease, multiple sclerosis (MS), amyotrophic lateral sclerosis (ALS), Alzheimer's disease, and, most prominently, in stroke.

Stroke

Estimates of dysphagia incidence in stroke range between 20% and 90% depending on the method of ascertainment [1]. Conservative estimates of dysphagia incidence in stroke patients suggest that it occurs acutely in about 50% of cases [2–4]. Dysphagia has been associated with increased stroke mortality, increased hospital length of stay, dehydration, and malnutrition [5–7]. Stroke patients with dysphagia have an increased risk for aspiration pneumonia (3-fold) [3]. This risk is markedly increased (20-fold) in cases with confirmed aspiration on videofluoroscopy [8]. Aspiration without a cough (silent aspiration) increases the risk of pneumonia and occurs in up to two thirds of stroke patients [9].

Parkinson's disease

Up to 77% of Parkinson's disease patients experience dysphagia [10]. Conservative estimates report a dysphagia incidence of about 50%

* Corresponding author.
E-mail address: mgonzal5@jhmi.edu (M. González-Fernández).

1047-9651/08/$ - see front matter © 2008 Elsevier Inc. All rights reserved.
doi:10.1016/j.pmr.2008.07.001

Table 1
Neurologic disorders associated with swallowing dysfunction

Central	Peripheral
Nondegenerative	*Anterior horn cell*
Vascular	ALS
Stroke	*Neuromuscular*
Trauma	Myasthenia gravis
Traumatic brain injury	Poliomyelitis and post-polio syndrome
Neoplastic	*Peripheral neuropathy*
Brain tumors	Chronic inflammatory
Congenital	Demyelinating polyneuropathy
Cerebral palsy	(Guillain-Barré)*Muscle disorders*
Iatrogenic	*Myopathies*
Medication-induced	OPMD
Tardive dyskinesia	Myotonic dystrophy
Degenerative	*Inflammatory muscle disorders*
Progressive course	PM
Dementia	DM
Alzheimer's disease	Inclusion body myositis
Frontotemporal dementia	
Lewy body dementia	
Vascular dementia	
Movement disorders	
Parkinson's disease	
Progressive supranuclear palsy	
Olivopontocerebellar atrophy	
Huntington's disease	
Wilson's disease	
Relapsing-remitting course	
MS	

[11,12]. Solids have been reported to be more problematic than liquids in Parkinson's disease patients [13]. Parkinson's disease patients experience delayed swallowing reflex, prolonged laryngeal movements, and prolonged esophageal phase [14].

Multiple sclerosis

Dysphagia is not as common in MS. Frequency of dysphagia in MS has been estimated to be between 33% and 43% [15–18]. De Pauw and colleagues conducted a large study which reported that 29% of patients had swallowing difficulties and 24%, permanent swallowing difficulties [19]. Dysphagia in MS has also been associated with increasing disability [15,18,19], depressed mood, and low vital capacity [15]. Abnormalities observed include impaired oral phase and delayed swallow reflex [19]. Abraham and Yum reported upper esophageal sphincter (UES) dysfunction in all MS patients studied (13 cases) [20]. A 10-item questionnaire for evaluation of dysphagia in MS has recently been developed [21]. This tool allows for overall assessment of dysphagia and characterization of dysphagia to solids or liquids.

Amyotrophic lateral sclerosis

ALS can affect both bulbar and spinal motor systems. Dysphagia occurs at onset in about one third of cases, although generally it occurs late in the disease [22]. ALS severity scales include swallowing as an important factor [23]. Mayberry and Atkinson [24] reported some feeding difficulty in 73% of surveyed patients with motor neuron disease. Dysphagia was reported in 87% of patients who had died of motor neuron disease versus 68% of surviving patients [24]. Aspiration pneumonia rates of 13% have been reported and have been associated with increased mortality (mean survival time postinfection, 2 months) [25].

Alzheimer's disease

Swallowing dysfunction in Alzheimer's disease has been reported extensively, but not many studies have reported the incidence of dysphagia in this population. Horner and colleagues [26] reported that aspiration occurred in 28.6% of Alzheimer's disease patients studied using videofluoroscopy. Pneumonia is the most common cause of death in this population [27–29]. Deficits in this population range from oral dysfunction to pharyngeal dysfunction with aspiration. Oral dysfunction is important in this population because it usually leads to eating dependency; a marker for poor outcome and mortality in institutionalized individuals [30].

Muscular dystrophies

Patients with muscular dystrophy can have a variety of deficits resulting in feeding and swallowing difficulties. Approximately 35% of individuals in a group of patients with myotonic dystrophy, spinal muscular atrophy, facioscapulohumeral muscular dystrophy (FSMD), Duchenne muscular dystrophy (DMD), or limb girdle muscular dystrophy reported problems with at least 1 aspect of feeding [31].

Patients with DMD have difficulties with mouth opening and chewing that are more frequent as they age and experience choking episodes on average once a week or less frequently [32]. As a result of these problems, patients modify their diet, opting for smaller pieces and softer foods and have increasing mealtime duration [32]. In DMD, the oral phase is affected, and although the pharyngeal phase is timely, it is weak, leaving pharyngeal residue [33]. Videofluoroscopic swallow study (VFSS) has been recommended for asymptomatic DMD patients in their teens because the possibility of dysphagia increases with age [34]. Aloysius and colleagues [33] suggest that for DMD cases with choking, the VFSS is of limited usefulness when compared with a careful feeding regimen.

Oculopharyngeal muscular dystrophy (OPMD) is a disorder among adults that is characterized by bilateral ptosis and dysphagia; it is more common in French Canadians. The overall incidence of OPMD is unclear because it usually manifests itself in the sixth decade of life, and genetic testing was not available until after 1998, when Brais and colleagues [35] determined the specific abnormality in chromosome 14 that causes the disease. Dysphagia in OPMD patients is aggravated by head retroflexion (astrologist's view), a compensation for ptosis [36]. Cricopharyngeal dysfunction with aspiration is common in OPMD, and treatment with cricopharyngeal myotomy is common [37,38].

Dysphagia is not a common symptom of FSMD and was once considered an exclusion criterion [39]. Recent studies suggest that dysphagia occurs in advanced cases of FSMD, but that involvement is mild and seldom life threatening [40].

Dysphagia is considered one of the most important symptoms of myotonic dystrophy because of its relationship with recurrent pulmonary infections [41]. The prevalence of dysphagia in this population has been reported to be between 25% and 80% [42]. Swallowing dysfunction in myotonic dystrophy is associated with asymmetric pharyngeal contraction and weak UES contraction [42].

Polymyositis and dermatomyositis

Swallowing dysfunction has been reported in 12% to 54% of patients with polymyositis/dermatomyositis (PM/DM) [43] and is more common in the acute inflammatory phase [31]. The first signs of dysphagia are usually lingual weakness and incoordination [44]. Cricopharyngeal muscle obstruction and esophageal dysmotility are the main abnormalities seen in PM/DM patients, causing aspiration when food backs up into the pharynx [44]. Dysphagia is related to poor prognosis in PM/DM patients. Cricopharyngeal myotomy has been useful in treatment of dysphagia in PM/DM patients, as have corticosteroids given during the acute phase [44,45].

Swallowing physiology

Functional swallowing occurs as a result of a series of purposeful movements that allow transport of food from the oral cavity into the stomach while avoiding passage of food into the airway.

Swallowing is divided into 4 stages: (1) oral preparatory—preparation of food for propulsion to the pharynx, (2) oral propulsive—the food is pushed by the tongue through the pharynx, (3) pharyngeal—specific movements transport the bolus to the UES, and (4) esophageal—the bolus is propelled through the esophagus and lower esophageal sphincter to the stomach [46]. The oral preparatory and oral propulsive stages are under volitional control [47]. Once oral propulsion occurs, the following processes are a series of involuntary movements designed to transport the food and protect the airway. Individuals with neurologic disease can have physiologic deficits in any of the swallowing stages.

Oral preparatory stage

The duration of the oral preparatory stage depends on food type and consistency [48]. When food is placed in the mouth, the bite is pulled back, followed by rotational movements of the tongue that place the food in the occlusal surface of the postcanine teeth [49]. Mastication reduces the food to the appropriate consistency for transport.

Oral phase dysfunction can be one of the first signs of dysphagia in neurologic patients. Difficulty in moving food to the pharynx was reported by more than 50% of patients with motor neuron disease [24]. Parkinson's disease patients develop difficulty in chewing and other oral complaints [50]. Altered feeding habit was the most common complaint in patients with MS [19].

Oral propulsive stage

When food has been processed and the consistency is appropriate for swallowing, the tongue contacts the hard palate and the area of tongue–palate contact expands posteriorly. This movement squeezes the bolus into the valleculae. Food transport occurs intermittently during processing, allowing for bolus accumulation in the oropharynx before the swallow occurs.

Neurologic disorders that directly affect tongue strength and coordination are more likely to affect oral propulsion. Decreased tongue pressures have been associated with higher incidence of dysphagia [51]. Impaired oral propulsion can result in delayed or absent swallow initiation.

Pharyngeal stage

The pharyngeal phase is a series of highly coordinated events. When the bolus is ready to be swallowed, the soft palate elevates to seal the nasopharynx while the tongue base retracts and the pharyngeal wall contracts to squeeze the bolus downward. Submental muscles contract pulling the hyoid and larynx superiorly and anteriorly and folding the epiglottis backward to seal the laryngeal vestibule. The vocal folds close to seal the glottis and breathing ceases briefly to prevent food inhalation. The cricopharyngeus muscle relaxes to allow for UES opening assisted by contraction of the suprahyoid muscles and the pressure of the descending bolus.

Pharyngeal dysfunction usually occurs later in the course of degenerative neurologic diseases and is associated with increased disease severity. Identifying pharyngeal dysfunction is critical in the prevention of aspiration and subsequent pneumonia.

Esophageal stage

After the bolus passes the UES, peristalsis carries the bolus down to the stomach, assisted by gravity. The lower esophageal sphincter relaxes, allowing bolus passage into the stomach.

Esophageal dysfunction is common is Parkinson's disease. Abnormalities include delayed transport, stasis, bolus redirection, and tertiary esophageal contractions [52].

Differences between eating and drinking

During drinking, the oral stage is modified to prevent premature spillage of liquids into the oropharynx. Before swallow initiation, the dorsal tongue is in contact with the soft palate, creating a posterior oral seal [53]. Even in normal individuals, this seal is often incomplete, allowing some liquid to enter the oropharynx. A posterior oral seal is not present in continuous sequential drinking (as in straw drinking), and the liquid usually is at or below the level of the valleculae at swallow onset [54]. Straws may increase the risk of aspiration in patients with an already compromised system due to neurologic disease. It would be a sensible approach to avoid their use in this population unless their safety has been confirmed during instrumental evaluation.

Neural control of swallowing function

Brain stem

The main center for swallowing control is located in the brain stem. The central pattern generator (CPG) is located in the rostral medulla within the nucleus tractus solitarius and the surrounding reticular formation [55,56]. The CPG controls 2 main functions: (1) the triggering and timing of the swallowing pattern and (2) the control of motor neurons involved in swallowing [55]. Sensory information to the CPG has been implicated in swallow response modulation and airway protection [1,55,57–59].

Disruption of the CPG results in severe dysphagia. This is most commonly seen in cases of lateral medullary strokes. It has been suggested that in lateral medullary strokes, swallowing function is globally affected because of an acute disconnection syndrome with the contralateral CPG [60].

ALS can cause swallowing dysfunction (bulbar ALS) but most commonly dysphagia develops several months after the onset of the disease [61]. Dysphagia in ALS cases is associated with abnormal UES opening, decreased coordination between the laryngeal elevator muscles and the cricopharyngeal sphincter, and a delayed swallow all related to bulbar dysfunction, and progressive corticobulbar degeneration [61].

Supramedullary control

Several supratentorial structures have been implicated in swallowing control, most prominently the cerebral cortex. The primary motor, motor supplementary, and primary somatosensory cortices (Brodmann areas [BA] 1, 2, 3, 4, and 6) have been implicated in swallowing motor regulation and execution, and sensorimotor control [62–65]. Other cortical areas have been implicated in swallowing, including the anterior cingulate (BA 24 and 32) [63–66], orbitofrontal cortex (BA 10, 11, 12, 44, 45, and 47) [67], parieto-occipital cortex (BA 7, 17, 18, and 40) [62,63,68,69], temporopolar cortex (BA 22 and 38) [67], and insular cortex [67,70–72].

Subcortical structures including the internal capsule [67,72,73], thalamus [9,62,67], basal ganglia [9,62,67], and cerebral peduncles [58] have also been implicated in swallowing control.

Even though the areas previously mentioned have been repeatedly implicated in swallowing control, a comprehensive model integrating the function of supratentorial and bulbar structures has not been described. Future research is necessary to determine how all of these areas integrate to produce functional swallowing.

Dysphagia related to dysfunction of supratentorial structures is the most common type seen in neurologic disease. Dysphagia related to nondegenerative diseases, such as stroke or traumatic brain injury, tends to remain stable or improve with time [7,74]. In degenerative diseases, dysphagia tends to worsen with time as global brain function deteriorates, interrupting the coordination of the multiple areas involved in swallowing control.

The evaluation of dysphagia in neurogenic disease

Cognitive and communication assessment

In patients with neurogenic disease, before evaluation of swallowing function, it is wise to screen cognitive and communication functioning (Table 2).

Table 2
Cognitive and neurologic screening elements for the dysphagic patient

- Level of consciousness
- Attention
  Focus/concentration
  Neglect
    Sensory neglect (inattention)
    Motor neglect (intention)
    Spatial neglect
    Awareness of deficits
- Memory
- Communication
  Auditory comprehension
  Verbal expression
  Motor speech
    Dysarthria
    Apraxia of speech
  Voice

This information will not only affect completion of the clinical swallowing evaluation (CSE) but will also impact the instrumental swallowing evaluation and subsequent treatment. Given the importance of supratentorial modulation of pharyngeal biomechanics, preoral phase deficits, such as decreased attention, may have substantial consequences for oral and pharyngeal swallowing efficiency [75]. The level to which a patient's cognition and communication are impaired depends on the location and extent of neural damage. A patient with right hemisphere damage or involvement of the parietal or prefrontal lobes is more likely to present with cognitive impairment as compared with the patient with occipital lobe damage. Likewise, a patient with left hemisphere damage is more likely to have aphasia than a person with right hemisphere damage.

Recent research has supported the notion that neglect is associated with dysphagia. Neglect is defined as failure to respond or orient to stimuli presented to the contralesional side in the presence of intact elemental sensory and motor functioning [76]. Neglect may be spatial or personal and is evidenced by sensory inattention, motor intention, spatial neglect, and/or unawareness of deficits. Parker and colleagues [77] reported that fewer than half of acute stroke patients were aware of their dysphagia symptoms (eg, coughing, drooling). Most of the patients who were diagnosed with dysphagia and were aware of symptoms did not acknowledge having a "swallowing problem." Patients with poor awareness of their dysphagic symptoms did not modify swallowing behavior, whereas patients who were aware of their dysphagia modified rate and volume of ingestion. Moreover, patients with poor awareness developed more medical complications at 3 months post-onset as compared with the group with good awareness of dysphagia symptoms. Spatial neglect has been associated with initial non-oral intake in acute stroke patients [78], and rehabilitation of dysphagia is longer in patients with neglect [79].

The clinical bedside swallowing evaluation

In patients with complaints of dysphagia or those patients with neurogenic disorders associated with a high frequency of dysphagia, a clinical bedside swallowing evaluation (CSE) should be completed. From the CSE, one can determine which patients warrant an instrumental examination, develop a hypothesis of the underlying swallowing pathophysiology, and develop plans concerning a management program. The CSE generally includes an examination of oral structural integrity, cranial nerve function, and swallowing.

Notation is made of the appearance of oral mucosa in terms of salivation and color. Pooling of saliva in the oral cavity generally does not indicate hypersalivation in patients with neurogenic disease; rather, it may indicate dysphagia. Dentition should be evaluated in terms of the number and appearance of the teeth, and the presence or absence of a dental prosthesis. Poor dental care in combination with decreased mobility, sensation, and awareness of dysphagia may increase the risk of pneumonia in stroke patients. Dental decay and dependence for oral care are significant contributors to the development of aspiration pneumonia [80].

A thorough cranial nerve examination will allow inference of potential swallowing pathophysiology. Evaluation of motor and sensory integrity of the face, lips, tongue, and palate will allow the examiner to link clinical observations of cranial nerve impairment with suspected oropharyngeal pathophysiology and thereby increase sensitivity for detecting dysphagia on the CSE [81].

The swallowing portion of the CSE includes administration of various consistencies (liquids, semi-solids, solids) and volumes over multiple trials. It is generally best to start the examination with small volumes of thin liquids to reduce the amount of aspiration, should it occur, and to prevent contaminating the pharynx with residue from a thicker consistency. In some patients, particularly those who have been without oral intake for a period of time or those with significant cognitive deficits, it may be wise to start by having the patient chew and swallow ice chips to "prime" the swallowing system and direct the patient's attention to the swallowing task.

From the CSE, particular features have been identified to determine which stroke patients are at risk for aspiration and warrant an instrumental examination. This is important, particularly after an acute stroke, as all patients may not warrant an instrumental examination. However, it should be noted that much of this focus is directed to identification of patients with risk of aspiration, not with risk of dysphagia. Many patients with neurologic disease may present with dysphagia without aspiration. Early studies relied on the presence of a cough or voice change after ingestion of 3 oz of water [82] to determine aspiration. Poor sensitivity, however, has decreased the usefulness of an isolated water swallow test, as the risk of false-negative results is high [83].

A cluster of symptoms and signs of aspiration in addition to coughing or voice change after swallowing have been evaluated in acute stroke patients to increase the ability to detect silent aspiration in acute stroke. Six clinical features (dysphonia, dysarthria, abnormal volitional cough, abnormal gag reflex, cough on trial swallow, and voice change on trial swallow) were associated with risk of aspiration (residual material in the larynx or aspiration) as identified using videofluoroscopy [9]. The presence of any 2 of these 6 clinical features correctly identified risk of aspiration with 92% accuracy [84]. Studies by other investigators have confirmed the usefulness of these 6 clinical features in the identification of risk of aspiration in acute stroke patients but have suggested that the presence of 4 clinical predictors increases specificity [84,85]. Others have indicated that the presence of 2 of these 6 features identified by Daniels and colleagues [84]. was not strongly related to aspiration as identified by endoscopic evaluation [86]. Contradictory findings may be related to different outcome measures, evaluation type, and evaluation protocol. Overall, research suggests that clinicians can rule in aspiration when it is truly present but that ruling out aspiration when it is absent is difficult to do [87].

Dysarthria may correlate with dysphagia in individuals with bulbar ALS. Individuals with ALS may not complain of dysphagia but may evidence reduced speech intelligibility. Progression of dysphagia parallels the progression of speech intelligibility in ALS [88]. Furthermore, dysphagia increases as respiratory capacity decreases regardless of the form of ALS [88]. As such, vital capacity should be consistently measured. Accurate and timely assessment of a clinically relevant decline in respiratory status seems crucial for determining the timing of feeding tube placement.

Instrumentation, such as pulse oximetry and cervical auscultation, has been added to the CSE to increase sensitivity and specificity. With pulse oximetry, oxygen saturation is measured before, during, and after swallowing, with decrease in saturation during and after swallowing purported to be associated with aspiration. Contradictory findings; however, have been reported, with some studies indicating a strong correlation between desaturation and aspiration [89,90], whereas others have shown poor association [91,92]. Such discrepancies may be attributed to the desaturation criteria and to the lack of an instrumental evaluation to confirm aspiration. Cervical auscultation is used to amplify either swallowing sounds or airway sounds during direct oral intake. Generally, a simple stethoscope is used, but a microphone [93] or accelerometer [94] may be added for improved fidelity and signal recording. Recent research identified reduced reliability among raters, which in turn yielded reduced ability to distinguish between stroke patients with and without aspiration [95,96]. Until reliability is established for cervical auscultation and pulse oximetry, neither adjunct can be assumed to provide additional value to the CSE.

Instrumental evaluation

The purpose of an instrumental swallowing study is to evaluate physiologic functioning of the oropharyngeal swallowing mechanism, determine swallowing safety, and identify the effects of compensatory strategies, such as posture and bolus consistency, on deglutition. By determining the exact cause of dysfunction, therapeutic intervention can be initiated to address the specific disorder. The 2 primary instrumental tools used to evaluate oropharyngeal dysphagia are VFSS and videoendoscopy. The advantages and disadvantages of each are listed in Table 3. As neurogenic dysphagia can impair all 3 stages of swallowing, VFSS is the preferred instrumental assessment tool for the neurogenic population. However, medical diagnosis and results from the cognitive evaluation and CSE may dictate which examination is done. For example, videoendoscopy may be useful in the evaluation of swallowing in patients with specific diagnoses, such as myasthenia gravis, in which dysphagia occurs with fatigue, or in patients with contractures, for whom positioning during the VFSS is suboptimal.

Table 3
Advantages and disadvantages for each instrumental assessment

Tool	Advantages	Disadvantages
Videofluoroscopy (VFSS)	Direct assessment of oral, pharyngeal, and esophageal stages Evaluate bolus flow, temporal and spatial structural measurements Determine the effects of compensatory strategies Direct assessment of UES opening and closing	Radiation exposure limits the length of the examination Difficulty with patient positioning, especially patients with hemiplegia or contractures Non-natural environment may exacerbate cognitive problems Use of barium as opposed to real food
Videoendoscopy (FEES)	Completed at bedside Use of real food No time constraints No radiation exposure Direct visualization of the larynx Evaluation of secretions	No visualization of the oral stage No visualization of the actual swallow due to "whiteout"; thus, details of oral and pharyngeal motility must be inferred. No ability to assess esophageal functioning Limited to no ability to evaluate bolus flow and analyze structural movement

Swallowing of liquids, semi-solids, and solids should be evaluated during the CSE. It is wise to start the evaluation with small, calibrated volumes of liquid and progress to larger volumes if possible. In addition to single swallows, sequential swallowing should be tested in patients who can safely ingest larger liquid volumes (eg, 10–20 mL). If aspiration is observed, the examination is not stopped. Rather, the clinician attempts to identify underlying pathophysiology and apply compensatory strategies. By applying the appropriate compensatory strategy during the instrumental examination, objective documentation can be made as to whether or not the therapeutic technique was successful in maintaining a safe and efficient swallow. The compensatory strategy can then be recommended during consumption of the specific consistency on which dysphagia was identified.

Treatment of dysphagia in neurologic disease

Behavioral

Treatment really begins during the evaluation. In the instrumental evaluation, specific compensatory strategies are confirmed as successful or not, and rehabilitative exercises are decided based on the identified pathophysiology. Before determining the appropriate swallowing treatment, it is important to understand the disease process as well as a patient's cognitive, motor, and sensory abilities, as any or all of these can affect swallowing recovery. For example, use of a chin tuck posture and thickened liquids may both decrease the risk of aspiration of liquids for a delayed pharyngeal swallow. However, in patients with reduced awareness of deficits and/or reduced attention and memory, thickened liquids may be more appropriate, as the individual may not remember to implement or cannot maintain a chin tuck posture without strict supervision.

Swallowing therapy may be thought of as compensatory, rehabilitative, or both. Compensatory strategies result in immediate benefit; however, the effects are not permanent. That is, once the strategy is removed, swallowing is no longer safe and efficient. Implementation of these strategies is intended to maintain some form of oral intake for the patient, and their benefit should be confirmed during the instrumental examination. However, rehabilitative strategies aim to positively alter swallowing physiology over time, resulting in permanent improvement in deglutitive function. Classification of treatment into 1 of these 2 categories is not always straightforward. Depending on how specific therapies are implemented, some can be considered as both compensatory and rehabilitative (Fig. 1). For example, the Mendelsohn maneuver may be compensatory if a patient uses this technique during mealtime to improve bolus transfer through the UES. Yet, repeated practice of this technique outside of mealtime may result in long-term improved UES opening and bolus clearance. Certain treatments have been studied in specific neurogenic populations, such as the Lee Silverman Voice Treatment in patients with Parkinson's disease [97] and thermal tactile stimulation in patients after stroke [98–101]. Further research is needed to confirm immediate and long-term effects of these specific strategies for the various neurologic diseases that are associated with dysphagia. The reader is referred to the article by Logemann in this issue for discussion on behavioral swallowing treatment.

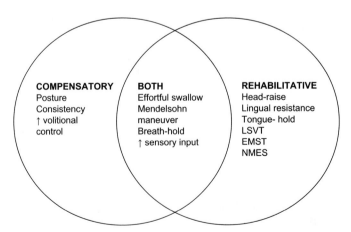

Fig. 1. Behavioral treatment approaches to dysphagia. ↑, Increase; LSVT, Lee Silverman Voice Treatment; EMST, expiratory muscle strength training; NMES, neuromuscular electrical stimulation.

Studies of the effects of behavioral treatment on dysphagia were generally limited to case studies or small case series. Over the last decade, larger studies and clinical trials have been completed. A recent study revealed that that the proportion of surviving stroke patients who returned to a normal diet at 6 months was greater for individuals who underwent high-intensity treatment (rehabilitative treatment) as compared with those who underwent low-intensity treatment (compensatory therapy), which, in turn, was greater than in patients who underwent usual care (physician recommendations) [102]. Return to functional swallowing was significantly greater in the active treatment groups, and chest infection and complications related to dysphagia were significantly less in these 2 treatment groups compared with the control group. Although not as rigorous as the randomized controlled clinical trial from Carnaby and colleagues [102], other studies over the past 15 years have provided evidence of benefits from behavioral swallowing intervention in patients with nonprogressive neurologic disease [79,103,104].

Most patients with dysphagia due to neurogenic disease warrant an attempt at aggressive rehabilitation. However, some individuals may not be candidates for rehabilitative treatment because of diagnosis, prognosis, and/or cognitive status. For example, a person in the late stage of Parkinson's disease will probably not benefit from active treatment but may benefit from compensatory strategies. However, a person in the early stages of the disease would benefit from rehabilitative swallowing treatment. Many individuals with neurogenic dysphagia are elderly and frail and will probably require treatment for a longer period of time to obtain the precision and endurance to complete a specified treatment regime.

Medical

Randomized, controlled clinical trials have not been conducted to determine the effectiveness of medical or surgical interventions on the rehabilitation of patients having neurogenic dysphagia.

Medical treatments for specific neurologic disease may facilitate swallowing. Some studies suggest that antiparkinsonism medication (levodopa, apomorphine) may improve swallowing in some patients [105,106], whereas others have found little consistent improvement in swallowing with these medications [107,108]. For patients with myasthenia gravis, cholinesterase inhibitors (eg, pyridostigmine, thymectomy, corticosteroids, plasmapheresis, and immunosuppressant medications) may improve symptoms, including dysphagia, but no empiric study of swallowing has been completed. It is suggested that the use of Mestinon in individuals with myasthenia gravis and dysphagia be timed with meals to provide optimal muscular strength [109].

Specific medical intervention has been proposed to target specific physiologic problems. Botulinum toxin type A (Botox) has been used in treating dysphagia due to UES dysfunction. Studies generally report improved swallowing on the instrumental examination and/or by patient report [110–112], with benefit lasting from 1 to 14 months postinjection [112]. However, these studies are typically retrospective, completed in heterogeneous populations, without use of a placebo control. Botox injection into the salivary glands (parotid, submandibular) has also been used to treat sialorrhea in neurogenic patients, including those with Parkinson's disease and ALS [113–116]. Subjective reductions in drooling were identified in patients receiving Botox, whereas the placebo group in both studies reported no change. It should be reiterated that in most patients with neurogenic disease, reduced saliva control is not related to increased production; rather, it is due to impaired ability to swallow the saliva.

Dilation, either pneumatic or through bougienage, may also be used to treat cricopharyngeal dysfunction; however, no study has specifically focused on this procedure in a group of patients having neurogenic dysphagia. Symptomatic response to cricopharyngeal disruption with either dilation or myotomy was studied in a heterogeneous group of subjects [117]. Results suggested that 58% of subjects who underwent dilation had a subjective improvement in swallowing.

Surgical

Cricopharyngeal myotomy is the most common surgery performed to alleviate oropharyngeal dysphagia [118]; however, evidence supporting its use for neurogenic dysphagia is limited. Although no controlled clinical trial has been completed to evaluate the effectiveness of cricopharyngeal myotomy for neurogenic dysphagia, such a trial has been completed after surgery for head and neck cancer, with results revealing no significant difference in swallowing between patients undergoing a myotomy and those who did not [118,119]. The exact nature of UES dysfunction must be understood before proceeding with a myotomy in patients with neurogenic dysphagia. Generally with neurogenic dysphagia, decreased anterior hyolaryngeal traction to open the UES is the etiology, rather than failure of the muscle to relax [46]. In this case, myotomy would not improve dysphagia. Patients with dysphagia due to muscular disease (eg, OPMD) may benefit from myotomy, as the pharyngeal propulsive force is minimal, and the UES acts as a barrier for bolus transfer into the esophagus [120]. VFSS and manometric evaluation of the UES should facilitate identification of patients who will respond favorably to myotomy. It has been suggested that in patients with nonprogressive diseases, such as stroke, a myotomy should not be completed until 6 months postinjury, as most patients recover function within that time frame [46].

Vocal fold medialization is the procedure generally performed to treat aspiration due to an incompetent larynx. If recovery of function is anticipated (eg, after stroke), augmentation of the vocal folds with an absorbable material, such as collagen or fat, is recommended [121]. In a recent study of a heterogeneous population, including poststroke patients, who underwent VFSS pre- and post-vocal fold medialization, the incidence of airway invasion did not significantly decrease after surgery [122].

A tracheostomy may be performed for neurologic patients with chronic aspiration. Although it will not improve swallowing and not completely eliminate aspiration, it will facilitate pulmonary toileting. Tracheostomy should be considered only on the most severe patients.

Oral versus non-oral feeding in neurologic dysphagia

As mentioned previously, a careful clinical evaluation is the first step in determining if oral feeding is safe for a particular individual (Fig. 2). When the clinical evaluation raises concerns of dysphagia, it should be followed by an instrumental examination to determine pathophysiology of the deglutitive disorder. If dysphagia and aspiration are identified, strategies such as diet modification, compensatory maneuvers, or postural changes are attempted to improve swallowing safety and efficiency. If the interventions are successful, oral feeding can continue with concomitant swallowing rehabilitation. Repeated instrumental examination should be performed to assess response to treatment and to determine if and when compensatory conditions can be discontinued.

When compensatory maneuvers, postural changes, and diet modifications are ineffective, it is important to examine the history of the underlying

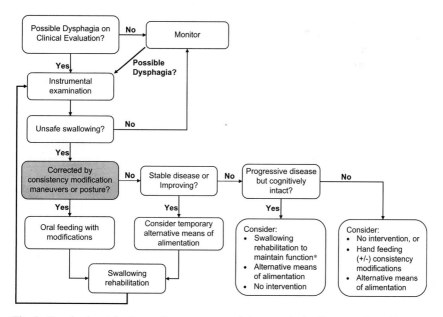

Fig. 2. Dysphagia evaluation and management of the neurologic disease patient. *Exercise might be contraindicated in certain diseases, such as amyotrophic lateral sclerosis.

neurologic disease. As an example, it is well known that dysphagia occurs in up to 90% of stroke patients [1] but that the recovery potential is high, with persistent dysphagia being present in only 11% to 13% of patients after 6 months [74,123]. For stroke patients in whom maneuvers, diet, or postural modifications fail to correct an unsafe swallow, temporary non-oral means of alimentation should be considered. The use of nasogastric (NG) tubes is sensible, because about half of dysphagic stroke patients will recover swallowing function within 7 days [74,123]. Attempts have been made to determine if there is a difference in mortality rate when using percutaneous endoscopic gastrostomy (PEG) versus NG tubes [124]. No statistically significant increase in mortality was found when PEG tubes were used, but an increased risk of 7.8% was found for the combined measure of death and poor outcome (defined as a modified Rankin score of 4–5). Gastrostomy placement should be considered when a long recovery time is expected, such as in cases of lateral medullary stroke (Wallenberg syndrome).

Evaluating cognitive status is critical to determine appropriate interventions for individuals with progressive disease. In cognitively intact individuals, such as those with ALS, patient involvement in the decision-making process is critical. Practice guidelines for ALS recommend placement of a gastrostomy tube early in the disease and before the vital capacity is below 50% [125]. Swallowing rehabilitation might be useful to maintain function or to slow progression of dysphagia. It is not recommended in all progressive neurologic diseases, such as ALS or myasthenia gravis, as active rehabilitation leads to fatigue.

The management of the cognitively impaired individual presents some challenges. When compensatory techniques fail to attain safe swallowing, the use of alternative means of alimentation, particularly PEG tubes, is controversial. A meta-analysis published by Finucane and colleagues [126] failed to identify any studies suggesting that PEG tubes improved survival, functional status, or patient comfort, or reduced infections, aspiration pneumonia, malnutrition, and incidence of pressure ulcers. Multiple reports suggest that demented patients managed with careful hand-feeding have no difference in survival when compared with individuals without dementia [127–130]. In the cognitive-impaired population, there is no evidence to suggest that alternative means of alimentation improve outcomes. In other progressive diseases associated with cognitive deterioration, the evidence as to the use of alternative means of alimentation is scarce. In those cases, decisions should be made by a multidisciplinary team taking into account patient and family wishes.

Summary

Dysphagia is very common in neurologic disease. Appropriate management needs to consider clinical findings, response to compensatory maneuvers, and the presence of deficits amenable to rehabilitation in the context of the underlying diseaseand its natural progression.

Acknowledgments

This work was supported, in part, by the National Institutes of Health (NICHD) award 5-T32-HD-007,414-13 (MGF) and the Department of Veterans Affairs, Rehabilitation Research and Development career development grant B4262K (SKD).

References

[1] Miller RM, Chang MW. Advances in the management of dysphagia caused by stroke. Phys Med Rehabil Clin N Am 1999;10:925–41.

[2] Groher ME, Bukatman R. The prevalence of swallow disorders in two teaching hospitals. Dysphagia 1986;1:3–6.

[3] Martino R, Foley N, Bhogal S, et al. Dysphagia after stroke: incidence, diagnosis, and pulmonary complications. Stroke 2005;36:2756–63.

[4] Paciaroni M, Mazzotta G, Corea F, et al. Dysphagia following stroke. Eur Neurol 2004;51: 162–7.

[5] Axelsson K, Asplund K, Norberg A, et al. Eating problems and nutritional status during hospital stay of patients with severe stroke. J Am Diet Assoc 1989;89:1092–6.

[6] Gordon C, Hewer RL, Wade DT. Dysphagia in acute stroke. Br Med J (Clin Res Ed) 1987; 295:411–4.

[7] Kidd D, Lawson J, Nesbitt R, et al. The natural history and clinical consequences of aspiration in acute stroke. QJM 1995;88:409–13.

[8] Teasell RW, McRae M, Marchuk Y, et al. Pneumonia associated with aspiration following stroke. Arch Phys Med Rehabil 1996;77:707–9.

[9] Daniels SK, Brailey K, Priestly DH, et al. Aspiration in patients with acute stroke. Arch Phys Med Rehabil 1998;79:14–9.

[10] Edwards LL, Quigley EM, Harned RK, et al. Characterization of swallowing and defecation in Parkinson's disease. Am J Gastroenterol 1994;89:15–25.

[11] Edwards LL, Pfeiffer RF, Quigley EM, et al. Gastrointestinal symptoms in Parkinson's disease. Mov Disord 1991;6:151–6.

[12] Eadie MJ, Tyrer JH. Alimentary disorder in parkinsonism. Australas Ann Med 1965;14: 13–22.

[13] Edwards LL, Quigley EM, Pfeiffer RF. Gastrointestinal dysfunction in Parkinson's disease: frequency and pathophysiology. Neurology 1992;42:726–32.

[14] Potulska A, Friedman A, Krolicki L, et al. Swallowing disorders in Parkinson's disease. Parkinsonism Relat Disord 2003;9:349–53.

[15] Thomas FJ, Wiles CM. Dysphagia and nutritional status in multiple sclerosis. J Neurol 1999;246:677–82.

[16] Merson RM, Rolnick MI. Speech-language pathology and dysphagia in multiple sclerosis. Phys Med Rehabil Clin N Am 1998;9:631–41.

[17] Hartelius L, Svensson P. Speech and swallowing symptoms associated with Parkinson's disease and multiple sclerosis: a survey. Folia Phoniatr Logop 1994;46:9–17.

[18] Calcagno P, Ruoppolo G, Grasso MG, et al. Dysphagia in multiple sclerosis—prevalence and prognostic factors. Acta Neurol Scand 2002;105:40–3.

[19] De Pauw A, Dejaeger E, D'hooghe B, et al. Dysphagia in multiple sclerosis. Clin Neurol Neurosurg 2002;104:345–51.

[20] Abraham SS, Yun PT. Laryngopharyngeal dysmotility in multiple sclerosis. Dysphagia 2002;17:69–74.

[21] Bergamaschi R, Crivelli P, Rezzani C, et al. The DYMUS questionnaire for the assessment of dysphagia in multiple sclerosis. J Neurol Sci 2008;269(1–2):49–53.

[22] Higo R, Tayama N, Nito T. Longitudinal analysis of progression of dysphagia in amyotrophic lateral sclerosis. Auris Nasus Larynx 2004;31:247–54.

[23] Hillel AD, Miller RM, Yorkston K, et al. Amyotrophic lateral sclerosis severity scale. Neuroepidemiology 1989;8:142–50.

[24] Mayberry JF, Atkinson M. Swallowing problems in patients with motor neuron disease. J Clin Gastroenterol 1986;8:233–4.

[25] Sorenson EJ, Crum B, Stevens JC. Incidence of aspiration pneumonia in ALS in Olmsted county, MN. Amyotroph Lateral Scler 2007;8:87–9.

[26] Horner J, Alberts MJ, Dawson DV, et al. Swallowing in Alzheimer's disease. Alzheimer Dis Assoc Disord 1994;8:177–89.

[27] Beard CM, Kokmen E, Sigler C, et al. Cause of death in Alzheimer's disease. Ann Epidemiol 1996;6:195–200.

[28] Burns A, Jacoby R, Luthert P, et al. Cause of death in Alzheimer's disease. Age Ageing 1990;19:341–4.

[29] Molsa PK, Marttila RJ, Rinne UK. Survival and cause of death in Alzheimer's disease and multi-infarct dementia. Acta Neurol Scand 1986;74:103–7.

[30] Siebens H, Trupe E, Siebens A, et al. Correlates and consequences of eating dependency in institutionalized elderly. J Am Geriatr Soc 1986;34:192–8.

[31] Willig TN, Paulus J, Lacau Saint Guily J, et al. Swallowing problems in neuromuscular disorders. Arch Phys Med Rehabil 1994;75:1175–81.

[32] Pane M, Vasta I, Messina S, et al. Feeding problems and weight gain in Duchenne muscular dystrophy. Eur J Paediatr Neurol 2006;10:231–6.

[33] Aloysius A, Born P, Kinali M, et al. Swallowing difficulties in Duchenne muscular dystrophy: indications for feeding assessment and outcome of videofluroscopic swallow studies. Eur J Paediatr Neurol 2008;12:239–45.

[34] Hanayama K, Liu M, Higuchi Y, et al. Dysphagia in patients with Duchenne muscular dystrophy evaluated with a questionnaire and videofluorography. Disabil Rehabil 2008;30:517–22.

[35] Brais B, Bouchard JP, Xie YG, et al. Short GCG expansions in the PABP2 gene cause oculopharyngeal muscular dystrophy. Nat Genet 1998;18:164–7.

[36] de Swart BJ, van der Sluijs BM, Vos AM, et al. Ptosis aggravates dysphagia in oculopharyngeal muscular dystrophy. J Neurol Neurosurg Psychiatry 2006;77:266–8.

[37] Dobrowski JM, Zajtchuk JT, LaPiana FG, et al. Oculopharyngeal muscular dystrophy: clinical and histopathologic correlations. Otolaryngol Head Neck Surg 1986;95:131–42.

[38] Brais B, Rouleau GA, Bouchard JP, et al. Oculopharyngeal muscular dystrophy. Semin Neurol 1999;19:59–66.

[39] Padberg GW, Lunt PW, Koch M, et al. Fascioscapulohumeral muscular dystrophy. In: Emery AEH, editor. Diagnostic criteria for neuromuscular disorders. Netherlands: European Neuromuscular Center; 1997. p. 9–15.

[40] Wohlgemuth M, de Swart BJ, Kalf JG, et al. Dysphagia in facioscapulohumeral muscular dystrophy. Neurology 2006;66:1926–8.

[41] Garrett JM, DuBose TD Jr, Jackson JE, et al. Esophageal and pulmonary disturbances in myotonia dystrophica. Arch Intern Med 1969;123:26–32.

[42] Bellini M, Biagi S, Stasi C, et al. Gastrointestinal manifestations in myotonic muscular dystrophy. World J Gastroenterol 2006;12:1821–8.

[43] Ertekin C, Secil Y, Yuceyar N, et al. Oropharyngeal dysphagia in polymyositis/dermatomyositis. Clin Neurol Neurosurg 2004;107:32–7.

[44] Sonies BC. Evaluation and treatment of speech and swallowing disorders associated with myopathies. Curr Opin Rheumatol 1997;9:486–95.

[45] Shapiro J, Martin S, DeGirolami U, et al. Inflammatory myopathy causing pharyngeal dysphagia: a new entity. Ann Otol Rhinol Laryngol 1996;105:331–5.

[46] Logemann JA. Evaluation and treatment of swallowing disorders. 2nd edition. Austin (TX): Pro-Ed; 1998.

[47] Palmer JB, Hiiemae KM, Matsuo K, et al. Volitional control of food transport and bolus formation during feeding. Physiol Behav 2007;91:66–70.

[48] Hiiemae KM, Palmer JB. Food transport and bolus formation during complete feeding sequences on foods of different initial consistency. Dysphagia 1999;14:31–42.

[49] Hiiemae KM, Palmer JB. Tongue movements in feeding and speech. Crit Rev Oral Biol Med 2003;14:413–29.

[50] Nakayama Y, Washio M, Mori M. Oral health conditions in patients with Parkinson's disease. J Epidemiol 2004;14:143–50.

[51] Yoshida M, Kikutani T, Tsuga K, et al. Decreased tongue pressure reflects symptom of dysphagia. Dysphagia 2006;21:61–5.

[52] Leopold NA, Kagel MC. Pharyngo-esophageal dysphagia in Parkinson's disease. Dysphagia 1997;12:11–8.

[53] Kahrilas PJ, Lin S, Logemann JA, et al. Deglutitive tongue action: volume accommodation and bolus propulsion. Gastroenterology 1993;104:152–62.

[54] Daniels SK, Foundas AL. Swallowing physiology of sequential straw drinking. Dysphagia 2001;16:176–82.

[55] Jean A. Brain stem control of swallowing: neuronal network and cellular mechanisms. Physiol Rev 2001;81:929–69.

[56] Broussard DL, Altschuler SM. Brainstem viscerotopic organization of afferents and efferents involved in the control of swallowing. Am J Med 2000;108(Suppl 4a):79S–86S.

[57] Ertekin C, Kiylioglu N, Tarlaci S, et al. Voluntary and reflex influences on the initiation of swallowing reflex in man. Dysphagia 2001;16:40–7.

[58] Miller AJ. Deglutition. Physiol Rev 1982;62:129–84.

[59] Miller AJ. Characteristics of the swallowing reflex induced by peripheral nerve and brain stem stimulation. Exp Neurol 1972;34:210–22.

[60] Aydogdu I, Ertekin C, Tarlaci S, et al. Dysphagia in lateral medullary infarction (Wallenberg's syndrome): an acute disconnection syndrome in premotor neurons related to swallowing activity? Stroke 2001;32:2081–7.

[61] Ertekin C, Aydogdu I, Yuceyar N, et al. Pathophysiological mechanisms of oropharyngeal dysphagia in amyotrophic lateral sclerosis. Brain 2000;123(Pt 1):125–40.

[62] Mosier K, Bereznaya I. Parallel cortical networks for volitional control of swallowing in humans. Exp Brain Res 2001;140:280–9.

[63] Hamdy S, Mikulis DJ, Crawley A, et al. Cortical activation during human volitional swallowing: an event-related fMRI study. Am J Physiol 1999;277:G219–25.

[64] Hamdy S, Rothwell JC, Brooks DJ, et al. Identification of the cerebral loci processing human swallowing with $H_2(15)O$ PET activation. J Neurophysiol 1999;81:1917–26.

[65] Martin RE, Goodyear BG, Gati JS, et al. Cerebral cortical representation of automatic and volitional swallowing in humans. J Neurophysiol 2001;85:938–50.

[66] Martin RE, MacIntosh BJ, Smith RC, et al. Cerebral areas processing swallowing and tongue movement are overlapping but distinct: a functional magnetic resonance imaging study. J Neurophysiol 2004;92:2428–43.

[67] Mosier KM, Liu WC, Maldjian JA, et al. Lateralization of cortical function in swallowing: a functional MR imaging study. AJNR Am J Neuroradiol 1999;20:1520–6.

[68] Kern M, Birn R, Jaradeh S, et al. Swallow-related cerebral cortical activity maps are not specific to deglutition. Am J Physiol Gastrointest Liver Physiol 2001;280:G531–8.

[69] Toogood JA, Barr AM, Stevens TK, et al. Discrete functional contributions of cerebral cortical foci in voluntary swallowing: a functional magnetic resonance imaging (fMRI) "go, no-go" study. Exp Brain Res 2005;161:81–90.

[70] Daniels SK, Corey DM, Fraychinaud A, et al. Swallowing lateralization: the effects of modified dual-task interference. Dysphagia 2006;21:21–7.

[71] Daniels SK, Foundas AL. The role of the insular cortex in dysphagia. Dysphagia 1997;12:146–56.

[72] Mosier K, Patel R, Liu WC, et al. Cortical representation of swallowing in normal adults: functional implications. Laryngoscope 1999;109:1417–23.

[73] Gonzalez-Fernandez M, Kleinman JT, Ky PKS, et al. Supratentorial regions of ischemia associated with clinically important swallowing disorders: a pilot study. Stroke 2008 [ePub ahead of print].

[74] Smithard DG, O'Neill PA, England RE, et al. The natural history of dysphagia following a stroke. Dysphagia 1997;12:188–93.

[75] Leopold NA, Kagel MC. Dysphagia—ingestion or deglutition?: a proposed paradigm. Dysphagia 1997;12:202–6.

[76] Heilman KM, Watson RT, Valenstein E. Neglect and related disorders. In: Heilman KM, Valenstein E, editors. Clinical neuropsychology. 4th edition. New York: Oxford University Press; 2003. p. 296–346.

[77] Parker C, Power M, Hamdy S, et al. Awareness of dysphagia by patients following stroke predicts swallowing performance. Dysphagia 2004;19:28–35.

[78] Schroeder MF, Daniels SK, McClain M, et al. Clinical and cognitive predictors of swallowing recovery in stroke. J Rehabil Res Dev 2006;43:301–10.

[79] Neumann S. Swallowing therapy with neurologic patients: results of direct and indirect therapy methods in 66 patients suffering from neurological disorders. Dysphagia 1993;8: 150–3.

[80] Langmore SE, Terpenning MS, Schork A, et al. Predictors of aspiration pneumonia: how important is dysphagia? Dysphagia 1998;13:69–81.

[81] Daniels SK, Huckabee ML. Dysphagia following stroke. San Diego (CA): Plural; 2008.

[82] DePippo KL, Holas MA, Reding MJ. Validation of the 3-oz water swallow test for aspiration following stroke. Arch Neurol 1992;49:1259–61.

[83] Garon BR, Engle M, Ormiston C. Reliability of the 3-oz water swallow test utilizing cough reflex as sole indicator of aspiration. Journal of Neurologic Rehabilitation 1995; 9:139–43.

[84] Daniels SK, McAdam CP, Brailey K, et al. Clinical assessment of swallowing and prediction of dysphagia severity. Am J Speech Lang Pathol 1997;6:17–24.

[85] McCullough GH, Wertz RT, Rosenbek JC. Sensitivity and specificity of clinical/bedside examination signs for detecting aspiration in adults subsequent to stroke. J Commun Disord 2001;34:55–72.

[86] Leder SB, Espinosa JF. Aspiration risk after acute stroke: comparison of clinical examination and fiberoptic endoscopic evaluation of swallowing. Dysphagia 2002;17:214–8.

[87] McCullough GH, Rosenbek JC, Wertz RT, et al. Utility of clinical swallowing examination measures for detecting aspiration post-stroke. J Speech Hear Res 2005;48:1280–93.

[88] Strand EA, Miller RM, Yorkston KM, et al. Management of oral-pharyngeal dysphagia symptoms in amyotrophic lateral sclerosis. Dysphagia 1996;11:129–39.

[89] Collins MJ, Bakheit AM. Does pulse oximetry reliably detect aspiration in dysphagic stroke patients? Stroke 1997;28:1773–5.

[90] Smith HA, Lee SH, O'Neill PA, et al. The combination of bedside swallowing assessment and oxygen saturation monitoring of swallowing in acute stroke: a safe and humane screening tool. Age Ageing 2000;29:495–9.

[91] Colodny N. Comparison of dysphagics and nondysphagics on pulse oximetry during oral feeding. Dysphagia 2000;15:68–73.

[92] Leder SB. Use of arterial oxygen saturation, heart rate, and blood pressure as indirect objective physiologic markers to predict aspiration. Dysphagia 2000;15:201–5.

[93] Cichero JA, Murdoch BE. Detection of swallowing sounds: methodology revisited. Dysphagia 2002;17:40–9.

[94] Takahashi K, Groher ME, Michi K. Methodology for detecting swallowing sounds. Dysphagia 1994;9:54–62.

[95] Borr C, Hielscher-Fastabend M, Lucking A. Reliability and validity of cervical auscultation. Dysphagia 2007;22:225–34.

[96] Leslie P, Drinnan MJ, Finn P, et al. Reliability and validity of cervical auscultation: a controlled comparison using videofluoroscopy. Dysphagia 2004;19:231–40.

[97] El Sharkawi A, Ramig L, Logemann JA, et al. Swallowing and voice effects of Lee Silverman voice treatment (LSVT): a pilot study. J Neurol Neurosurg Psychiatry 2002;72:31–6.

[98] Lazzara G, Lazarus C, Logemann JA. Impact of thermal stimulation on the triggering of the swallowing reflex. Dysphagia 1986;1:73–7.

[99] Rosenbek JC, Robbins J, Fishback B, et al. Effects of thermal application on dysphagia after stroke. J Speech Hear Res 1991;34:1257–68.

[100] Rosenbek JC, Robbins J, Willford WO, et al. Comparing treatment intensities of tactile-thermal application. Dysphagia 1998;13:1–9.

[101] Rosenbek JC, Roecker EB, Wood JL, et al. Thermal application reduces the duration of stage transition in dysphagia after stroke. Dysphagia 1996;11:225–33.

[102] Carnaby G, Hankey GJ, Pizzi J. Behavioural intervention for dysphagia in acute stroke: a randomised controlled trial. Lancet Neurol 2006;5:31–7.

[103] Bartolome G, Prosiegel M, Yassouridis A. Long-term functional outcome in patients with neurogenic dysphagia. NeuroRehabilitation 1997;9:195–204.

[104] Neumann S, Bartolome G, Buchholz D, et al. Swallowing therapy of neurologic patients: correlation of outcome with pretreatment variables and therapeutic methods. Dysphagia 1995;10:1–5.

[105] Bushmann M, Dobmeyer SM, Leeker L, et al. Swallowing abnormalities and their response to treatment in Parkinson's disease. Neurology 1989;39:1309–14.

[106] Fuh JL, Lee RC, Wang SJ, et al. Swallowing difficulty in Parkinson's disease. Clin Neurol Neurosurg 1997;99:106–12.

[107] Calne DB, Shaw DG, Spiers AS, et al. Swallowing in parkinsonism. Br J Radiol 1970;43:456–7.

[108] Hunter PC, Crameri J, Austin S, et al. Response of parkinsonian swallowing dysfunction to dopaminergic stimulation. J Neurol Neurosurg Psychiatry 1997;63:579–83.

[109] Sanders DB, Howard JF Jr. Disorders of neuromuscular transmission. In: Bradley WG, Daroff RB, Fenichel GM, et al, editors. Neurology in clinical practice: the neurological disorders, vol. 2. 4th edition. Philadelphia: Butterworth-Heinemann; 2004. p. 2441–61.

[110] Alberty J, Oelerich M, Ludwig K, et al. Efficacy of botulinum toxin A for treatment of upper esophageal sphincter dysfunction. Laryngoscope 2000;110:1151–6.

[111] Parameswaran MS, Soliman AM. Endoscopic botulinum toxin injection for cricopharyngeal dysphagia. Ann Otol Rhinol Laryngol 2002;111:871–4.

[112] Shaw GY, Searl JP. Botulinum toxin treatment for cricopharyngeal dysfunction. Dysphagia 2001;16:161–7.

[113] Giess R, Naumann M, Werner E, et al. Injections of botulinum toxin A into the salivary glands improve sialorrhoea in amyotrophic lateral sclerosis. J Neurol Neurosurg Psychiatry 2000;69:121–3.

[114] Mancini F, Zangaglia R, Cristina S, et al. Double-blind, placebo-controlled study to evaluate the efficacy and safety of botulinum toxin type A in the treatment of drooling in parkinsonism. Mov Disord 2003;18:685–8.

[115] Ondo WG, Hunter C, Moore W. A double-blind placebo-controlled trial of botulinum toxin B for sialorrhea in Parkinson's disease. Neurology 2004;62:37–40.

[116] Pal PK, Calne DB, Calne S, et al. Botulinum toxin A as treatment for drooling saliva in PD. Neurology 2000;54:244–7.

[117] Ali GN, Wallace KL, Laundl TM, et al. Predictors of outcome following cricopharyngeal disruption for pharyngeal dysphagia. Dysphagia 1997;12:133–9.

[118] Cook IJ, Kahrilas PJ. AGA technical review on management of oropharyngeal dysphagia. Gastroenterology 1999;116:455–78.

[119] Jacobs JR, Logemann J, Pajak TF, et al. Failure of cricopharyngeal myotomy to improve dysphagia following head and neck cancer surgery. Arch Otolaryngol Head Neck Surg 1999;125:942–6.

[120] Duranceau A. Cricopharyngeal myotomy in the management of neurogenic and muscular dysphagia. Neuromuscular Disorders 1997;7(Suppl 1):S85–9.

[121] Ergun GA, Kahrilas PJ. Medical and surgical treatment interventions in deglutitive dysfunction. In: Perlman AL, Schulze-Delreiu K, editors. Deglutition and its disorders. San Diego (CA): Singular; 1997. p. 463–90.

[122] Bhattacharyya N, Kotz T, Shapiro J. Dysphagia and aspiration with unilateral vocal cord immobility: incidence, characterization, and response to surgical treatment. Ann Otol Rhinol Laryngol 2002;111:672–9.

[123] Mann G, Hankey GJ, Cameron D. Swallowing function after stroke: prognosis and prognostic factors at 6 months. Stroke 1999;30:744–8.

[124] Dennis MS, Lewis SC, Warlow C. FOOD trial collaboration. Effect of timing and method of enteral tube feeding for dysphagic stroke patients (FOOD): a multicentre randomised controlled trial. Lancet 2005;365:764–72.

[125] Miller RG, Rosenberg JA, Gelinas DF, et al. Practice parameter: the care of the patient with amyotrophic lateral sclerosis (an evidence-based review): report of the quality standards subcommittee of the American Academy of Neurology: ALS practice parameters task force. Neurology 1999;52:1311–23.

[126] Finucane TE, Christmas C, Travis K. Tube feeding in patients with advanced dementia: a review of the evidence. JAMA 1999;282:1365–70.

[127] Franzoni S, Frisoni GB, Boffelli S, et al. Good nutritional oral intake is associated with equal survival in demented and nondemented very old patients. J Am Geriatr Soc 1996; 44:1366–70.

[128] Volicer L, Seltzer B, Rheaume Y, et al. Eating difficulties in patients with probable dementia of the Alzheimer type. J Geriatr Psychiatry Neurol 1989;2:188–95.

[129] DiBartolo MC. Careful hand feeding: a reasonable alternative to PEG tube placement in individuals with dementia. J Gerontol Nurs 2006;32:25–33, quiz 34–5.

[130] Garrow D, Pride P, Moran W, et al. Feeding alternatives in patients with dementia: examining the evidence. Clin Gastroenterol Hepatol 2007;5:1372–8.

PHYSICAL MEDICINE
AND REHABILITATION
CLINICS OF
NORTH AMERICA

ELSEVIER
SAUNDERS

Phys Med Rehabil Clin N Am
19 (2008) 889–928

Rehabilitation of Dysphagia Following Head and Neck Cancer

Barbara R. Pauloski, PhD, CCC-SP

Communication Sciences and Disorders, Northwestern University,
2240 Campus Drive, Suite 3-331, Evanston, IL 60208-3540, USA

This article provides information concerning the rehabilitation of dysphagia following treatment of cancer of the head and neck. It is divided into two major sections. The first describes the types of swallowing disorders that are observed in patients after cancer treatment; the second identifies the various intervention strategies available to the clinician to treat the disordered swallow in treated head and neck cancer patients.

Dysphagia after treatment of head and neck cancer

Patients who have cancerous tumors of the oral cavity, pharynx, or larynx are usually treated for their disease with surgical removal of the tumor, radiotherapy, chemotherapy, or a combination of these procedures. Each type of cancer treatment may result in some degree of dysphagia. The type and severity of dysphagia depends on the size and location of the original tumor, the structures involved, and the treatment modality used for cure.

Swallowing function after surgery for cancer of the head and neck

Surgical removal of tumors of the head and neck is a long-standing and well-established treatment modality that is still in wide use today [1,2]. Swallow dysfunction is often observed after surgical excision of tumors in the head and neck; swallow disorders may occur in the oral preparatory, oral propulsive, and pharyngeal stages of the swallow. The type and degree of

---

This work was supported by grant R01CA95576 from the National Cancer Institute and grant R01DC007659 from the National Institute on Deafness and Other Communication Disorders.

E-mail address: pauloski@northwestern.edu

swallow disorder depend on the site and stage of the tumor, the extent of surgical resection, and the nature of the surgical reconstruction. In general, the larger the resection, the greater the impairment of swallowing function [3–11]; however, the degree of resection of structures vital to bolus formation, bolus transit, and airway protection (such as oral tongue, tongue base, or arytenoid cartilages) has a greater impact on postsurgical swallow function than the extent of involvement of other structures (such as lateral floor of mouth or alveolar ridge) [3,9,12,13].

Swallow function after surgery for oral and pharyngeal tumors

Impact of structures resected and extent of resection on swallow function

The impact of resection of the oral tongue on swallowing function has been well reported in the literature. Patients who have a portion of the oral tongue removed exhibit worsened swallow function characterized by prolonged oral preparatory time [14], slowed oral transit time [14–17], increased oral residue [15,16], and increased pharyngeal residue [15]. Oral-stage swallowing disorders tend to worsen for these patients as bolus viscosity increases [8,15]. As the extent of resection of the oral tongue increases, swallowing function also worsens [18]. Patients who have resection of the oral tongue demonstrate increased oral transit time and increased oral and pharyngeal residue as the extent of resection increases [16,17]. The increased bolus residue is at greater risk of being aspirated after the swallow in patients who undergo a total glossectomy.

Patients who have resection of the tongue base may experience severe impairment of swallow function [10]. Those who have resections of the tongue base have increased oral preparatory time, increased oral transit time, increased oral residue, along with increased pharyngeal transit time [5,8,11,19], increased pharyngeal residue, and reduced oropharyngeal swallow efficiency [19,20]. Resection of greater than 25% of the tongue base is associated with inability to trigger a pharyngeal swallow, difficulty clearing the bolus from the pharynx, and severe postsurgical aspiration [6,8]. Swallowing disorders tend to worsen for these patients as bolus viscosity increases [8,15].

Surgical excision of oropharyngeal structures that do not contribute to normal swallowing function have little impact on swallow in the postsurgical patient [21]. Resection of the floor of mouth has been found to have limited impact on swallowing function [3,12,13], except when the resection extends to the geniohyoid or mylohyoid muscles [5]. With resection of the floor-of-mouth muscles, patients may experience problems with hyolaryngeal elevation, resulting in residue in the pyriform sinuses that may be aspirated after the swallow.

Some tumors may infiltrate the alveolar ridge and mandible, requiring resection for disease control. A rim or marginal resection of the mandible may be all that is required when tumor invasion is limited to the alveolar ridge. A marginal resection does not disrupt the continuity of the mandibular arch and has little impact on swallowing function. More invasive tumors require segmental mandibular resection, that is, removal of a section of the mandible that separates the remaining mandible bone into two sections. Although some investigators have found that the resected mandible is not functionally different from the intact mandible [22,23], more research indicates that segmental mandibular resection without reconstruction has a profound negative impact on oropharyngeal swallow efficiency, oral residue [13], and mastication [24–27].

Nature of reconstruction

The swallow function of postsurgical cancer patients may also be influenced by the type of surgical reconstruction. Surgical closure or reconstruction after ablation of head and neck tumors falls into four general categories: (1) primary closure (approximation and surgical closure of the edges of the resection); (2) skin grafts (transplantation of a superficial layer of skin from another site such as the thigh into the surgical resection); (3) pedicled flaps (flaps of tissue lifted from a donor site and migrated into the surgical defect, with a pedicle or stem of tissue attached to the donor site to maintain the blood supply); and (4) microvascular free flaps (flaps of tissue lifted from a donor site and sutured into the surgical defect with the blood vessels and sometimes nerves anastomosed to the existing supply at the excision site).

Some research indicates that patients closed primarily or with skin grafts have better postsurgical swallowing function than those reconstructed with pedicled or free flaps. [20,28–32]. The use of primary closure, however, may result in some restriction in tongue movement when a large amount of the tongue is resected or when the tongue is sutured to the floor of mouth or alveolar ridge after a composite resection. Some patients reconstructed with skin grafts demonstrate superior tongue mobility compared with those closed primarily [30]. Skin grafts are often not viable in the oropharynx, however, especially when the patient received radiotherapy, which may disrupt the blood supply to the area.

Patients reconstructed with pedicled flaps, such as the pectoralis major myocutaneous flap, have been shown to demonstrate impaired tongue mobility scores [30], excessively long oral transit times, increased oral residue after the swallow [15,33], and reduced oropharyngeal swallow efficiency [15]. Pedicled flap reconstruction is often used in the head and neck population to close a large surgical defect [28]. These flaps are often considered to be bulky, which may interfere with movement of the remaining oral tissues [28,29]. Swallow impairment in patients reconstructed with pedicled flaps may also be related to the adynamic nature of the flap: use of this type of flap introduces tissue that has no sensation or motor control into an area in which range, rate, and coordination are critical to normal swallow function [15,33].

Microvascular free flaps such as the radial forearm free flap have the advantage of being thin yet viable flaps that can be used to repair a surgical defect without adding excessive bulk to the oropharyngeal structures. This type of flap is flexible enough to permit lining of the floor of mouth without tethering the tongue. Adequate flap design permits the appropriate degree of closure without sacrificing tongue movement [34–41]. Some comparative studies have indicated no difference in swallow function after reconstruction with a radial forearm free flap or a pedicled pectoralis major flap [18], whereas others have shown that the ability to swallow in patients reconstructed with free flaps is superior to that of patients reconstructed with pectoralis major myocutaneous pedicled flaps [42–44]. Nevertheless, swallow function is still impaired after resection and free flap reconstruction. Some studies have indicated worse levels of oropharyngeal functioning in patients who have free flap reconstruction compared with primary closure [45,46]. In addition, oropharyngeal swallow efficiency has been shown to be severely reduced, and pharyngeal transit time and excessive oral and pharyngeal residues increased, in patients reconstructed with free flaps [19,21], with no recovery of preoperative function by 1-year post-treatment [19,21,47].

Sensate flaps are microvascular free flaps that have not only their blood supply but also their innervation joined to the remaining supplies at the surgical resection site. Few objective swallow data are available for sensate flaps; some data indicate swallowing function is superior in patients who have a re-innervated flap [48], whereas other research does not indicate the superiority of sensate flaps over nonsensate mirovascular free flaps in improving swallow function [47], oropharyngeal swallow efficiency [49], or oral sensation [47].

Reconstruction of the mandible after segmental mandibular resection can be achieved using microvascular free flaps containing bone. Reports of functional outcome after mandibular reconstruction are mixed. Some studies have demonstrated a clear advantage for patients who have mandibular reconstruction in most oropharyngeal functions [26], whereas others have indicated that reconstruction of mandibular continuity does not contribute to improved swallow function [12,32].

Assessing the relative impact of the various surgical closure procedures on swallowing function can be difficult because of the profound impact of extent of resection on swallow function. In addition, not all closures may be used with all resections. In the one study that controlled for extent of resection of the oral tongue and tongue base, no significant differences were observed on swallow function between those reconstructed with pedicled and microvascular free flaps. Those closed primarily or with skin grafts had higher oropharyngeal swallow efficiencies and less pharyngeal residue than those reconstructed with flaps [50].

Swallow disorders after surgery for laryngeal tumors

Cancerous tumors of the larynx may need to be removed surgically. Surgical excision of cancers of the larynx may also have a profound impact on swallowing function (primarily the risk of aspiration), depending on the site of the tumor, the structures resected, and the resulting reconstruction. Many tumors may be removed without complete removal of the larynx, that is, a total laryngectomy. Partial laryngectomy procedures such as the supraglottic laryngectomy and hemilaryngectomy are performed with the intent to maintain as much normal laryngeal function as possible while controlling the disease.

Supraglottic laryngectomy

For lesions involving the epiglottis, aryepiglottic folds, or false vocal folds with no involvement of the vocal folds, a supraglottic laryngectomy is the standard surgical intervention. A supraglottic laryngectomy, also referred to as a horizontal partial laryngectomy, includes resection of the epiglottis, aryepiglottic folds, false vocal folds, and the superior aspect of the thyroid cartilage, sparing the true vocal folds and arytenoids [51–53]. Preservation of the hyoid bone, when possible, may help swallowing function postoperatively [54]. Classically, supraglottic surgery also included removal of the hyoid bone [55]. Some of these patients may present with swallow difficulties decades later, especially if they had received postoperative radiotherapy [56], so it is possible that clinicians currently practicing may come in contact with patients who underwent supraglottic laryngectomy and do not have a hyoid bone. Because structures involved in the protective mechanism of the airway are resected, patients who have received a supraglottic laryngectomy are at risk for aspiration during the swallow [51,57–59]. Rates of aspiration during the swallow as high as 74% have been reported [59]. The base of tongue and arytenoid cartilages play an important role in compensating for the supragottic structures resected in the surgery [60]. Patients who are able to achieve good contact between the tongue base and the arytenoid after supraglottic laryngectomy are able to prevent material from entering the airway during the swallow [58]. When the supraglottic laryngectomy procedure needs to be extended into the tongue base or to the arytenoid, this potential compensatory mechanism is compromised, and aspiration during the swallow is the likely consequence [57,59,61]. Patients who have extended supraglottic laryngectomy, especially into the base of tongue, demonstrate increased pulmonary complications due to aspiration [62] and take significantly longer to achieve preoperative diet and normal swallowing than those who have limited resections [63].

Tumors limited to a true vocal fold may be treated with a hemilaryngectomy, also referred to as vertical partial laryngectomy. This resection includes one false vocal fold, one ventricle, and one true vocal fold, excluding the arytenoids but usually taking the vocal process and a portion of the thyroid cartilage on the same side as the lesion [52,53,55]. Because the hyoid bone, epiglottis, and arytenoids are left in place, a patient receiving a standard hemilaryngectomy should not have difficulty with airway closure when properly reconstructed with bulk tissue on the operated side [53,64]. Various techniques exist for creating a pseudocord from pedicled and free flaps [53,65,66]; the goal of reconstruction is to provide enough bulk to allow the remaining vocal cord to make contact with the reconstructed site and permit protection of the airway [53]. Patients who undergo a hemilaryngectomy usually have fewer incidents of aspiration [67] and achieve oral intake and return to a normal diet sooner than those who have had any type of supraglottic laryngectomy [63]. When the resection is extended posteriorly to include the arytenoid cartilage, however, an important component of airway closure is affected, and the risk of aspiration during the swallow increases [64,68]. Aspiration rates of up to 91% during the swallow have been reported [59,69].

Total laryngectomy

Total laryngectomy may be used as the primary treatment in cases of advanced laryngeal carcinoma. Generally, aspiration is not a risk for those who have received a total laryngectomy unless there is leakage around or though a tracheoesophageal fistula that is created for voice restoration or that results from healing complications [59]. In addition, patients who have received a total laryngectomy may experience other difficulties with their swallow. Manometric studies of patients who have total laryngectomy have indicated that the postlaryngectomy swallow is characterized by significantly lower resting pressures in the pharyngoesophageal segment, lower peak pressures after swallow, greater numbers of swallows with discoordination between contraction of the pharyngeal constrictors and relaxation of the pharyngoesophageal segment [70,71], a loss of the normal negative pressure preceding the bolus, reduced pharyngeal clearing force [60,72,73], and loss of asymmetric contractile forces [74] compared with subjects who have normal anatomy. Bolus clearance through the oral cavity and pharyngocervical esophagus is often impaired in this group of patients [75–77], especially when resection is extended to the tongue base.

At the present time, total laryngectomy is used most often as a salvage procedure—after recurrence or in the case of intractable aspiration [78]. The incidence of pharyngocutaneous fistula formation is higher after salvage laryngectomy than primary laryngectomy, especially in irradiated patients [59,79,80]. Completion laryngectomy for patients treated with chemoradiation who experience intractable aspiration may not result in improved swallow function. Patients who have total laryngectomy must typically generate pressures greater than normal during the swallow to achieve bolus transit [72]. Adequate tongue-base motion is important in this pressure generation. Patients who have received chemoradiation to the head and neck often experience reduced tongue-base retraction, as is discussed in the following section. Completion laryngectomy may eliminate aspiration in these patients, but they may not be able to advance their diet beyond pureed consistencies if they are unable to produce sufficient bolus driving pressure [16,76].

The impact of postoperative radiotherapy on swallow function

Radiotherapy is commonly used in conjunction with surgical excision of tumors of the head and neck to control for microscopic disease. Preoperative radiation has classically been used to reduce the size of the primary tumor before surgery; this modality generally has been replaced with induction chemotherapy. Postoperative radiotherapy is often focused on the lymph nodes of the neck to prevent spread of disease. Although radiotherapy provides important curative benefits, it also induces damage in normal tissues and may result in mucositis, xerostomia, fibrosis, soft tissue necrosis, and osteoradionecrosis of the mandible [81–85]. The swallowing disorders observed during the first few months after surgery are the result of the surgical procedure; additional dysfunction or lack of improvement in swallow function observed after the initial postoperative period is the result of radiation damage to the tissues.

Many investigators have found that oropharyngeal functioning is worse in patients receiving postoperative radiotherapy than in those receiving surgical excision only [8,10,16,45]. Multiple logistic regression has shown that radiotherapy is one of the main predictors of poor swallowing function after surgical excision of oral and oropharyngeal cancer [46]. Radiation treatments affect the oral and the pharyngeal stages of swallowing. Irradiated patients experience significantly increased oral and pharyngeal transit times (especially for boluses of thicker consistency), greater pharyngeal residue, lower oropharyngeal swallow efficiency, and shorter duration of cricopharyngeal opening [8,86]. Increased oral transit time is most likely the result of xerostomia. Increased pharyngeal residue, decreased oropharyngeal swallow efficiency, and shortened cricopharyngeal opening duration in irradiated patients suggest a reduction in pharyngeal bolus driving pressure [86]. This reduction in pharyngeal driving force is the result of radiation-induced fibrosis of the oropharyngeal musculature, resulting in reduced tongue-base retraction, decreased bulging of the posterior pharyngeal wall, and reduced duration of tongue-base contact to the posterior pharyngeal wall [87].

In longitudinal studies of swallowing function in patients treated surgically for oral or oropharyngeal tumors, patients who received postoperative radiotherapy had worse swallow function characterized by lower swallow efficiencies and a significantly different course of recovery of swallow function over time. Those who did not have any postoperative radiotherapy demonstrated a steady improvement in swallow efficiency between 3 and 12 months postsurgery, whereas those who received postoperative radiotherapy did not show any improvement in function [8,88].

Patients who have been treated for laryngeal cancer also experience the adverse effects of postoperative radiotherapy. A greater incidence of tracheostomy dependence, delayed independent swallowing function, and an increased incidence of aspiration pneumonia are noted in patients requiring radiotherapy after supraglottic laryngectomy [52]. Patients who have partial laryngectomy procedures have delayed recovery of swallowing function when they have not achieved oral intake by the time their postoperative radiotherapy begins [63].

Summary: swallowing function after surgery for cancer of the head and neck

Swallowing problems after surgery for head and neck cancer depend on the extent of the resection, the specific structures resected, and to a limited extent, the nature of reconstruction. Patients who have resections involving the oral tongue experience difficulty with bolus formation, slowed oral transit, and increased oral residue. As food viscosity increases, these swallowing problems tend to be more problematic. Aspiration is not usually a problem in patients who have resections limited to the anterior oral cavity unless resection extends into the tongue base. When resection involves the tongue base or arytenoid cartilage, the risk of aspiration increases. The nature of reconstruction of the surgical defect also may have an impact on postsurgical swallowing problems; however, because the type of reconstruction is often dictated by the extent of resection, it is not clear how much of an impact reconstruction type has on postoperative swallow function. The few available multivariate studies of surgical parameters on swallowing function [6,10,13,89] suggest that extent of resection (more specifically, extent of resection of the tongue base) has a greater impact on postsurgical swallowing function than the nature of reconstruction. Postoperative radiotherapy has an additional negative impact on swallowing function by increasing fibrosis of the irradiated head and neck tissues.

Swallowing function after primary radiation or chemoradiation

There has been an increase over the past 20 years in the use of radiotherapy with or without chemotherapy as a primary treatment modality for cancer of the head and neck [90–100]. Although the primary goal of treatment is cure, a perceived additional benefit of this modality is the preservation of the organs of the head and neck, with the underlying assumption being that preservation of structure will result in preservation of function [101,102]. The current literature on swallowing function in patients treated with radiotherapy with or without chemotherapy for cancer of the head and neck indicates that despite preservation of the structures of the head and neck, swallow function is not maintained at normal levels after treatment [103–114]. Reported rates of posttreatment aspiration range considerably, from 5% to 89% [107,109,112,114–124], with silent aspiration reported at rates of 22% to 42% [117,120,121,123,124].

Studies of swallow function in patients treated with chemoradiation for cancers of the head and neck have focused on early and late effects. A body of literature indicates significant functional abnormality during the first year post treatment completion. Swallow motility disorders reported at frequencies of greater than 50% for patients treated with chemoradiotherapy to various sites in the head and neck include reduced anterior-to-posterior tongue movement [125], reduced tongue strength [118], reduced tongue-base retraction [103,105,107,109,118,125,126], increased oral residue [118], increased velopharyngeal closure duration [118], reduced epiglottic inversion [103,106,126], slowed or reduced laryngeal elevation [105–107,109,126], impaired pharyngeal constrictor motility [106], increased pharyngeal residue [118], delayed pharyngeal swallow [103], and delayed laryngeal vestibule closure [105,106,109,125].

Chemoradiated patients tend to exhibit similar swallowing disorders regardless of the site of the primary tumor. Patients treated for nasopharyngeal tumors exhibit problems with the oral stage (increased oral stasis and residue [122], reduced tongue control [115,118], impaired bolus transit [115]) and the pharyngeal stage of the swallow (reduced tongue-base retraction [118], reduced pharyngeal contraction [115], increased pharyngeal residue [115,122]), despite having the primary tumor confined to the nasal cavity. Patients who have tumors of the oropharynx demonstrate the expected pharyngeal motility disorders such as reduced tongue-base retraction [56,107,109,118], reduced pharyngeal contraction [109], and increased pharyngeal residue requiring multiple swallows to clear [107,109]; however, they also have problems with laryngeal mobility (reduced laryngeal elevation [56,107,109], reduced laryngeal vestibule closure [56,109,125], and reduced true cord closure [56]). In addition to reduced laryngeal elevation [121], patients treated with chemoradiation for cancer of the larynx also demonstrate difficulty during the oral preparatory and oral propulsive stages of the swallow (impaired bolus formation [121], reduced tongue control leading to premature spillage [112], reduced tongue strength [118], reduced anterior-to-posterior tongue movement [121,125], increased oral cavity stasis [121], reduced tongue-base retraction [118]) and demonstrate increased pharyngeal residue in the vallecula and pyriform sinuses [112,121]. Patients treated with traditional external-beam radiotherapy to most sites in the head and neck have similar structures involved in the treatment volume [56,107,112,118,122]. Radiation-induced fibrosis in the irradiated structures results in limited mobility of the oral tongue, tongue base, pharynx, and larynx [56,104,117,121]; therefore, the observed swallow disorders after treatment are similar despite the site of the primary tumor.

Swallow disorders that are evident early after treatment with chemoradiation appear to persist with little if any recovery of function by the end of the first year posttreatment [108,115,125] or in the long-term. Severe impairments of swallowing function are observed years after completion of treatment, including reduced tongue control resulting in premature spillage into the pharynx [112,122,127], reduced tongue-base retraction [56,116], impaired pharyngeal contraction [117,122,123,127], increased vallecula and pyriform sinus residue [112,116,122,123], impaired epiglottic function [122,127], reduced laryngeal elevation [56,117], and reduced laryngeal vestibule and true cord closure [56]. Dysphagia persists decades after treatment [117], and a longer duration after treatment does not yield a more proficient swallow [112]; in fact, there is evidence of continued deterioration of swallowing function for years after chemoradiation as a result of progressive fibrosis in irradiated tissues of the head and neck [122,127].

Attempts have been made to minimize the amount of damage to normal tissues and reduce the adverse effects of treatment on swallowing function. A comparison of two groups of patients treated with altered doses of radiotherapy to the primary tumor (74.4 Gy versus 60.0 Gy) for lesions of the oropharynx or hypopharynx indicated a significant reduction in odynophagia, aspiration, and gastrostomy use at 4 and 12 months posttreatment with the lowered dosage [128]. The intensity of the radiation beam can also be modulated to decrease the doses to normal structures without compromising the doses to the target. Intensity-modulated radiotherapy (IMRT) is an advanced form of three-dimensional conformal radiation therapy with the ability to precisely target and escalate radiation doses to the tumor while reducing radiation exposure to surrounding normal structures. Initially studied in terms of its impact on salivary flow and xerostomia (the perception of "dry mouth"), IMRT has proved to be successful in reducing damage to the parotid gland and in preserving salivary flow [129,130]. The impact of IMRT on posttreatment swallowing function has also been investigated. Patients treated with tissue-sparing techniques demonstrate less-severe ratings of dysphagia [131,132], significantly fewer days of tube feeding [132], increased oral intake, lower pharyngeal residue, and better oropharyngeal swallowing efficiency [131]. There has been particular interest in applying IMRT techniques to reduce the dose to structures specifically related to swallowing function, especially the pharyngeal constrictors, supraglottic larynx, and glottic larynx [133,134]. With lower doses to the pharyngeal constrictor muscles, fewer problems with dysphagia are observed [134]. Reduced epiglottic inversion, reduced laryngeal elevation, and aspiration are related to significantly higher doses to the pharyngeal constrictors, glottis, and supraglottic larynx [135]. There is obvious benefit in reducing the radiation dose to normal tissues, especially in those structures contributing to swallow function. Future refinement of techniques to reduce radiation dosage to normal structures should yield additional improvement in swallowing function.

Other adverse effects of chemoradiation that may impact swallowing function

In addition to inducing fibrosis, which appears to be the primary reason for swallowing dysfunction after treatment, chemoradiation causes other side effects that may have an impact on swallowing function.

Reduced salivary flow and xerostomia

Radiation for cancers of the head and neck often includes the salivary glands in the treatment volume; damage to the salivary glands results in significantly reduced salivary flow [85,129,136,137]. The parotid gland is especially sensitive to the effects of radiotherapy; radiation doses in excess of 55 Gy to 64 Gy appear to result in permanent damage with no anticipated long-term recovery of salivary function [136,137]. Studies of saliva flow after treatments designed to reduce the dose to the parotid gland indicate that with doses below 24 Gy to 26 Gy, saliva flow is preserved and will increase toward pretreatment levels over the first year. Glands receiving a mean dose higher than the threshold produce little saliva, with no recovery over time [129].

The relationships among reduced salivary flow, xerostomia (or the perception of dry mouth), and swallow function are not clear. Although patients who have significantly reduced saliva production after radiotherapy also have increased reports of perceived difficulty swallowing, dry mouth, needing water while eating, food sticking in the mouth or throat, and changes in taste [85,138], patients who have objective improvement in salivary flow over time may still complain of xerostomia [136]. Reduced saliva weight does not correlate with slowed or inefficient swallow. Instead, reduced saliva weight seems to change the patient's perception of swallowing ability and, on that basis, affects diet choices [85,138].

Mucositis

Mucositis is a frequent and severe consequence of radiotherapy to the head and neck [84]. Oral mucositis is defined as an injury to the oral mucosa characterized by erythema (redness) and ulcerative lesions [139,140]. Mucositis is limited to the tissues in the field of radiation, with nonkeratinized tissues such as buccal and labial mucosa, ventral and lateral surfaces of the tongue, floor of mouth, and soft palate affected more often than other tissues [139,140]. Mucositis also may affect other sites along the digestive tract as a result of high-dose chemotherapy [84,141].

Nearly all patients receiving conventional (once daily) radiotherapy (97%) or chemoradiotherapy (90%) experience mucositis. It is reported that 100% of patients who receive altered fractionation (twice-daily treatments) have mucositis, with more than half experiencing the highest grades (worst level) of this toxicity [84]. The severity of oral mucositis is directly proportional to the dose of radiation administered to the head and neck [139,142]. The first mucosal reaction can be observed as a white discoloration after a cumulative radiation dose of 10 Gy to 20 Gy. Deepening erythema is usually visible after 20 Gy of cumulative radiation, and ulcerations, often covered with a pseudomembranous layer, develop after about 30 Gy, usually occurring after 3 weeks of conventional radiotherapy. After completion of radiotherapy, mucositis generally declines after 2 to 6 weeks [139,143].

Pain is a common side effect of mucositis; the ulcerative stage is especially painful [84,139]. Ulceration of the oral mucosa and the resulting pain can impair a patient's ability to swallow and eat [84,139,144]. In the few studies that report dietary-related outcomes, there is a high and significant correlation between severity of mucositis and the incidence of gastrostomy tube feeding and weight loss [84].

Any irritants to the oral mucosa such as spicy foods or alcohol should be avoided while mucositis is present. There is great need for education of the patient and family on proper oral care during mucositis [144]. The dysphagia rehabilitation specialist (commonly a speech-language pathologist) can play an important role in reinforcing oral care procedures with the patient suffering from mucositis.

Stricture

Stricture, a segment of narrowing or complete closure in the pharynx or esophagus, occurs at reported rates of 8% to 24% after chemoradiation and has a profound impact on swallowing function by limiting or blocking the passage of food or liquid [110,114,124,127,145]. The average time after treatment completion to diagnosis is 6 to 7 months. Strictures rarely develop until the radiation dose to the hypopharynx or esophagus exceeds 60 Gy to 70 Gy [126,146], so the proximal esophagus is another organ to consider sparing with IMRT techniques.

The hypothesized pathophysiology of stricture formation begins with ulceration after severe mucositis, along with a relatively immobile larynx secondary to radiation-induced fibrosis and the lack of passage of food or liquid through lumen possibly due to use of gastrostomy tubes. These conditions lead to healing of the opposing anterior and posterior mucosal surfaces, resulting in adhesions that lead to narrowing and possible obstruction [126,147]. The hypopharynx is especially susceptible to stricture formation because of the close proximity of the mucosal membranes in the posterior cricoid area and posterior pharyngeal wall [145].

It has been suggested that use of gastrostomy tubes may contribute to the development of strictures [148]. Patients who have gastrostomy tubes may be at increased risk of stricture formation because of the relative inactivity of the upper esophageal/hypopharyngeal musculature. Those who have gastrostomy tubes are likely to cease all efforts at passage of food or liquid, especially when suffering from mucositis. Therefore, formation of stricture may not be related to radiation dose but to whether the patient swallowed during the course of treatment, resulting in less significant muscular fibrosis in the treated area compared with those patients who did not swallow routinely throughout the course of treatment [145,147]. Lack of swallowing may result in atrophy of hypopharyngeal muscles. Patients undergoing chemoradiation should be strongly encouraged to swallow orally even if they have gastrostomy tubes or other supplemental feeding tubes in place. The use of the swallow mechanism should limit adhesion formation and disuse atrophy of pharyngeal muscles [147].

Summary: swallowing function after primary radiation or chemoradiation for cancer of the head and neck

The use of radiotherapy with or without chemotherapy for treatment of cancer of the head and neck as a primary treatment modality has increased significantly over the past 20 years. Despite preservation of the structures of the head and neck, swallow function is not maintained at normal levels after treatment. Aspiration rates approaching 90% have been reported in the literature for patients after treatment with primary chemoradiotherapy. Dysfunction is observed across all stages of the swallow in most tumor sites treated with standard external-beam radiation. The uniformity of swallow disorders after this treatment modality is related to the wide field of radiation required for effective cure. Fibrosis of the irradiated tissue of the head and neck results in impaired movement of the oral tongue, tongue base, pharyngeal constrictors, and larynx, leading to dysfunction. Swallow disorders persist through the first year post treatment and may be present many years after completion of radiotherapy.

Reduced salivary flow, xerostomia, mucositis, and hypopharyngeal or esophageal strictures are also side effects of chemoradiotherapy that may have a profound and negative impact on posttreatment swallow function.

Attempts have been made to minimize the amount of damage to normal tissues and reduce the adverse effects of treatment on swallowing function by reducing radiation dose to swallow-critical structures. Less swallow impairment is observed when the dose to the pharyngeal constrictors, supraglottic and glottic larynx, and proximal esophagus is reduced.

Diagnosis and treatment planning

The management of dysphagia after treatment of cancers of the head and neck begins with an imaging procedure to properly diagnose the pathophysiology of the swallow. Given the reported rates of silent aspiration, especially in those treated with chemoradiation, the use of an imaging procedure is vital in the proper diagnosis of dysphagia.

The most useful imaging techniques for diagnosing swallowing disorders are (1) the modified barium swallow (MBS) procedure with videofluorography and (2) fiberoptic endoscopic examination of swallow (FEES). Both procedures are thoroughly addressed in this issue of the *Physical Medicine and Rehabilitation Clinics of North America*. During the MBS, patients are administered calibrated boluses of radiopaque material of varying consistency. The patient's swallow is viewed in the lateral plane with videofluorography so that disorders of the swallow during oral preparation, the oral propulsive stage of swallow, and the pharyngeal stage of swallow may be observed and documented. FEES visualizes the pharynx from above by placing an endoscopic tube transnasally such that the end of the tube is suspended over the end of the soft palate. This procedure gives a view of the pharynx that is different from the videofluoroscopic view and permits observation of true cord closure; however, FEES does not provide information concerning the oral stage of swallow, which may be the most problematic for some head and neck cancer patients who have been treated surgically for oral cavity tumors. MBS is therefore the most commonly used technique to observe the swallow, diagnose dysphagia, and develop a treatment plan for patients who have impaired swallow function [149–154]. It is especially suited to determining the effects of trial therapy. After the dysphagia rehabilitation specialist documents the specific swallowing disorders observed on MBS, he or she can introduce interventions to treat the disorder or to compensate for the swallow impairment.

Interventions during the modified barium swallow

The goal of the MBS assessment is to define the presence and cause of any aspiration and motility disorders and to determine whether there are interventions that will eliminate or reduce the aspiration and improve swallow function. Therefore, patients should be given trial therapy to determine the effectiveness of strategies such as postures, maneuvers, and modifications to bolus size or consistency.

Postures

Postures are used to control the flow of the bolus and to reduce or eliminate aspiration. There are a number postures that are effective in treated head and neck cancer patients. After determining the cause of aspiration or swallow dysfunction, the clinician should attempt under fluoroscopy an appropriate posture (or postures) to determine the effect in each individual patient. Changes in head or body position have been shown to eliminate aspiration of at least one liquid bolus volume in 77% of patients who have various medical diagnoses [155] and in 81% of postsurgical head and neck cancer patients [156]. The efficacy of postures varies depending on the swallowing disorder identified as causing the aspiration [157].

Chin-down

The chin-down posture (also referred to as chin tuck or neck flexion) is useful for patients who have a delayed pharyngeal swallow, reduced tongue-base retraction, or reduced laryngeal elevation. The patient is instructed to touch the chin to the neck while swallowing. This action pushes the anterior pharyngeal wall posteriorly and the tongue base and epiglottis closer to the posterior pharyngeal wall, thereby narrowing the airway entrance. This posterior shift with the chin-down posture improves airway protection, so it is useful for patients who have reduced laryngeal elevation or laryngeal vestibule closure. The vallecular space is also widened, giving a potentially larger place for the bolus to set before the pharyngeal swallow is initiated [158,159].

The chin-down posture, alone or combined with other postures or maneuvers such as head rotation, head-back to chin-down movement, or voluntary airway protection (to be discussed later) has been reported as successful in eliminating aspiration in 72% of patients who have various medical diagnoses [157]; success with postsurgical head and neck cancer patients ranges from 50% in patients who have tongue-base resection [8] to 81% in esophagectomy patients [160] and 90% in patients who have oral or laryngeal resections [156]. The chin-down posture has been shown to significantly reduce depth of bolus penetration into the larynx and trachea [161]. Patients prefer the simple chin-down posture technique to other interventions such as thickening liquids [162], and most find it easy to perform correctly [160,161].

Head back

The head-back posture uses gravity to clear the bolus from the oral cavity in patients who have difficulty with oral transit of the bolus [16,149]. When there is a question about adequate airway protection, the patient may be instructed in various voluntary airway protection maneuvers (discussed later). In appropriately selected patients, the head-back posture has been shown to be 100% effective in transporting the bolus out of the oral cavity and into the pharynx [156].

Head rotation

Head rotation toward the weak or damaged side of the pharynx or larynx closes the damaged side so that the bolus flows down the side that is more nearly normal. This posture is useful for patients who have unilateral pharyngeal wall impairment or unilateral vocal fold weakness. Head rotation to the weaker side causes the bolus to lateralize away from the direction of rotation and increases upper esophageal sphincter (UES) opening diameter while causing a significant reduction in UES pressure [163]. During head rotation, compensatory movement of the arytenoid on the healthy side has been observed on videofluoroscopy [164]. Serial CT of the pharynx in a patient who had lateral medullary syndrome using head rotation indicated that hemipharyngeal closing occurs at the level of the hyoid bone and in the hypopharyngeal cavity above the pyriform sinus [165].

Head rotation performed alone or in combination with other postures or maneuvers is effective in reducing aspiration in postsurgical head and neck cancer patients 71% of the time [156]. Because head rotation may cause compensatory movement of the arytenoid on the healthy side [164], this posture may be effective in patients who have undergone hemilarygectomy and who have difficulty achieving closure of the remaining vocal fold against the reconstructed pseudocord. In addition, because UES opening diameter is increased and resting pressure is decreased during head rotation, patients who have cricopharyngeal dysmotility problems may also benefit from the posture.

Lateral head-tilt

The lateral head-tilt posture may be used for a patient who has unilateral oral and pharyngeal impairment on the same side. The patient tilts the head to the stronger side so that gravity drains the bolus along the stronger side and avoids the weaker side [149]. There are no reports in the literature on the efficacy of this posture in the head and neck population, but the clinician may find it useful to try this procedure in patients who have unilateral impairment.

Swallow maneuvers

Swallow maneuvers are designed to place specific aspects of the oropharyngeal swallow under voluntary control. Maneuvers should be checked fluoroscopically to verify that the patient is performing them properly and to determine the impact on aspiration and swallow motility disorders.

Supraglottic and supersupraglottic swallow maneuvers

The goal of the supraglottic and supersupraglottic swallow maneuvers, also referred to as voluntary airway closure techniques, is to close the vocal folds before and during the swallow to prevent aspiration [149,166]. For the supraglottic swallow, the patient is instructed to take a deep breath and hold it, swallow while continuing to hold the breath, and cough immediately after the swallow to expel any residue from the airway entrance. The supersupraglottic swallow is designed to close the entrance to the airway voluntarily by tilting the arytenoid cartilage anteriorly to contact the base of the epiglottis before and during the swallow and by closing the false vocal folds tightly. The patient is instructed to inhale and hold his or her breath very tightly, bearing down. The patient should keep holding his or her breath and bearing down while swallowing, and then cough when finished. Videofluoroscopic and videoendoscopic evaluations have demonstrated that airway closure duration is prolonged during the supraglottic and supersupraglottic swallow maneuvers in normal subjects and in treated head and neck cancer patients [167,168]. Normal subjects also experience earlier cricopharyngeal opening, prolonged pharyngeal swallow, some degree of laryngeal valving before swallow, and change in extent of vertical laryngeal position before swallow. These changes in swallow physiology are more pronounced with the supersupraglottic swallow [168].

The supraglottic swallow was originally conceptualized for use with patients who underwent supraglottic laryngectomy, to improve the ability to protect the airway and prevent aspiration during the swallow [169].

Endoscopic studies have demonstrated that true cord closure may not always be achieved during the supraglottic swallow, so the airway may not be protected in all patients using this procedure. The supersupraglottic swallow, however, provides an additional level of airway protection by tilting the arytenoid cartilages anteriorly to contact the base of the epiglottis (or tongue base if the epiglottis has been resected) [166]. The supersupraglottic swallow also influences aspects of the swallow other than airway protection. In irradiated head and neck cancer patients, the supersupraglottic swallow not only closes the airway entrance earlier than without the maneuver but also results in improved tongue-base motion [170], greater hyoid and laryngeal elevation at the time of cricopharyngeal opening, and increased maximal hyoid and laryngeal elevation [171]. These results suggest that the supersupraglottic swallow not only improves airway closure at the entrance but also improves tongue-base movement and the speed and extent of hyolaryngeal movement, especially early in the swallow.

Based on the observed effects of the supersupraglottic swallow on oropharyngeal biomechanics, this technique is useful for patients who have reduced laryngeal airway closure and for those who have reduced tongue-base retraction and reduced laryngeal elevation. It has been shown to be effective in eliminating aspiration in patients who have undergone supraglottic laryngectomy [58] and in those treated with a full course of radiotherapy to the head and neck [171].

Effortful swallow maneuver

The effortful swallow is designed to increase tongue-base retraction and pharyngeal pressure during the swallow to improve bolus clearance from the valleculae [149]. The patient is instructed to squeeze hard with all their muscles as they swallow.

The effortful swallow is believed to increase pharyngeal pressures, thus pushing the bolus through the pharynx and cricopharyngeous, leaving less residue in the pharynx after the swallow. Studies designed to measure oral, pharyngeal, and esophageal pressures during the effortful swallow maneuver provide conflicting information concerning the pressures generated with the procedure.

Effortful swallows performed by healthy normal adults are characterized by significantly higher oral pressures; diminished oral residue; longer laryngeal vestibule closure, hyoid excursion, and extent of hyoid elevation [172]; and longer pharyngeal pressure duration and UES relaxation duration [173]. The effortful swallow also has an effect on the esophageal phase of swallow, with significantly increased peristaltic amplitudes within the distal smooth muscle region of the esophagus, possibly as a result of overflow effort from the maneuver [174].

There are limited data on the effortful swallow in patient populations. In patients who have pharyngeal dysfunction, the effortful swallow does not alter peak amplitude or duration of the intrabolus pressure [175]; however, the use of the effortful swallow in these patients significantly reduces depth of contrast penetration into the larynx and trachea. Although there is no impact on pharyngeal residue, the hyoid is held in a more superior position before onset of the swallow [161]. In treated head and neck cancer patients, the effortful swallow is associated with higher pharyngeal pressure amplitudes and longer pressure durations than are observed with swallows using no maneuver; compared with other maneuvers, the effortful swallow produces the highest pharyngeal pressure and results in slightly less pharyngeal residue [170].

Although the effortful swallow was conceived to increase pharyngeal pressure during the swallow to improve bolus clearance from the vallecula, data indicate that the maneuver also has an impact on other aspects of the oral and pharyngeal stages of the swallow. Therefore, the effortful swallow may be appropriate to use in treated head and neck cancer patients who demonstrate reduced tongue strength, reduced pharyngeal contraction, reduced laryngeal elevation, reduced laryngeal vestibule closure, and cricopharyngeal dysmotility.

Mendelsohn maneuver

The Mendelsohn maneuver is a voluntary prolongation of laryngeal excursion at the midpoint of the swallow intended to increase the extent and duration of laryngeal elevation and thereby increase the duration of cricopharyngeal opening [176]. Patients are instructed to swallow normally, and when they feel their voice box go up, to grab it with the throat muscles and not let it go down. Patients are instructed to hold it for three counts and then let it go. This maneuver can be practiced without food, and then food may be introduced with the maneuver after the patient has learned to perform it correctly.

Videomanometric data confirm that use of the Mendelsohn maneuver in healthy adults results in increased peak pharyngeal contraction and duration [177] and increased duration of anterior and superior excursion of the larynx and hyoid (and consequently prolonged cricopharyngeal opening) by maintaining traction on the anterior sphincter wall [170]. Significantly longer bolus transit times also occur, as would be expected when the subject is instructed to prolong laryngeal elevation.

In treated head and neck cancer patients, swallows performed with the Mendelsohn maneuver have been shown to exhibit higher tongue-base pressure amplitudes, longer pressure durations, and less pharyngeal residue compared with swallows with no maneuver [170]. Use of the Mendelsohn maneuver can improve coordination and timing of pharyngeal swallow events, including timing of posterior movement of the tongue base to the pharyngeal wall in relation to airway closure and cricopharyngeal opening, with elimination of aspiration [167].

Prolonged cricopharyngeal opening times associated with the Mendelsohn maneuver may allow passage of a larger amount of the bolus into the esophagus. The improvement in laryngeal elevation may also reduce residue in the pyriform sinus after the swallow. Increased duration and magnitude of pharyngeal pressure might result in improved propulsion of bolus into the esophagus. The Mendelsohn maneuver is therefore a useful technique for patients who have reduced laryngeal movement, delayed or reduced cricopharyngeal opening, or discoordinated swallow.

Tongue-hold maneuver

The tongue-hold maneuver is a technique for enhancing posterior pharyngeal wall movement. Contact between the tongue base and posterior pharyngeal wall is important for applying pressure on the bolus to aid in transport through the pharynx [178]. Head and neck cancer patients who have had resection of the tongue base or radiation to the oropharynx may experience difficulty achieving contact between the tongue base and pharyngeal wall. The tongue-hold maneuver was designed to augment posterior pharyngeal wall movement.

The patient is instructed to protrude the tongue and hold it between the central incisors while swallowing. Young adult subjects demonstrate a significant increase in posterior pharyngeal wall bulging while performing this maneuver [178]. Treated head and neck cancer patients produce higher pressure at the level of the tongue base and pharyngeal wall while performing this maneuver [170].

It is unfortunate that the tongue-hold maneuver also results in increased pharyngeal residue (especially in the vallecula), reduced laryngeal vestibule closure, and delayed triggering of the pharyngeal swallow [178]. Although as originally conceptualized the tongue-hold maneuver is to be used with a bolus, it is advisable to use the tongue-hold maneuver as an exercise without food for treated head and neck cancer patients because of the significant risk of aspirating vallecular residue during a swallow delay. A trial of the tongue-hold maneuver under fluoroscopy is recommended to see whether the posterior pharyngeal wall responds as anticipated.

Bolus size and consistency modifications

Modification of bolus size and consistency may also be effective in eliminating aspiration in patients treated for head and neck cancer. These changes should be observed under fluoroscopy so that the clinician can determine their impact on swallow physiology. For some patients, a larger-volume bolus may be more effective at eliciting a more rapid pharyngeal swallow. Larger volumes may provide greater sensory input for the patient and increase awareness of the bolus in the oral cavity [179,180]; however, patients who require multiple swallows to clear a single bolus will probably benefit from smaller bolus sizes to reduce residue and the risk of aspiration [181].

Patients who have oral-stage problems such as reduced tongue range of motion (ROM), coordination, or strength will have the greatest difficulty with thick foods. Patients who have a delayed pharyngeal swallow or reduced airway closure may benefit from eliminating thin liquids or thickening them to a more viscous consistency. Those who have swallowing disorders that result in retention of bolus in the pharynx (such as reduced tongue-base retraction, reduced laryngeal elevation, and cricopharyngeal dysfunction) will have greater difficulty with thicker, higher-viscosity foods [182].

Removal of specific food consistencies from the diet should be the last strategy to be contemplated [149]. Elimination of certain food consistencies from the diet, such as liquids, can be difficult for the patient and may have an impact on the patient's nutritional status. Modification of bolus consistency should be considered when postures and maneuvers are not feasible or are unsuccessful.

Therapy procedures

Aspiration may be eliminated through the use of postures, maneuvers, and modifications to bolus size and consistency; however, until the swallow physiology can be improved, a patient will need to use these techniques consistently while eating to maintain oral intake. The following are active therapy procedures that have been designed to improve impaired swallow function after treatment of cancer of the head and neck.

Range of motion exercises

The normal ROM of the lips, jaw, tongue, and larynx is often disrupted after treatment of cancer of the head and neck as a result of surgical resection and reconstruction of the structures, fibrosis induced by radiation, or both. ROM exercises are designed to improve the movement by extending the target structure in a desired direction until a strong stretch is felt. The stretched position is held for 1 second and then the structure is relaxed [149]. It has been shown that postsurgical patients who perform ROM exercises in the first 3 months after surgery have significantly better swallowing function than those who do not perform these exercises [183]. ROM exercises can be used for the lips, jaw, oral tongue, tongue base, larynx, and hyoid-related musculature. Although the optimal frequency and duration of ROM exercises is not yet determined, 5 to 10 repetitions of each exercise for 5 to 10 sessions per day are generally recommended [149,183,184].

Jaw range-of-motion exercises

Restricted mouth opening, often referred to as trismus, may result from surgical resection of the muscles of mastication, scarring after ablation of a portion of the mandible, or fibrosis of irradiated tissues. Current methods used to increase mouth opening include unassisted jaw ROM exercises, finger-assisted stretching exercises, stacked tongue depressors, and mechanical assistance with a device such as the TheraBite (Atos Medical Inc., Milwaukee, WI).

The jaw may be exercised by instructing the patient to open the mouth as widely as possible without causing pain and to hold this position for 2 seconds. The patient should next move the jaw to the right side as far as possible, hold for 2 seconds, then relax, and repeat the same movement on the left side. Finally, the patient should move the jaw in a circular movement, relaxing after completing a full circle. The patient should repeat the preceding exercises 5 to 10 times per session, with the goal of 5 to 10 sessions per day.

Patients who have very restricted oral aperture may assist jaw opening by stacking wooden tongue blades and inserting them between the teeth, adding additional tongue blades as ROM increases. Mechanical devices such as the TheraBite may provide assistance with mouth opening. A mechanical device may increase jaw opening more than other methods of stretching [185]; however, research indicates that unassisted stretching exercises, the use of stacked tongue depressors, and assistance by mechanical devices are all effective at increasing jaw opening in treated head and neck cancer patients [186,187].

Tongue range-of-motion exercises

Scarring of the tongue after surgery may prevent sufficient ROM to clear the bolus from the oral cavity; reconstruction procedures that tether the tongue anteriorly negatively impact tongue-base retraction. Fibrosis after radiotherapy also reduces the tongue's ability to move normally. ROM exercises may be used for the oral tongue and tongue base to improve movement.

Oral tongue range-of-motion exercises. Tongue ROM exercises for the oral tongue include extension, lateralization, elevation, and retraction [149]. Instruct the patient to stick out the tongue as far as possible past the lips without feeling pain, hold for 2 seconds, and then relax. Next have the patient move the tongue to the right corner of the mouth (stretching as far as possible), hold for 2 seconds, and then relax. Repeat this extension on the left side. To elevate the front of the tongue, instruct the patient to lift the tip of the tongue and place it behind the top teeth along the alveolar ridge, hold the position for 2 seconds, and then relax. To elevate the back of the tongue, instruct the patient to raise the tongue as if to produce /k/ or /g/, hold the position for 2 seconds, and then relax. As the patient's tongue elevation improves, extend the stretch by instructing the patient to lower the jaw as far as possible while holding the elevated tongue positions. For tongue retraction, instruct the patient to pull the tongue straight back in the mouth as far as it will go, hold for 2 seconds, and then relax. Suggesting imagery of gargling or yawning may elicit greater retraction [188]. Have the patient repeat the preceding exercises 5 to 10 times.

Bolus manipulation exercises. Bolus manipulation exercises are a form of ROM exercise intended to enhance tongue movements required for chewing, bolus formation, and bolus transport [149]. The exercises may be performed with a strip of gauze soaked in water or beverage, a flexible licorice stick or similar candy, or a small lollipop on a stick.

Tongue cupping is an exercise to practice holding a bolus in the oral cavity. Instruct the patient to take a piece of soaked gauze (or licorice stick or lollipop) and place it on the middle of the tongue, holding on to the other end outside the mouth. The patient is asked hold the gauze against the roof of the mouth so that the tip of the tongue is sealed behind the alveolar ridge and the sides of the tongue are against the roof of the mouth near the molars (or gums if the patient has no teeth). The patient should hold the position for 5 seconds and then relax. Have the patient repeat this exercise 5 to 10 times.

Tongue side-to-side movement is an exercise to practice moving the bolus back and forth onto the teeth or gums for chewing. Instruct the patient to take the gauze and place it on the tongue, holding the end of the gauze outside the mouth. The patient should maneuver the gauze around in the mouth over to the left, then to the middle, then to the right, and back again, repeating this circuit 5 to 10 times. As the patient improves with lateralizing the gauze, he or she may be challenged by using a piece of loose hard candy.

Tongue posterior movement is an exercise to practice transporting the bolus through the oral cavity. Instruct the patient to take a piece of gauze and place it on the tongue, holding the other end outside the mouth. The patient should move the gauze up and back with the tongue, as if attempting to swallow the gauze. If the gauze is soaked in a beverage, ask the patient to try to squeeze the liquid from the gauze and swallow (if it is safe for the patient to swallow). Have the patient repeat this task 5 to 10 times.

Tongue-base range-of-motion exercises. Retraction of the tongue as far back as possible in the oral cavity will exercise the tongue base. Other exercises for tongue-base ROM include pretending to gargle and pretending to yawn, as discussed in the oral-tongue ROM section. Although the gargle task has been demonstrated to elicit the most tongue-base retraction compared with pretending to yawn and pulling the tongue back as far as possible [188], it is wise for the individual patient to try several techniques to determine which is the most effective. If reduced tongue-base retraction is identified on MBS, it is wise to determine the effects of tongue retraction, yawn, and gargle imagery under fluoroscopy so that the most effective procedure may be integrated into the patient's swallow therapy plan.

Some maneuvers are also effective at increasing tongue-base ROM. As discussed in the "Interventions during the modified barium swallow" section, the Mendelsohn maneuver, effortful swallow, and supersupraglottic swallow are not only effective at producing their intended target move but also result in increased tongue-base retraction [167,170]. Practicing these maneuvers with or without food as indicated for swallow safety may exercise the tongue base and enhance retraction.

Laryngeal range-of-motion exercises

Reduced laryngeal elevation is often reported in treated head and neck cancer patients, especially in those who have been irradiated. It has been demonstrated that reduced laryngeal elevation is significantly correlated with limitations in oral intake and diet during the first year after cancer treatment [189], so improving laryngeal ROM is a very important goal when formulating a swallow therapy plan for treated head and neck cancer patients.

Falsetto voice exercise. A falsetto voice exercise may be useful in improving laryngeal ROM for elevation. During falsetto voice production, the larynx elevates nearly as much as it does during the swallow. The patient is asked to slide up the pitch scale as high as possible, into a high squeaky voice. At the top of the scale, the patient should hold the note for several seconds with as much effort as possible. The clinician may manually assist the patient in raising the larynx if necessary, with the ultimate aim to eventually eliminate the manual assist.

Mendelsohn maneuver. As previously discussed in the "Interventions during the modified barium swallow" section, the Mendelsohn maneuver is a voluntary prolongation of laryngeal excursion at the midpoint of the swallow intended to increase the extent and duration of laryngeal elevation and thereby increase the duration of cricopharyngeal opening. Research has indicated that it is effective at increasing the extent and duration of laryngeal elevation and the duration of cricopharyngeal opening [167,176]. The Mendelsohn maneuver may be practiced with or without a bolus as dictated for safety.

Shaker exercise for hyolaryngeal range of motion. Another exercise that holds promise for patients who have cricopharyngeal dysfunction is the Shaker exercise. Because the suprahyoid muscle group responsible for displacement of the hyolaryngeal complex and opening of the UES appears responsive to external influences, a simple isometric/isokinetic head-lift exercise aimed at these muscles was developed and tested [190].

The Shaker exercise consists of 3 repetitive 1-minute sustained head raisings in the supine position, interrupted by a 1-minute rest period. Sustained head-raising exercises are followed by 30 consecutive repetitions of head raisings in the same supine position. For the sustained and repetitive head raisings, subjects are instructed to raise the head high and forward enough to be able to see their toes without raising shoulders off the ground. The rationale for the exercise is to build strength in the suprahyoid musculature, thus enhancing hyoid and laryngeal elevation, which may permit longer and wider opening of the UES.

The Shaker exercise has produced encouraging results in remedying or improving UES-related dysphagia [191,192], although its efficacy for treating dysphagia after treatment of head and neck cancer has not yet been demonstrated.

Neuromuscular electrical stimulation. Surface neuromuscular electrical stimulation (NMES) has recently been proposed as a treatment option for pharyngeal dysphagia [193]. Surface electrical stimulation is applied through electrodes placed on the neck, with the goal of promoting increased hyoid or laryngeal elevation. If surface NMES, commonly referred to as E-stim, can stimulate the deep strap muscles of the head and neck, then it could benefit treated head and neck cancer patients who experience reduced laryngeal elevation. Because surface NMES is intended to improve hyolaryngeal elevation, it can be considered an ROM exercise and is therefore discussed in this section.

NMES for dysphagia has become a widely used clinical procedure yet is accompanied by considerable controversy because of a lack of physiologic rationale and limited published efficacy data. The available literature yields mixed results concerning the ability of NMES to improve swallow function. Reported success rates after treatment with surface NMES range from 40% in patients who have severe dysphagia [194] to 98% in patients who have dysphagia after stroke [193]. Significant improvements also have been reported in swallow function in a long-term acute care setting [195].

Conversely, research investigations have shown that 85% of subjects failed to exhibit gain in myoelectrical activity in the submental muscles after 10 1-hour sessions of NMES [196]. Videofluoroscopic evaluation of hyolaryngeal movement during surface NMES revealed that contrary to the intended goal of treatment, NMES (provided through nine recommended electrode placement loci) significantly lowered the hyoid and larynx. Stimulated swallows were also judged as less safe than nonstimulated swallows using the National Institutes of Health Swallowing Safety Scale [197].

Meta-analyses indicate that there is a small but significant summary effect size for surface NMES for swallowing, but that the small number of available studies and their poor methodology indicate the need for more rigorous research in the area [198]. Implementation of NMES in clinical rehabilitation settings is premature [199].

Stroke is the most common etiology of dysphagia treated with surface NMES [200]. No published efficacy data on the use of NMES for treated head and neck cancer patients are available. Given the potential for surface NMES to depress the hyoid and larynx, the clinician should proceed with caution when considering use of this technique in treated head and neck cancer patients. When the clinician chooses to try this procedure, it is advisable to observe the effects of NMES under fluoroscopy.

Laryngeal closure exercises

Patients who have received surgical intervention or radiation to the larynx may have difficulty protecting the airway. Laryngeal closure exercises may be used to improve airway closure at the level of the true cords or higher at the vestibule.

Vocal cord adduction exercises such as producing hard glottal attacks may be used to improve ROM and enhance true cord closure [149]. As discussed earlier, the supersupraglottic swallow is designed to close the entrance to the airway voluntarily by tilting the arytenoid cartilage anteriorly to contact the base of the epiglottis before and during the swallow and by closing the false vocal folds tightly. The patient may practice this maneuver with or without food as needed for swallow safety to enhance closure of the laryngeal vestibule.

Tongue resistance or strengthening exercises

Oral-tongue strength may be reduced in patients who have cancer of the head and neck [201,202]. Resistance or strengthening exercises are used to build or maintain strength in the oral tongue with the rationale that stronger muscles will function better during the swallow. Strengthening exercises usually involve pushing the target structure against some type of resistance and holding it for several seconds [149]. Instruct the patient to extend the tongue and push it against the tongue depressor (or another item such as the back of a spoon) as hard as possible without causing pain. The patient should resist the force of the tongue with the tongue depressor, hold for two seconds, and then relax. Proceed to the side of the tongue. Depending on the patient's ROM, the tongue may be extended outside the corner of the mouth to the right or left side and pushed against the tongue depressor as hard as possible, held for 2 seconds, and relaxed. If tongue ROM is very limited, the patient may place the tongue inside the cheek, making it bulge. Instruct the patient to press against the bulged cheek with a finger, hold for 2 seconds, and relax. This exercise should be repeated on the opposite side. Finally, instruct the patient to push down on the tongue with the tongue depressor while simultaneously pushing up with the tongue. The patient should push against the resistance for 2 seconds and then relax. Each strengthening exercise should be repeated 5 to 10 times per session, with the goal of 5 to 10 sessions per day.

A biofeedback instrument such as the Iowa Oral Pressure Instrument (IOPI) may be useful to the patient in monitoring maximum pressure during tongue strengthening exercises [203], although a study of the effects of tongue strengthening exercises in young healthy adults indicated that there were no significant differences in tongue strength after using a tongue depressor or the IOPI [204]. As with ROM exercises, the optimal frequency and intensity of tongue strengthening exercises has not been determined. The efficacy of tongue strengthening exercises for patients treated for cancer of the head and neck has not yet been demonstrated.

Thermal/tactile stimulation

Delayed triggering of the pharyngeal swallow has been observed in treated head and neck cancer patients. Thermal/tactile stimulation is designed to sensitize or stimulate the area of the oral cavity where the swallow reflex is thought to trigger. The procedure consists of applying cold pressure to the base of the anterior faucial arches [205]. The clinician may perform thermal/tactile stimulation on the patient or may instruct the patient on how to perform the technique for home practice. Instruct the patient to dip a laryngeal mirror into a cup of ice and ice water for 10 seconds. The patient should firmly rub vertically up and down on the anterior faucial arch approximately five times on each side, making sure that the metal side of the mirror is against the tissue (this rubbing should be repeated on the other side only if it is anatomically intact). The patient should remove the mirror, pipette a few drops of water at the faucial arch, and swallow. This procedure should be repeated 10 times.

The effects of thermal/tactile stimulation have been investigated primarily in healthy adults and neurologically impaired patients who have delayed pharyngeal swallow, with some data indicating that thermal/tactile stimulation has no impact on the swallow [180,206–208] and other studies supporting the use of the technique for improving swallow physiology [205,209–212]. There are currently no published data demonstrating the efficacy of thermal/tactile stimulation for treated head and neck cancer patients.

Intraoral prosthestics

Intraoral prosthetics are developed by a maxillofacial prosthodontist with input from the surgeon and a speech pathologist for patients who receive surgical resection in the oral cavity for head and neck tumors. Several varieties of intraoral prostheses may be constructed to compensate for the loss of oropharyngeal structures in postsurgical oral cancer patients. Maxillary reshaping prostheses, also known as palatal drop or palatal-lowering prostheses, are used to recontour and lower the palatal vault so that the remaining portion of the resected tongue can make contact with the palate for speech and swallowing [213–215]. Obturators fill a palatal defect to create separation of the oral and nasal cavities, thereby preventing loss of bolus into the nasopharynx and reestablishing intraoral pressure [214,216,217]. An intraoral prosthesis may incorporate an obturator and a maxillary reshaping component. The use of intraoral prosthetics may result in a marked reduction in oral residue [213,218,219]. The maxillary reshaping/lowering prosthesis allows the patient to clear more of the bolus from the oral cavity because the resected tongue is able to make contact with the prosthesis, thereby reducing the inaccessible portions of the palate. Obturation of a soft palate defect restores the continuity of the oral cavity chamber required for bolus transport and adequate intraoral pressure, thereby permitting the patient to build sufficient pressure to improve clearance of the bolus from the oral cavity while preventing passage of the bolus into the nasal cavity.

Table 1 summarizes the types of swallowing disorders most often reported for patients treated for head and neck cancer. Associated with each disorder are postures, maneuvers, exercises, and other interventions that have some evidence in the literature for being effective in alleviating the disorder or reducing its negative impact on swallowing. This table should not be considered all-inclusive. As understanding of swallow physiology and the effects of cancer treatment evolves, more interventions will be developed and become available to the clinician.

Timing of dysphagia rehabilitation for patients who have head and neck cancer

The speech pathologist or other dysphagia rehabilitation specialist who works with head and neck cancer patients is part of a multidisciplinary team that may include surgeons, radiation and medical oncologists, dentists or maxillofacial prosthodontists, nurses, physical therapists, and social workers. Ideally, the clinician has the opportunity to provide pretreatment counseling to inform the patient and family of the possible swallowing problems that may occur during and after treatment and to provide information concerning posttreatment swallow rehabilitation. Because surgical patients are often admitted to the hospital on the day of surgery, the clinician may not have an opportunity for pretreatment counseling in person but may communicate necessary information by phone. Patients who are to be treated with chemoradiotherapy may be counseled at bedside just before the onset of treatment [220].

Because fibrosis of irradiated tissues is related to many of the swallowing problems experienced by treated head and neck cancer patients, exercises for preventing or reducing the effects of fibrosis should be provided before treatment. ROM and resistance exercises may be used as a strategy for preventing swallowing disorders before they develop in patients undergoing treatment of cancer of the head and neck. Use of tongue and jaw ROM exercises during primary or postoperative radiotherapy may help prevent trismus, reduce the formation of fibrotic tissue, and improve pharyngeal clearance by maintaining adequate contact between the tongue base and pharyngeal wall. Some limited data indicate that patients who perform ROM exercises before and during chemoradiation have significantly greater quality of life for swallowing than those who perform the exercises post treatment only [221]. Patients should also be encouraged to keep using the swallow mechanism for oral intake even if there is a gastrostomy tube in place. As discussed in the section on adverse effects of chemoradiation,

Table 1
Swallowing disorders and their associated interventions

Swallow-related disorder	Possible interventions
Reduced mouth opening	Jaw ROM exercises
Reduced tongue control/shaping	Chin-down posture
	Supersupraglottic swallow
	Tongue ROM exercises
	Bolus manipulation exercises
	Tongue strengthening exercises
Reduced vertical tongue movement	Tongue ROM exercises
	Maxillary reshaping prosthesis
Reduced anterior-to-posterior tongue movement	Head-back posture
	Multiple swallows
	Alternate liquids and solids
	Tongue ROM exercises
	Bolus manipulation exercises
	Maxillary reshaping prosthesis
Reduced tongue strength	Effortful swallow
	Tongue strengthening exercises
Delayed pharyngeal swallow	Chin-down posture
	Supersupraglottic swallow
	Thermal/tactile stimulation
Reduced tongue-base retraction	Chin-down posture
	Effortful swallow
	Supersupraglottic swallow
	Tongue-hold maneuver
	Mendelsohn maneuver
	Tongue ROM exercises
	Gargle/yawn for tongue-base retraction
Reduced laryngeal vestibule closure	Chin-down posture
	Supersupraglottic swallow
	Effortful swallow
	Mendelsohn maneuver
	Gargle/yawn for tongue-base retraction
Reduced laryngeal elevation	Mendelsohn maneuver
	Chin-down posture
	Supersupraglottic swallow
	Effortful swallow
	Laryngeal ROM exercises
	Shaker exercise
Reduced glottic closure	Head rotation to weaker side
	Supersupraglottic swallow
	Thickened liquids
	Vocal-fold adduction exercises
Reduced pharyngeal constriction/clearance	Head rotation to weaker side
	Effortful swallow
	Mendelsohn maneuver
	Multiple swallows
	Alternate liquids and solids
	Gargle/yawn for tongue-base retraction
	Tongue-hold maneuver
Reduced/impaired cricopharyngeal opening	Head rotation to weaker side
	Mendelsohn maneuver
	Shaker exercise
	Effortful swallow

strictures are more likely to develop in the hypopharynx or proximal esophagus when a gastrostomy tube is in place rather than a nasogastric tube because of disuse atrophy and secondary healing of opposing ulcerated tissue in the postcricoid hypoharynx [145,147,148]. It is possible that patients who continue to use the swallowing mechanism, even just a small amount, may reduce the potential for stricture development.

Patients should be encouraged to perform their exercises every day; however, as radiotherapy progresses, most patients feel that they do not have the energy to practice. Also, signs of mucositis may appear as early as the first couple of weeks into radiotherapy [139,143]. The pain associated with mucositis also impacts a patient's desire to work with ROM and resistance exercises. Although this reluctance is understandable, the clinician should continue to encourage the patient to practice as much as possible during the course of treatment to reduce the severity of posttreatment swallow disorders.

After treatment is completed, the dysphagia rehabilitation specialist should evaluate the patient's swallow function and formulate a plan for therapy as soon as the patient is medically cleared to begin work on swallowing function. Early initiation of swallowing therapy is generally advocated [126,145,222], although there is little research available demonstrating the optimal timing, intensity, or duration of such treatment. A randomized study of swallow therapy initiated more than a year after completion of cancer treatment revealed no significant improvement in swallowing function [184], suggesting that amelioration of long-standing dysphagia may not be possible. Because fibrosis of irradiated tissues may continue to develop years after completion of cancer treatment [117,122,127], patients should continue to practice ROM and resistance exercises regularly for the rest of their lives to keep the negative effects of fibrosis on swallowing function at a minimum.

Efficacy of swallowing therapy procedures for patients who have head and neck cancer

Throughout this article, the efficacy of individual postures, maneuvers, and other therapy procedures reported in the literature has been noted. Although there is considerable evidence that these interventions work with treated head and neck cancer patients, there are still many unanswered questions concerning (1) the relative contributions of the various therapy techniques to improve swallow function; (2) the optimal frequency, timing, and intensity of swallow rehabilitation programs; and (3) the impact of patient practice and feedback strategies. Randomized clinical trials are the gold standard in treatment efficacy studies. A number of randomized clinical trials have been instituted in the past few years that address some of these issues and may demonstrate the superiority of various therapy procedures in treated head and neck cancer patients [223]. One study funded by the

National Institute of Diabetes and Digestive and Kidney Diseases compared the effects of the Shaker exercise with ROM exercise in treated head and neck cancer patients and poststroke patients. A second study, funded by the National Cancer Institute, compared a program of ROM exercises with postural/sensory intervention in treated head and neck cancer patients. Both trials were completed in 2007; the results have not been published at this time. A third clinical trial funded by the National Cancer Institute will compare surface NMES combined with ROM exercises with ROM exercises alone in irradiated head and neck cancer patients. This trial will begin accrual in 2008. The results of these and future randomized clinical trials for swallowing therapy procedures will aid the clinician in choosing the most effective approaches for rehabilitating dysphagia after treatment of cancer of the head and neck.

Summary

Patients who have cancers of the head and neck may be treated with surgery, radiotherapy, chemotherapy, or a combination. Each treatment modality may have a negative impact on posttreatment swallowing function. The clinician has a number of rehabilitative procedures available to reduce or eliminate swallowing disorders in patients treated for cancer of the head and neck. After diagnosing the swallowing disorder with the MBS procedure, the clinician can use postures, maneuvers, and exercises to treat the swallow disorder and to help the patient achieve optimal function. The efficacy of various treatment procedures for dysphagia still needs to be examined in carefully controlled randomized clinical trials. The field of dysphagia rehabilitation will continue to grow as novel approaches for cancer treatment are developed, possibly resulting in new manifestations of swallow dysfunction. Dysphagia rehabilitation specialists will continue to meet these challenges by developing new interventions to reduce the adverse effects of cancer treatment on swallowing function.

References

[1] Day TA, Davis BK, Gillespie MB, et al. Oral cancer treatment. Curr Treat Options Oncol 2003;4:27–41.

[2] Andry G, Hamoir M, Leemans CR. The evolving role of surgery in the management of head and neck tumors. Curr Opin Oncol 2005;17(3):241–8.

[3] McConnel FM, Logemann JA, Rademaker AW, et al. Surgical variables affecting postoperative swallowing efficiency in oral cancer patients: a pilot study. Laryngoscope 1994;104: 87–90.

[4] Martini DV, Har-El G, Lucente FE, et al. Swallowing and pharyngeal function in postoperative pharyngeal cancer patients. Ear Nose Throat J 1997;76:450–6.

[5] Hirano M, Kuroiwa Y, Tanaka S, et al. Dysphagia following various degrees of surgical resection for oral cancer. Ann Otol Rhinol Laryngol 1992;101:138–41.

[6] Fujimoto Y, Hasegawa Y, Nakayama B, et al. Usefulness and limitation of cricopharyngeal myotomy and laryngeal suspension after wide resection of the tongue or oropharynx. Nippon Jibiinkoka Gakkai Kaiho 1998;101:307–11.

[7] Gagnebin J, Jaques B, Pasche P. [Reconstruction of the anterior floor of mouth by surgical flap microanastomosis: oncologic and functional results]. Schweiz Med Wochenschr Suppl 2000;116:39S–42S [in French].

[8] Zuydam AC, Rogers SN, Brown JS, et al. Swallowing rehabilitation after oropharyngeal resection for squamous cell carcinoma. Br J Oral Maxillofac Surg 2000;38:513–8.

[9] Konsulov SS. Surgical treatment of anterolateral tongue carcinoma. Folia Med (Plovdiv) 2005;47(3–4):20–3.

[10] Nicoletti G, Soutar DS, Jackson MS, et al. Chewing and swallowing after surgical treatment for oral cancer: functional evaluation in 196 selected cases. Plast Reconstr Surg 2004;114:329–38.

[11] Leder SB, Joe JK, Ross DA, et al. Presence of a tracheostomy tube and aspiration status in early, postsurgical head and neck cancer patients. Head Neck 2005;27:757–61.

[12] Jacobson MC, Franssen E, Fliss DM, et al. Free forearm flap in oral reconstruction. Arch Otolaryngol Head Neck Surg 1995;121:959–64.

[13] Pauloski BR, Rademaker AW, Logemann JA, et al. Surgical variables affecting swallowing in treated oral/oropharyngeal cancer patients. Head Neck 2004;26:625–36.

[14] Logemann JA, Bytell DE. Swallowing disorders in three types of head and neck surgical patients. Cancer 1979;81:469–78.

[15] Pauloski BR, Logemann JA, Rademaker AW, et al. Speech and swallowing function after anterior tongue and floor of mouth resection with distal flap reconstruction. J Speech Hear Res 1993;36:267–76.

[16] Furia CL, Carrara-de Angelis E, Martins NM, et al. Videofluoroscopic evaluation after glossectomy. Arch Otolaryngol Head Neck Surg 2000;126:378–83.

[17] Krappen S, Remmert S, Gehrking E, et al. Cinematographic functional diagnosis of swallowing after plastic reconstruction of large tumor defects of the mouth cavity and pharynx. Laryngorhinootologie 1997;76:229–34.

[18] Su WF, Hsia YJ, Chang YC, et al. Functional comparison after reconstruction with a radial forearm free flap or a pectoralis major flap for cancer of the tongue. Otolaryngol Head Neck Surg 2003;128(3):412–8.

[19] Borggreven PA, Verdonck-de Leeuw I, Rinkel RN, et al. Swallowing after major surgery of the oral cavity or oropharynx: a prospective and longitudinal assessment of patients treated by microvascular soft tissue reconstruction. Head Neck 2007;29:638–47.

[20] Logemann JA, Pauloski BR, Rademaker AW, et al. Speech and swallow function after tonsil/base of tongue resection with primary closure. J Speech Hear Res 1993;36:918–26.

[21] Tei K, Maekawa K, Kitada H, et al. Recovery from postsurgical swallowing dysfunction in patients with oral cancer. J Maxillofac Surg 2007;65:1077–83.

[22] Marchetta FC. Function and appearance following surgery for intraoral cancer. Clin Plast Surg 1976;3:471–9.

[23] Christopoulos E, Carrau R, Segas J, et al. Transmandibular approaches to the oral cavity and oropharynx. A functional assessment. Arch Otolaryngol Head Neck Surg 1992;118:1164–7.

[24] Schliephake H, Ruffert K, Schneller T. Prospective study of the quality of life of cancer patients after intraoral tumor surgery. J Oral Maxillofac Surg 1996;54:664–9.

[25] Haribhakti VV, Kavarana NM, Tibrewala AN. Oral cavity reconstruction: an objective assessment of function. Head Neck 1993;15:119–24.

[26] Urken ML, Buchbinder D, Weinberg H, et al. Functional evaluation following microvascular oromandibular reconstruction of the oral cancer patient: a comparative study of reconstructed and nonreconstructed patients. Laryngoscope 1991;101:935–50.

[27] Curtis DA, Plesh O, Miller AJ, et al. A comparison of masticatory function in patients with or without reconstruction of the mandible. Head Neck 1997;19:287–96.

[28] Schramm VL, Johnson JT, Myers EN. Skin grafts and flaps in oral cavity reconstruction. Arch Otolaryngol 1983;109:175–7.

[29] Baek S, Lawson W, Biller H. An analysis of 133 pectoralis major myocutaneous flaps. Plast Reconstr Surg 1982;69:460–7.

[30] Teichgraeber J, Bowman J, Goepfert H. New test series for the functional evaluation of oral cavity cancer. Head Neck Surg 1985;8:9–20.

[31] Anain SA, Yetman RJ. The fate of intraoral free muscle flaps: is skin necessary? Plast Reconstr Surg 1993;91:1027–31.

[32] Schliephake H, Neukam FW, Schmelzeisen R, et al. Long-term quality of life after ablative intraoral tumour surgery. J Craniomaxillofac Surg 1995;23:243–9.

[33] Hamlet S, Jones L, Patterson R, et al. Swallowing recovery following anterior tongue and floor of mouth surgery. Head Neck 1991;13:334–9.

[34] Soutar DS, McGregor IA. The radial forearm flap in intraoral reconstruction: the experience of 60 consecutive cases. Plast Reconstr Surg 1986;78:1–8.

[35] Song R, Gao Y, Song Y, et al. The forearm flap. Clin Plast Surg 1982;9:21–6.

[36] McGregor IA. Fasciocutaneous flaps in intraoral reconstruction. Clin Plast Surg 1985;12: 453–61.

[37] Lovie MJ, Duncan GM, Glasson DW. The ulnar artery forearm free flap. Br J Plast Surg 1984;37:486–92.

[38] Christie DRH, Duncan GM, Glasson DW. The ulnar artery free flap: the first 7 years. Plast Reconstr Surg 1994;93:547–51.

[39] Urken ML, Biller HF. A new bilobed design for the sensate radial forearm flap to preserve tongue mobility following significant glossectomy. Arch Otolaryngol Head Neck Surg 1994;120:26–31.

[40] Salibian AH, Allison GR, Krugman ME, et al. Reconstruction of the base of the tongue with the microvascular ulnar forearm flap: a functional assessment. Plast Reconstr Surg 1995;96:1081–9.

[41] Uwiera T, Seikaly H, Rieger J, et al. Functional outcomes after hemiglossectomy and reconstruction with a bilobed radial forearm free flap. J Otolaryngol 2004;33(6):356–9.

[42] Civantos FJ, Burkey B, Lu FL, et al. Lateral arm microvascular flap in head and neck reconstruction. Arch Otolaryngol Head Neck Surg 1997;123:830–6.

[43] Hsiao HT, Leu YS, Lin CC. Primary closure versus radial forearm flap reconstruction after hemiglossectomy: functional assessment of swallowing and speech. Ann Plast Surg 2002;49: 612–6.

[44] Hsiao HT, Leu YS, Chang SH, et al. Swallowing function in patients who underwent hemiglossectomy: comparison of primary closure and free radial forearm flap reconstruction with videofluoroscopy. Ann Plast Surg 2003;50:450–5.

[45] Rogers SN, Lowe D, Patel M, et al. Clinical function after primary surgery for oral and oropharyngeal cancer: an 11-item examination. Br J Oral Maxillofac Surg 2002;40:1–10.

[46] Zuydam AC, Lowe D, Brown JS, et al. Predictors of speech and swallowing function following primary surgery for oral and oropharyngeal cancer. Clin Otolaryngol 2005;30: 428–37.

[47] Markkanen-Leppanen M, Isotalo E, Makitie AA, et al. Swallowing after free-flap reconstruction in patients with oral and pharyngeal cancer. Oral Oncol 2006;42:501–9.

[48] Yu P. Reinnervated anterolateral thigh flap for tongue reconstruction. Head Neck 2004;26: 1038–44.

[49] Mah SM, Durham JS, Anderson DW, et al. Functional results in oral cavity reconstruction using reinnervated versus nonreinnervated free fasciocutaneous grafts. J Otolaryngol 1996; 25:75–81.

[50] McConnel FMS, Pauloski BR, Logemann JA, et al. The functional results of primary closure versus flaps in oropharyngeal reconstruction: a prospective study of speech and swallowing. Arch Otolaryngol Head Neck Surg 1998;124:625–30.

[51] Rinaldo A, Ferlito A. Open supraglottic laryngectomy. Acta Otolaryngol 2004;124:768–71.

[52] Wein RO, Weber RS. The current role of vertical partial laryngectomy and open supraglottic laryngectomy. Curr Probl Cancer 2005;29(4):201–14.

[53] Yeager LB, Grillone GA. Organ preservation surgery for intermediate size (T2 and T3) laryngeal cancer. Otolaryngol Clin North Am 2005;38:11–20.

[54] Bocca E. Supraglottic cancer. Laryngoscope 1975;85:1318–26.

[55] Ogura J, Biller H, Calcaterra T, et al. Surgical treatment of carcinoma of the larynx, pharynx, base of tongue and cervical esophagus. Int Surg 1969;52:29–40.

[56] Lazarus CL. Effects of radiation therapy and voluntary maneuvers on swallow functioning in head and neck cancer patients. Clin Commun Disord 1993;3:11–20.

[57] Litton W, Leonard J. Aspiration after partial laryngectomy: cineradiographic studies-Laryngoscope 1969;79:888–908.

[58] Logemann JA, Gibbons PJ, Rademaker AW, et al. Mechanisms of recovery of swallow after supraglottic laryngectomy. J Speech Hear Res 1994;37:965–74.

[59] Kreuzer SH, Schima W, Schober E, et al. Complications after laryngeal surgery: videofluoroscopic evaluation of 120 patients. Clin Radiol 2000;55:775–81.

[60] McConnel FMS, Mendelsohn MS, Logemann JA. Manofluorography of deglutition after supraglottic laryngectomy. Head Neck Surg 1987;9:142–50.

[61] Staple T, Ogura J. Cineradiography of the swallowing mechanism following supraglottic subtotal laryngectomy. Radiology 1966;87:226–30.

[62] Prades JM, Simon PG, Timoshenko AP, et al. Extended and standard supraglottic laryngectomies: a review of 110 patients. Eur Arch Otorhinolaryngol 2005;262:947–52.

[63] Rademaker AW, Logemann JA, Pauloski BR, et al. Recovery of postoperative swallowing in patients undergoing partial laryngectomy. Head Neck 1993;15:325–34.

[64] Sessions D, Zill R, Schwartz J. Deglutition after conservation surgery for cancer of the larynx and hypopharynx. Otolaryngol Head Neck Surg 1979;87:779–96.

[65] Jacob R, Zorowka P, Welkoborsky HJ, et al. [Long-term functional outcome of Laccourreye hemipharyngectomy-hemilaryngectomy with reference to oncologic outcome]. Laryngorhinootologie 1998;77(2):93–9 [in German].

[66] Hagen R. [Functional long-term results following hemipharyngo-hemilaryngectomy and microvascular reconstruction using the radial forearm flap]. Laryngorhinootologie 2002; 81(3):233–42 [in German].

[67] Jovic R, Majdevac Z. [Swallowing and breathing after partial resection of the larynx]. Srp Arh Celok Lek 1994;122(11–12):319–22 [in Serbian].

[68] Tufano R. Organ preservation surgery for laryngeal cancer. Otolaryngol Clin North Am 2002;35:1067–80.

[69] DiSantis DJ, Balfe DM, Koehler RE, et al. Barium examination of the pharynx after vertical hemilaryngectomy. AJR Am J Roentgenol 1983;141(2):335–9.

[70] Duranceau A, Jamieson G, Hurwitz AL, et al. Alteration in esophageal motility after laryngectomy. Am J Surg 1976;131:30–5.

[71] Hanks JB, Fisher SR, Meyers WC, et al. Effect of total laryngectomy on esophageal motility. Ann Otol Rhinol Laryngol 1981;90:331–4.

[72] McConnel FM, Mendelsohn MS, Logemann JA. Examination of swallowing after total laryngectomy using manofluorography. Head Neck Surg 1986;9:3–12.

[73] McConnel FM, Cerenko D, Mendelsohn MS. Dysphagia after total laryngectomy. Otolaryngol Clin North Am 1988;21:721–6.

[74] Gates G. Upper esophageal sphincter: pre and post-laryngectomy—a normative study-Laryngoscope 1980;90:454–64.

[75] Pauloski BR, Blom ED, Logemann JA, et al. Functional outcome after surgery for prevention of pharyngospasms in tracheoesophageal speakers. Part II: swallow characteristics. Laryngoscope 1995;105:1104–10.

[76] Lazarus CL, Logemann JA, Shi G, et al. Does total laryngectomy improve swallowing after primary treatment of radiotherapy and chemotherapy?—A case study. Arch Otolaryngol Head Neck Surg 2002;128:54–7.

[77] Lewin JA, Barringer DA, May AH, et al. Functional outcomes after circumferential pharyngoesophageal reconstruction. Laryngoscope 2005;115:1266–71.

[78] Genden EM, Ferlito A, Silver CE, et al. Evolution of the management of laryngeal cancer. Oral Oncol 2007;43(5):431–9.

[79] Ganly I, Patel S, Matsuo J, et al. Postoperative complications of salvage total laryngectomy. Cancer 2005;103:2073–81.

[80] Grau C, Johansen LV, Hansen HS, et al. Salvage laryngectomy and pharyngocutaneous fistulae after primary radiotherapy for head and neck cancer: a national survey from DAHANCA. Head Neck 2003;25:711–6.

[81] Jansma J, Vissink A, Bouma J, et al. A survey of prevention and treatment regimens for oral sequelae resulting from head and neck radiotherapy used in Dutch radiotherapy institutes. Int J Radiat Oncol Biol Phys 1992;24:359–67.

[82] Jansma J, Vissink A, Spijkervet FK, et al. Protocol for the prevention and treatment of oral sequelae resulting from head and neck radiotherapy. Cancer 1992;70:2171–80.

[83] Nguyen NP, Sallah S, Karlsson U, et al. Combined chemotherapy and radiation therapy for head and neck malignancies: quality of life issues. Cancer 2002;94:1131–41.

[84] Trotti A, Bellm LA, Epstein JB, et al. Mucositis incidence, severity and associated outcomes in patients with head and neck cancer receiving radiotherapy with or without chemotherapy: a systematic literature review. Radiother Oncol 2003;66(3):253–62.

[85] Logemann JA, Pauloski BR, Rademaker AW, et al. Xerostomia: 12-month changes in saliva production and its relationship to perception of swallow function, oral intake and diet after chemoradiation. Head Neck 2003;25:432–7.

[86] Pauloski BR, Rademaker AW, Logemann JA, et al. Speech and swallowing in irradiated and nonirradiated postsurgical oral cancer patients. Otolaryngol Head Neck Surg 1998; 118:616–24.

[87] Pauloski BR, Logemann JA. Impact of tongue base and posterior pharyngeal wall biomechanics on pharyngeal clearance in irradiated postsurgical oral and oropharyngeal cancer patients. Head Neck 2000;22:120–31.

[88] Pauloski BR, Logemann JA, Rademaker AW, et al. Speech and swallowing function after oral and oropharyngeal resections: one year follow-up. Head Neck 1994;16:313–22.

[89] Hara I, Gellrich NC, Duker J, et al. Evaluation of swallowing function after intraoral soft tissue reconstruction with microvasular free flaps. Int J Oral Maxillofac Surg 2003;32: 593–9.

[90] Wolf G, Hong K, Fisher S, et al. Department of Veterans Affairs laryngeal cancer study group. Induction chemotherapy plus radiation compared with surgery plus radiation in patients with advanced laryngeal cancer. N Engl J Med 1991;324:1685–90.

[91] Robbins KT, Vicario D, Seagren S, et al. A targeted supradose cisplatin chemoradiation protocol for advanced head and neck cancer. Am J Surg 1994;168:419–22.

[92] Lefebvre JL, Chevalier D, Luboinski B, et al. EORTC Head and Neck Cancer Cooperative Group. Larynx preservation in pyriform sinus cancer: preliminary results of a European Organization for Research and Treatment of Cancer phase III trial. J Natl Cancer Inst 1996;88:890–9.

[93] Browman GP, Hodson DI, Mackenzie RJ, et al. Cancer Care Ontario Practice Guideline Initiative Head and Neck Cancer Disease Site Group. Choosing a concomitant chemotherapy and radiotherapy regimen for squamous cell head and neck cancer: a systematic review of the published literature with subgroup analysis. Head Neck 2001;23:579–89.

[94] Kies MS, Haraf DJ, Rosen F, et al. Concomitant infusional paclitaxel and fluorouracil, oral hydroxyurea and hyperfractionated radiation for locally advanced squamous cell head and neck cancer. J Clin Oncol 2001;19:1961–9.

[95] Rosen FR, Haraf DJ, Kies MS, et al. Multicenter randomized phase II study of paclitaxel (1-hour infusion), fluorouracil, hydroxyurea, and concomitant twice daily radiation with or without erythropoietin for advanced head and neck cancer. Clin Cancer Res 2003;9: 1689–97.

[96] Vokes EE, Stenson K, Rosen FR, et al. Weekly carboplatin and paclitaxel followed by concomitant paclitaxel, fluorouracil, and hydroxyurea chemoradiotherapy: curative and organ-preserving therapy for advanced head and neck cancer. J Clin Oncol 2003;21:320–6.

[97] Weber RS, Berkey BA, Forastiere A, et al. Outcome of salvage total laryngectomy following organ preservation therapy: the Radiation Therapy Oncology Group trial 91-11. Arch Otolaryngol Head Neck Surg 2003;129:44–9.

[98] Kitamoto Y, Akimoto T, Ishikawa H, et al. Acute toxicity and preliminary clinical outcomes of concurrent radiation therapy and weekly docetaxel and daily cisplatin for head and neck cancer. Jpn J Clin Oncol 2005;35(11):639–44.

[99] Allal AS, Zwahlen D, Becker M, et al. Phase I trial of concomitant hyperfractionated radiotherapy with docetaxel and cisplatin for locally advanced head and neck cancer. Cancer J 2006;12(1):63–8.

[100] Allen AM, Elshaikh M, Worden FP, et al. Acceleration of hyperfractionated chemoradiation regimen for advanced head and neck cancer. Head Neck 2007;29(2):137–42.

[101] Moyer JS, Wolf GT, Bradford CR. Current thoughts on the role of chemotherapy and radiation in advanced head and neck cancer. Curr Opin Otolaryngol Head Neck Surg 2004;12:82–7.

[102] Schwarz JK, Giese W. Organ preservation in patients with squamous cancers of the head and neck. Surg Oncol Clin N Am 2004;13:187–99.

[103] Eisbruch A, Lyden T, Bradford CR, et al. Objective assessment of swallowing dysfunction and aspiration after radiation concurrent with chemotherapy for head and neck cancer. Int J Radiat Oncol Biol Phys 2002;53:23–8.

[104] Eisele DW, Koch DG, Tarazi AE, et al. Aspiration from delayed radiation fibrosis of the neck. Dysphagia 1991;6:120–2.

[105] Graner DE, Foote RL, Kasperbauer JL, et al. Swallow function in patients before and after intra-arterial chemoradiation. Laryngoscope 2003;113:573–9.

[106] Kotz T, Abraham S, Beitler JJ, et al. Pharyngeal transport dysfunction consequent to an organ-sparing protocol. Arch Otolaryngol Head Neck Surg 1999;125:410–3.

[107] Lazarus CL, Logemann JA, Pauloski BR, et al. Swallowing disorders in head and neck cancer patients with radiotherapy and adjuvant chemotherapy. Laryngoscope 1996;106:1157–66.

[108] Smith RV, Kotz T, Beitler JJ, et al. Long-term swallowing problems after organ preservation therapy with concomitant radiation therapy and intravenous hydroxyurea. Arch Otolaryngol Head Neck Surg 2000;126:384–9.

[109] Kotz T, Costello R, Li Y, et al. Swallowing dysfunction after chemoradiation for advanced squamous cell carcinoma of the head and neck. Head Neck 2004;26:365–72.

[110] Nguyen NP, Vos P, Smith HJ, et al. Concurrent chemoradiation for locally advanced Oropharyngeal cancer. Am J Otolaryngol 2007;28:3–8.

[111] Rieger JM, Zalmanowitz JG, Wolfaardt JF. Functional outcomes after organ preservation treatment in head and neck cancer: a critical review of the literature. Int J Oral Maxillofac Surg 2006;35:581–7.

[112] Dworkin JP, Hill SL, Stachler RJ, et al. Swallowing function outcomes following nonsurgical therapy for advanced-stage laryngeal carcinoma. Dysphagia 2006;21:66–74.

[113] Shiley SG, Hargunani CA, Skoner JM, et al. Swallowing function after chemoradiation for advanced oropharyngeal cancer. Otolaryngol Head Neck Surg 2006;134:455–9.

[114] Nguyen NP, Moltz CC, Frank C, et al. Evolution of chronic dysphagia following treatment for head and neck cancer. Oral Oncol 2006;42:374–80.

[115] Ku PK, Yuen EH, Cheung DM, et al. Early swallowing problems in a cohort of patients with nasopharyngeal carcinoma: symptomatology and videofluoroscopic findings. Laryngoscope 2007;117:142–6.

[116] Jensen K, Lambertsen K, Grau C. Late swallowing dysfunction and dysphagia after radiotherapy for pharynx cancer: frequency, intensity and correlation with dose and volume parameters. Radiother Oncol 2007;85:74–82.

[117] Hughes PJ, Scott PJS, Kew J, et al. Dysphagia in treated nasopharyngeal cancer. Head Neck 2000;22:393–7.

[118] Logemann JA, Rademaker AW, Pauloski BR, et al. Site of disease and treatment protocol as correlates of swallowing function in patients with head and neck cancer treated with chemoradiation. Head Neck 2006;28:64–73.

[119] Nguyen NP, Moltz CC, Frank C, et al. Aspiration rate following nonsurgical therapy for laryngeal cancer. ORL J Otorhinolaryngol Relat Spec 2007;69(2):116–20.

[120] Nguyen NP, Moltz CC, Frank C, et al. Effectiveness of the cough reflex in patients with aspiration following radiation for head and neck cancer. Lung 2007;186:243–8.

[121] Carrara-de Angelis E, Feher O, Barros APB, et al. Voice and swallowing in patients enrolled in a larynx preservation trial. Arch Otolaryngol Head Neck Surg 2003;129:733–8.

[122] Chang YC, Chen SY, Lui LT, et al. Dysphagia in patients with nasopharyngeal cancer after radiation therapy: a videofluoroscopic swallowing study. Dysphagia 2003;18:135–43.

[123] Wu C, Hsiao TY, Ko JY, et al. Dysphagia after radiotherapy: endoscopic examination of swallowing in patients with nasopharyngeal carcinoma. Ann Otol Rhinol Laryngol 2000; 109:320–5.

[124] Goguen LA, Posner M, Norris CM, et al. Dysphagia after sequential chemoradiation therapy for advanced head and neck cancer. Otolaryngol Head Neck Surg 2006;134:916–22.

[125] Logemann JA, Pauloski BR, Rademaker AW, et al. Swallowing disorders in the first year after radiation and chemoradiation. Head Neck 2008;30:148–58.

[126] Sullivan CA, Jaklitsch MT, Haddad R, et al. Endoscopic management of hypopharyngeal stenosis after organ sparing therapy for head and neck cancer. Laryngoscope 2004;114: 1924–31.

[127] Bleier BS, Levine MS, Mick R, et al. Dysphagia after chemoradiation: analysis by modified barium swallow. Ann Otol Rhinol Laryngol 2007;116:837–41.

[128] Smith RV, Goldman Y, Beitler JJ, et al. Decreased short- and long-term swallowing problems with altered radiotherapy dosing used in an organ-sparing protocol for advanced pharyngeal carcinoma. Arch Otolaryngol Head Neck Surg 2004;130:831–6.

[129] Eisbruch A, TenHaken RK, Kim HM, et al. Dose, volume, and function relationships in parotid salivary glands following conformal and intensity-modulated irradiation of head and neck cancer. Int J Radiat Oncol Biol Phys 1999;45(3):577–87.

[130] Eisbruch A, Kim HM, Terrell JE, et al. Xerostomia and its predictors following parotid-sparing irradiation of head and neck cancer. Int J Radiat Oncol Biol Phys 2001;50:695–704.

[131] Mittal BB, Kepka A, Mahadevan A, et al. Tissue/dose compensation to reduce toxicity from combined radiation and chemotherapy for advanced head and neck cancers. Int J Cancer 2001;96(Suppl):61–70.

[132] Fua TF, Corry J, Milner AD, et al. Intensity-modulated radiotherapy for nasopharyngeal carcinoma: clinical correlation of dose to the pharyngo-esophageal axis and dysphagia. Int J Radiat Oncol Biol Phys 2007;67(4):976–81.

[133] Eisbruch A, Schwartz M, Rasch C, et al. Dysphagia and aspiration after chemoradiotherapy for head and neck cancer: which anatomic structures are affected and can they be spared by IMRT? Int J Radiat Oncol Biol Phys 2004;60:1425–39.

[134] Levendag PC, Teguh DN, Voet P, et al. Dysphagia disorders in patients with cancer of the oropharynx are significantly affected by the radiation therapy dose to the superior and middle constrictor muscle: a dose-effect relationship. Radiother Oncol 2007;85:64–73.

[135] Feng FY, Kim HM, Lyden TH, et al. Intensity-modulated radiotherapy of head and neck cancer aiming to reduce dysphagia: early dose-effect relationships for the swallowing structures. Int J Radiat Oncol Biol Phys 2007;68:1289–98.

[136] Franzen L, Funegard U, Ericson T, et al. Parotid gland function during and following radiotherapy of malignancies in the head and neck. A consecutive study of salivary flow and patient discomfort. Eur J Cancer 1992;28(2–3):457–62.

[137] Kaneko M, Shirato H, Nishioka T, et al. Scintigraphic evaluation of long-term salivary function after bilateral whole parotid gland irradiation in radiotherapy for head and neck tumour. Oral Oncol 1998;34(2):140–6.

[138] Logemann JA, Smith CH, Pauloski BR, et al. Effects of xerostomia on perception and performance of swallow function. Head Neck 2001;23(4):317–21.

[139] Lalla RV, Peterson DE. Treatment of mucositis, including new medications. Cancer J 2006; 12(5):348–54.

[140] Stokman MA, Spijkervet FK, Boezen HM, et al. Preventive intervention possibilities in radiotherapy- and chemotherapy-induced oral mucositis: results of meta-analyses. J Dent Res 2006;85(8):690–700.

[141] Rubenstein EB, Peterson DE, Schubert M, et al. Clinical practice guidelines for the prevention and treatment of cancer therapy-induced oral and gastrointestinal mucositis. Cancer 2004;100(Supplement):2026–46.

[142] Mantini G, Manfrida S, Cellini F, et al. Impact of dose and volume on radiation-induced mucositis. Rays 2005;30(2):137–44.

[143] Spijkervet FK, van Saene HK, Panders AK, et al. Scoring irradiation mucositis in head and neck cancer patients. J Oral Pathol Med 1989;18(3):167–71.

[144] Silverman S. Diagnosis and management of oral mucositis. J Support Oncol 2007; 5(Supplement 1):13–21.

[145] Lee WT, Akst LM, Adelstein DJ, et al. Risk factors for hypopharyngeal/upper esophageal stricture formation after concurrent chemoradiation. Head Neck 2006;28:808–12.

[146] Laurell G, Kraepelien T, Mavroidis P, et al. Stricture of the proximal esophagus in head and neck carcinoma patients after radiotherapy. Cancer 2003;97:1693–700.

[147] Franzmann EJ, Lundy DS, Abitbol AA, et al. Complete hypopharyngeal obstruction by mucosal adhesions: a complication of intensive chemoradiation for advanced head and neck cancer. Head Neck 2006;28:663–70.

[148] Mekhail TM, Adelstein DJ, Rybicki LA, et al. Enteral nutrition during the treatment of head and neck carcinoma: is a percutaneous endoscopic gastrostomy tube preferable to a nasogastric tube? Cancer 2001;91:1785–90.

[149] Logemann JA. Evaluation and treatment of swallowing disorders. 2nd edition. Austin (TX): Pro—Ed; 1998.

[150] Ott DJ, Hodge RG, Pikna LA, et al. Modified barium swallow: clinical and radiographic correlation and relation to feeding recommendations. Dysphagia 1996;11:187–90.

[151] Cook IJ, Kahrilas PJ. AGA Technical review on management of oropharyngeal dysphagia. Gastroenterology 1999;116:455–78.

[152] Mathers-Schmidt BA, Kurlinski M. Dysphagia evaluation practices: inconsistencies in clinical assessment and instrumental examination decision-making. Dysphagia 2003;18: 114–25.

[153] Doggett DL, Turkelson CM, Coates V. Recent developments in diagnosis and intervention for aspiration and dysphagia in stroke and other neuromuscular disorders. Curr Atheroscler Rep 2002;4:304–11.

[154] Martin-Harris B, Logemann JA, McMahon S, et al. Clinical utility of the modified barium swallow. Dysphagia 2000;15:136–41.

[155] Rasley A, Logemann JA, Kahrilas PJ, et al. Prevention of barium aspiration during videofluoroscopic swallowing studies: value of change in posture. AJR Am J Roentgenol 1993; 160(5):1005–9.

[156] Logemann JA, Rademaker AW, Pauloski BR, et al. Effects of postural change on aspiration in head and neck surgical patients. Otolaryngol Head Neck Surg 1994;110:222–7.

[157] Ohmae Y, Karaho T, Hanyu Y, et al. [Effect of posture strategies on preventing aspiration]. Nippon Jibiinkoka Gakkai Kaiho 1997;100(2):220–6 [in Japanese].

[158] Welch MV, Logemann JA, Rademaker AW, et al. Changes in pharyngeal dimensions effected by chin tuck. Arch Phys Med Rehabil 1993;74:178–81.

[159] Shanahan TK, Logemann JA, Rademaker AW, et al. Effects of chin down posture on aspiration in dysphagic patients. Arch Phys Med Rehabil 1993;74:178–81.

[160] Lewin JS, Hebert TM, Putnam JB Jr, et al. Experience with the chin tuck maneuver in post-esophagectomy aspirators. Dysphagia 2001;16(3):216–9.

[161] Bulow M, Olsson R, Ekberg O. Videomanometric analysis of supraglottic swallow, effort-ful swallow, and chin tuck in patients with pharyngeal dysfunction. Dysphagia 2001;16: 190–5.

[162] Logemann JA, Gensler G, Robbins J, et al. A randomized study of three interventions for aspiration of thin liquids in patients with dementia or Parkinson's disease. J Speech Hear Res 2008;51(1):173–83.

[163] Logemann J, Kahrilas P, Kobara M, et al. The benefit of head rotation on pharyngo—esophageal dysphagia. Arch Phys Med Rehabil 1989;70:767–71.

[164] Kawai S, Tsukuda M, Mochimatu I, et al. [The benefit of head rotation on pharyngoeso-phageal dysphagia from three cases of paraganglioma in the parapharyngeal space]. Nippon Jibiinkoka Gakkai Kaiho 1999;102(3):311–6 [in Japanese].

[165] Tsukamoto Y. CT study of closure of the hemipharynx with head rotation in a case of lat-eral medullary syndrome. Dysphagia 2000;15(1):17–8.

[166] Martin BJW, Logemann JA, Shaker R, et al. Normal laryngeal valving patterns during three breath hold maneuvers: a pilot investigation. Dysphagia 1993;8:11–20.

[167] Lazarus C, Logemann JA, Gibbons P. Effects of maneuvers on swallow functioning in a dysphagic oral cancer patient. Head Neck 1993;15:419–24.

[168] Ohmae Y, Logemann JA, Kaiser P, et al. Effects of two breath-holding maneuvers on oro-pharyngeal swallow. Ann Otol Rhinol Laryngol 1996;105(2):123–31.

[169] Ogura J, Kawasaki M, Takenouchi S. Neurophysiologic observations on the adaptive mechanism of deglutition. Ann Otol Rhinol Laryngol 1964;73:1062–81.

[170] Lazarus CL, Logemann JA, Song CW, et al. Effects of voluntary maneuvers on tongue base function for swallowing. Folia Phoniatr Logop 2002;54:171–6.

[171] Logemann JA, Pauloski BR, Rademaker AW, et al. Super-supraglottic swallow in irradi-ated head and neck cancer patients. Head Neck 1997;19:535–40.

[172] Hind JA, Nicosia MA, Roecker EB, et al. Comparison of effortful and noneffortful swallows in healthy middle-aged and older adults. Arch Phys Med Rehabil 2001; 82(12):1661–5.

[173] Hiss SG, Huckabee ML. Timing of pharyngeal and upper esophageal sphincter pressures as a function of normal and effortful swallowing in young healthy adults. Dysphagia 2005; 20(2):149–56.

[174] Lever TE, Cox KT, Holbert D, et al. The effect of an effortful swallow on the normal adult esophagus. Dysphagia 2007;22(4):312–25.

[175] Bulow M, Olsson R, Ekberg O. Supraglottic swallow, effortful swallow, and chin tuck did not alter hypopharyngeal intrabolus pressure in patients with pharyngeal dysfunction. Dys-phagia 2002;17(3):197–201.

[176] Kahrilas PJ, Logemann JA, Krugler C, et al. Volitional augmentation of upper esophageal sphincter opening during swallowing. Am J Physiol 1991;260:G450–6.

[177] Boden K, Hallgren A, Witt Hedstrom H. Effects of three different swallow maneuvers analyzed by videomanometry. Acta Radiol 2006;47(7):628–33.

[178] Fujiu M, Logemann JA. Effect of a tongue holding maneuver on posterior pharyngeal wall movement during deglutition. Am J Speech Lang Pathol 1996;5:23–30.

[179] Lazarus CL, Logemann JA, Rademaker AW, et al. Effects of bolus volume, viscosity and repeated swallows in nonstroke subjects and stroke patients. Arch Phys Med Rehabil 1993; 74:1066–70.

[180] Bisch EM, Logemann JA, Rademaker AW, et al. Pharyngeal effects of bolus volume, vis-cosity, and temperature in patients with dysphagia resulting from neurologic impairment and in normal subjects. J Speech Hear Res 1994;37:1041–9.

[181] Logemann JA. Behavioral management for oropharyngeal dysphagia. Folia Phoniatr Logop 1999;51:199–212.

[182] Kuhlemeier KV, Palmer JB, Rosenberg D. Effect of liquid bolus consistency and delivery method on aspiration and pharyngeal retention in dysphagia patients. Dysphagia 2001; 16:119–22.

[183] Logemann JA, Pauloski BR, Rademaker AW, et al. Speech and swallowing rehabilitation for head and neck cancer patients. Oncology 1997;11:651–9.

[184] Waters TM, Logemann JA, Pauloski BR, et al. Beyond efficacy and effectiveness: conducting economic analyses during clinical trials. Dysphagia 2004;19:109–19.

[185] Buchbinder D, Currivan RB, Kaplan AJ, et al. Mobilization regimens for the prevention of jaw hypomobility in the radiated patient: a comparison of three techniques. J Oral Maxillofac Surg 1993;51:863–7.

[186] Dijkstra PU, Sterken MW, Pater R, et al. Exercise therapy for trismus in head and neck cancer. Oral Oncol 2007;43:389–94.

[187] Cohen EG, Deschler DG, Walsh K, et al. Early use of a mechanical stretching device to improve mandibular mobility after composite resection: a pilot study. Arch Phys Med Rehabil 2005;86:1416–9.

[188] Veis S, Logemann JA, Colangelo L. Effects of three techniques on maximum posterior movement of the tongue base. Dysphagia 2000;15:142–5.

[189] Pauloski BR, Rademaker AW, Logemann JA, et al. Relationship between swallow motility disorders on VFG and oral intake in patients treated for head and neck cancer with radiotherapy ± chemotherapy. Head Neck 2006;28:1069–76.

[190] Shaker R, Kern M, Bardan E, et al. Augmentation of deglutitive upper esophageal sphincter opening in the elderly by exercise. Am J Physiol 1997;272(Gastrointestinal Liver Physiology, 35):G1518–22.

[191] Easterling C, Kern M, Nitschke T, et al. A novel rehabilitative exercise for dysphagic patients: effect on swallow function and biomechanics. Gastroenterology 1998;114(Suppl 1):A747.

[192] Shaker R, Easterling C, Kern M, et al. Rehabilitation of swallowing by exercise in tube-fed patients with pharyngeal dysphagia secondary to abnormal UES opening. Gastroenterology 2002;122:1314–21.

[193] Freed ML, Freed L, Chatburn RL, et al. Electrical stimulation for swallowing disorders caused by stroke. Respir Care 2001;46(5):466–74.

[194] Shaw GY, Sechtem PR, Searl J, et al. Transcutaneous neuromuscular electrical stimulation (VitalStim) curative therapy for severe dysphagia: myth or reality? Ann Otol Rhinol Laryngol 2007;116(1):36–44.

[195] Blumenfeld L, Hahn Y, Lepage A, et al. Transcutaneous electrical stimulation versus traditional dysphagia therapy: a nonconcurrent cohort study. Otolaryngol Head Neck Surg 2006;135(5):754–7.

[196] Suiter DM, Leder SB, Ruark JL. Effects of neuromuscular electrical stimulation on submental muscle activity. Dysphagia 2006;21(1):56–60.

[197] Humbert IA, Poletto CJ, Saxon KG, et al. The effect of surface electrical stimulation on hyolaryngeal movement in normal individuals at rest and during swallowing. J Appl Physiol 2006;101(6):1657–63.

[198] Carnaby-Mann GD, Crary MA. Examining the evidence on neuromuscular electrical stimulation for swallowing: a meta-analysis. Arch Otolaryngol Head Neck Surg 2007;133(6): 564–71.

[199] Steele CM, Thrasher AT, Popovic MR. Electric stimulation approaches to the restoration and rehabilitation of swallowing: a review. Neurol Res 2007;29(1):9–15.

[200] Crary MA, Carnaby-Mann GD, Faunce A. Electrical stimulation therapy for dysphagia: descriptive results of two surveys. Dysphagia 2007;22(3):165–73.

[201] Lazarus CL, Logemann JA, Pauloski BR, et al. Swallowing and tongue function following treatment for oral and oropharyngeal cancer. J Speech Hear Res 2000;43:1011–23.

[202] Lazarus C, Logemann JA, Pauloski BR, et al. Effects of radiotherapy with or without chemotherapy on tongue strength and swallowing in patients with oral cancer. Head Neck 2007;29(7):632–7.

[203] Robin DA, Goel A, Somodi LB, et al. Tongue strength and endurance: relation to highly skilled movements. J Speech Hear Res 1992;35:1239–45.

[204] Lazarus C, Logemann JA, Huang CF, et al. Effects of two types of tongue strengthening exercises in young normals. Folia Phoniatr Logop 2003;55:199–205.

[205] Lazzara G, Lazarus C, Logemann JA. Impact of thermal stimulation on the triggering of the swallowing reflex. Dysphagia 1986;1:73–7.

[206] Bove M, Mansson I, Eliasson I. Thermal oral-pharyngeal stimulation and elicitation of swallowing. Acta OtoLaryngol 1998;118(5):728–31.

[207] Ali GN, Laundl TM, Wallace KL, et al. Influence of cold stimulation on the normal pharyngeal swallow response. Dysphagia 1996;11(1):2–8.

[208] Rosenbek JC, Robbins J, Fishback B, et al. Effects of thermal application on dysphagia after stroke. J Speech Hear Res 1991;34(6):1257–68.

[209] Kaatzke-McDonald MN, Post E, Davis PJ. The effects of cold, touch, and chemical stimulation of the anterior faucial pillar on human swallowing. Dysphagia 1996;11(3):198–206.

[210] Sciortino K, Liss JM, Case JL, et al. Effects of mechanical, cold, gustatory, and combined stimulation to the human anterior faucial pillars. Dysphagia 2003;18(1):16–26.

[211] Hamdy S, Jilani S, Price V, et al. Modulation of human swallowing behaviour by thermal and chemical stimulation in health and after brain injury. Neurogastroenterol Motil 2003; 15(1):69–77.

[212] Rosenbek JC, Roecker EB, Wood JL, et al. Thermal application reduces the duration of stage transition in dysphagia after stroke. Dysphagia 1996;11(4):225–33.

[213] Davis JW, Lazarus C, Logemann J, et al. Effect of a maxillary glossectomy prosthesis on articulation and swallowing. J Prosthet Dent 1987;57:715–9.

[214] Light J. A review of oral and oropharyngeal prostheses to facilitate speech and swallowing. Am J Speech Lang Pathol 1995;4:15–21.

[215] Weber RS, Ohlms L, Bowman J, et al. Functional results after total or near total glossectomy with laryngeal preservation. Arch Otolaryngol Head Neck Surg 1991;117:512–5.

[216] DaBreo EL, Chalian VA, Lingeman R, et al. Prosthetic and surgical management of osteogenic sarcoma of the maxilla. J Prosthet Dent 1990;63:316–20.

[217] Yontchev E, Karlsson S, Lith A, et al. Orofacial functions in patients with congenital and acquired maxillary defects: a fluoroscopic study. J Oral Rehabil 1991;18:483–9.

[218] Wheeler RL, Logemann JA, Rosen MS. Maxillary reshaping prostheses: effectiveness in improving speech and swallowing of postsurgical oral cancer patients. J Prosthet Dent 1980;43:313–9.

[219] Pauloski BR, Logemann JA, Colangelo LA, et al. Effect of intraoral prostheses on swallowing function in postsurgical oral and oropharyngeal cancer patients. American Journal of Speech-Language Pathology 1996;5(3):31–46.

[220] Lazarus CL. Management of swallowing disorders in head and neck: optimal patterns of care. Semin Speech Lang 2000;21:293–309.

[221] Kulbersh BD, Rosenthal EL, McGrew BM, et al. Pretreatment, preoperative swallowing exercises may improve dysphagia quality of life. Laryngoscope 2006;116:883–6.

[222] Denk DM, Swoboda H, Schima W, et al. Prognostic factors for swallowing rehabilitation following head and neck cancer surgery. Acta Otolaryngol 1997;117:760–74.

[223] Logemann JA. Update on clinical trials in dysphagia. Dysphagia 2006;21:116–20.

ELSEVIER
SAUNDERS

Phys Med Rehabil Clin N Am
19 (2008) 929–938

PHYSICAL MEDICINE
AND REHABILITATION
CLINICS OF
NORTH AMERICA

Dysphagia Rehabilitation in Japan

Mikoto Baba, MD, DMSc[a],*,
Eiichi Saitoh, MD, DMSc[b],
Sumiko Okada, SLP, MS[a]

[a]*School of Health Science, Fujita Health University, 1-98 Dengakugakubo Kutsukake Toyoake Aichi, 470-1192 Japan*
[b]*Department of Rehabilitation Medicine, School of Medicine, Fujita Health University, 1-98 Dengakugakubo Kutsukake Toyoake Aichi, 470-1192 Japan*

Dysphagia is one of the most important targets for rehabilitation in Japan. The Japanese have the highest rates of life expectancy in the world, at 79 years for men and 85 years for women in 2007. Elderly people (aged 60 or over) comprised 26.3% of the Japanese population in 2005, and that figure is expected to grow to 41.7% by 2050 (Table 1). The population covered by long-term care insurance was 2,259,000 in 2004. The aging of the Japanese population is expected to raise the prevalence of dysphagia.

The top four causes of death in Japanese are malignant neoplasm (30.1%), heart disease (16%), stroke (12.3%), and pneumonia (9.9%). Stroke is one of the most common causes of dysphagia. Fig. 1 shows the disease of patients who underwent videofluorographic examinations in the authors' department over the past 10 years. As causes of dysphagia, stroke accounts for 45% of them.

The prevalence of stroke in Japan is higher than in the United States, at approximately 400 per 100,000 [1] or 1.6 times that of the United States [2]. The rate of ischemic stroke in Japan is about 78%, and hemorrhage is 15.5% [3]. In the case of infarction, we have many cases of brainstem disorders [4]. Therefore, many patients have dysphagia due to bulbar palsy. When pneumonia is the cause of death, aspiration pneumonia of the elderly is the most important factor. The authors believe that not fewer than 50% of cases of pneumonia in the elderly are caused by aspiration [5].

Clinical circumstance in Japanese rehabilitation

When we compare Japanese dysphagia rehabilitation with that of Europe and the Unites States, we should think about the difference of length of

* Corresponding author.
E-mail address: mbaba@fujita-hu.ac.jp (M. Baba).

1047-9651/08/$ - see front matter © 2008 Elsevier Inc. All rights reserved.
doi:10.1016/j.pmr.2008.07.002

pmr.theclinics.com

Table 1
Japan and United States populations and percentage older than 60: 2005 and 2050

	Japan		United States	
Year	2005	2050	2005	2050
Population 60+[a] (%)	128,085 (26.3)	115,710 (41.7)	298,213 (16.7)	350,103 (26.4)

[a] Thousands.

Data from Population Division of the Department of Economic and Social Affairs of the United Nations Secretariat. World population prospects: the 2004 revision. New York: United Nations; 2005.

hospital stay. The Japanese insurance system covers long periods of inpatient treatment. For example, in the case of stroke, the Japanese insurance system allows acute care for 2 or 3 weeks, after which care in the rehabilitation unit is covered for up to 180 days if necessary. The legally approved rehabilitation unit provides up to 180 minutes of exercise per day. In this way, Japanese rehabilitation consists of an inpatient system from the acute phase to the subacute phase and dysphagia rehabilitation is managed under these circumstances. In contrast, for cases of chronic disease such as Parkinson disease or neuromuscular diseases, the insurance system does not cover treatment in the rehabilitation unit. It is difficult to manage dysphagia rehabilitation for chronic patients.

In 2006, the Japanese Ministry of Health, Labor and Welfare introduced a new insurance system for the care of dysphagia called "eating function therapy." The insurance covers exercise or care for 30 minutes by nurses, dental hygienists, or therapists. This change was significant because the insurance pays for exercise therapy done by nontherapists and the insurance can cover the rehabilitation exercise done by therapists and the eating function therapy together, so that the insurance-covered exercise time for the dysphagic patient became 30 minutes longer.

Although dysphagia rehabilitation in the United States is managed mainly by speech language pathologists, it is different from that in the

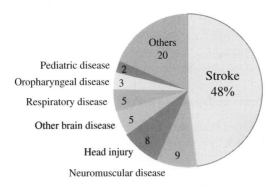

Fig. 1. Diseases of patients who underwent videofluorography in the Department of Rehabilitation, Fujita Health University between 1995 and 2007 (N = 1264).

authors' country. In Japan, many kinds of professionals join dysphagia rehabilitation clinics and research. Although speech therapists undertake an important role, nurses also take a major role in the dysphagia rehabilitation associated with the eating function therapy. The Japanese Nursing Association has managed the Training School for Dysphagia Rehabilitation Nursing since 2007. They offer paid educational lectures and clinical training for 1 year and provide a certification program as a certified dysphagia rehabilitation nurse through evaluation tests. Sixty nurses are certified every year.

Dentists and dental hygienists also play an important role in dysphagia rehabilitation. Some dentists make a diagnosis and evaluation of dysphagia using videoendoscopy or videofluorography. The importance of oral care is well known in Japan. Some acute care units or rehabilitation units have dental treatment teams. They treat oral problems to reduce the incidence of aspiration pneumonia and cooperate with medical doctors to improve eating function. Otolaryngologists in Japan have done extensive research on dysphagia and swallowing for a long time. They offer aggressive surgical treatment of dysphagia.

Physiatrists play a primary role in the evaluation and management of dysphagia rehabilitation from the viewpoint of kinesiology with the use of videofluorography. Speech therapy involves intensive exercise treatment, as in other countries. Fig. 2 shows the composition of the Japanese Society of Dysphagia Rehabilitation (JSDR) members. It reflects the features of an actual transdisciplinary rehabilitation team.

Diagnostic techniques

Several diagnostic techniques have been developed in Japan to detect swallowing problems without videofluorography or videoendoscopy.

The repetitive saliva swallowing test (RSST) is one of the most well known methods [6,7]. This screening test detects patient who have

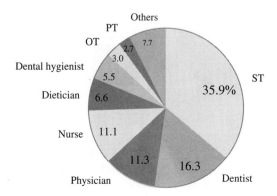

Fig. 2. Composition of membership in the Japanese Society of Dysphagia Rehabilitation in July 2007 (5181 members). OT, occupational therapist; PT, physical therapist; ST, speech therapist.

aspiration. The patient is asked to do saliva (dry) swallows as many times as possible in 30 seconds. If the patient does not swallow three times repetitively, he or she is likely to have dysphagia associated with aspiration. The sensitivity and specificity of the RSST to detect aspiration diagnosed by videofluorography are 0.98 and 0.66, respectively [7].

The modified water swallowing test and the food test were also developed in Japan [8]. These tests are easy and safe methods to evaluate swallowing function or a temporal change in the function.

The authors consider videofluorography to be the most important technique for the diagnosis and evaluation of dysphagia and in formulating a plan of dysphagia rehabilitation. The JSDR provides a guide for standardized performance of videofluorography. The standard method emphasizes that one should use an appropriate chair to control the examinee's posture, should prepare appropriate test foods, and must know the compensatory swallowing maneuvers. A physician or dentist does the videofluorography, and therapists often join it. The fee for videofluorography is up to $60, which is inexpensive compared with that in the United States.

The authors often apply transnasal flexible videoendoscopy for evaluation at the bedside or in a home visit but this procedure may be performed only by physicians or dentists in Japan (Fig. 3). Although dentists are permitted to do videoendoscopy by law, insurance sometimes does not cover it. The fee for videofluorography done by a physician is approximately $60.

Treatment or exercise

Nutrition management

The importance of nutritional management during the acute phase of illness is understood, so many hospitals have introduced nutrition support teams. But dysphagia rehabilitation on these teams is less well understood.

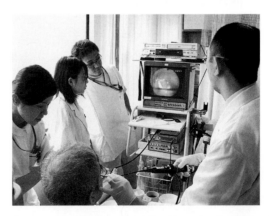

Fig. 3. Bedside swallowing evaluation using portable videoendoscopy system. Videoendoscopic biofeedback during direct therapy. From the left, speech therapist, dentist, nurse, and physiatrist.

Currently, the JSDR and the Japanese Society for Parental and Enteral Nutrition (JSPEN) are collaborating to improve this situation. The JSDR conducts a lecture about dysphagia rehabilitation at the annual meeting of the JSPEN, and the JSPEN conducts a lecture about nutritional management at the annual JSDR meeting.

The important methods of enteral nutrition are nasogastric tube and percutaneous endoscopic gastrostomy (PEG). PEG has become a common method in Japan but some misunderstanding exists. PEG is not a goal of nutritional management but rather, just a method of nutritional management. When PEG is completed and nutritional status is improved, one then has to begin constructive rehabilitation programs. The authors have extensive experience indicating that patients who have undergone PEG placement can subsequently improve their swallowing function through appropriate rehabilitation and nutritional control after PEG, and are finally able to quit the gastrostomy feeding. Although PEG has become common, the timing of PEG placement is comparatively late in Japan (several months after the onset of dysphagia), so a long period of nutritional management is done by nasogastric tube.

Intermittent catheterization is a unique method of nutritional management in Japan. This method is one in which the patient inserts his or her own feeding tube on demand per oral or nasal route, infuses an enteral nutrient, and, when finished infusing, immediately removes the tube. If the patient has good mental status and communication, this method can be applied easily without risk for aberrant tube placement in the airway. If the patient has a good esophageal function shown by videofluorography, a tip of the tube can be put at the middle of the esophagus, causing secondary peristalsis in the esophagus. The authors believe that this peristalsis induces the esophagogastric reflex and must be more physiologic than PEG tube feeding. This technique will work to reduce gastroesophageal reflux or diarrhea. The greatest benefit of this method is the opportunity to be tube free for periods during each day, and direct therapy exercise can be managed easily for intermittent catheterization patients.

Oral care

Oral care is recognized as an essential aspect of dysphagia rehabilitation in Japan. The Japanese Dental Association works to help dentists and dental-associated persons understand the importance of oral care for disabled persons, and it has educational programs on this topic in the community. Several important studies have been managed by collaborations between Japanese dentists and physicians. One important study showed that the oral hygiene of disabled people admitted to a subacute rehabilitation hospital was poor, and treatment by a dentist and dental hygienist led to improvements not only in the patients' oral condition but also in their activities of daily living and eating ability [9]. Another article reported that the oral care treatment of the disabled elderly in nursing homes reduced the incidence of aspiration pneumonia [10]. A study regarding the effects of oral care and functional training on entirely tube-fed patients showed that professional oral care and indirect therapy by a dental hygienist once weekly was sufficient to maintain oral hygiene and reduce the incidence of pneumonia [11].

Indirect therapy

Indirect therapy for dysphagia is widely practiced, as discussed elsewhere in this issue. The authors apply many kinds of methods, including respiratory exercise or range-of-motion exercise for the neck or around the shoulder. These days, they often apply the head-raising exercise developed by Shaker and colleagues [12] to many kinds of dysphagia (with some technical modifications). The authors understand that the exercise strengthens the hyolaryngeal elevator muscles as demonstrated by Shaker's randomized control study. They now call the exercise "Shaker exercise" and it is quite popular in Japan.

The authors sometimes apply balloon expansion of the upper esophageal sphincter (UES) for dysphagia in cases with large amounts of pharyngeal retention after swallowing [13]. The pharyngeal retention generally results from UES dysfunction or poor pharyngeal constriction. Therefore, when the authors find pharyngeal retention on videofluorography, they sometimes stretch the UES using a catheter that has a balloon (as in a standard urethral catheter) placed through the oral cavity. This method has a diagnostic usefulness; when a floppy UES is identified, they know that the retention may be caused by poor pharyngeal constrictors, but if the UES is tight, the retention may be caused by UES dysfunction. In any case, when the authors find that the balloon-expanding method reduces retention after swallowing, and the patient has no difficulty (such as pain or gagging), they apply balloon expansion as an indirect therapy for dysphagia (Fig. 4). Although the long-term effect of this method may vary from case to case, some cases show obvious benefit, and the authors know of no reported ill effects with this method when treating functional dysphagia. Therefore, they do not hesitate to try this method.

Direct therapy

Direct therapy is conducted not only by speech therapists but also by nurses certified in dysphagia treatment, or other well-trained nurses in Japan. In direct therapy during the early stage, the authors often use jelly food or paste food. Many Japanese food companies develop thickeners, easy-to-swallow foods, or easy-to eat-foods for dysphagic patients, which can also be used in therapy. Recently, special jelly food for dysphagia was developed that does not change its viscosity in room temperature or in the oral cavity, and it is useful for therapeutic feeding trials in people who

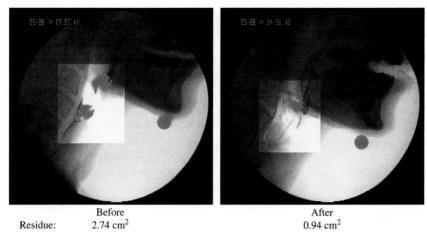

Before   After
Residue: 2.74 cm²   0.94 cm²

Fig. 4. The change of pharyngeal residue by the balloon expanding method. This sample case is a 52-year-old woman who has traumatic subarachnoid hemorrhage. Before treatment, the case shows a large amount of residue in the vallecula and piriform sinus. Just after treatment, two-dimensional analysis shows the residue is reduced.

have severe pharyngeal dysphagia with prolonged oral transit because the jelly does not melt into liquid. Moreover, it is useful for the test food for bedside videoedoscopy because it can be brought to the bedside without a cooler box.

The principal diet of the Japanese is rice, even now. The rice produced in Japan has some viscosity; therefore, well-done rice porridge is good for many dysphagic patients. On the other hand, some habitual Japanese eating behaviors are dangerous for individuals who have dysphagia. The Japanese like to eat high-temperature food with much liquid, such as miso soup or udon noodles, and they eat those dishes from the bowel with sucking behavior to reduce the liquid temperature or to ingest long noodles. Some Japanese, especially the elderly, use sucking behavior even when eating with a spoon. These eating behaviors will act adversely for dysphagic people because they can produce actual aspiration, so one has to pay attention to this sucking style of eating.

In actual direct therapy, the authors think that changing posture is an important technique to facilitate swallowing. The reclining posture changes the inlet of the larynx position higher than the inlet of the esophagus and this change works to keep the pharyngeal retention in the piriform sinus and inhibit aspiration after the swallow. One can then proceed safely with a second or third swallow, or apply some swallowing maneuvers to improve pharyngeal clearance. Thus, the authors often apply this posture in the management of aspiration after the swallow. The reclining posture helps the dysphagic patients hold a bolus in the pharynx without aspiration.

The authors often introduce the neck rotation posture in cases of bulbar palsy that have obvious laterality. These cases often have intact pharyngeal function on the unaffected side. At that time, the patient is asked to rotate the neck to the affected side. This neck rotation to the affected side shifts the bolus passage to the unaffected side, improving pharyngeal clearance. Even if no immediate improvement is apparent, patients are trained in that posture because it may help severe dysphagia to improve gradually.

When the reclining position and the head rotation are applied simultaneously, one must consider the gravity effect resulting from reclining and rotation. With neck rotation to the affected side in a reclining position, the affected side may become lower than the unaffected side, which may oppose the effect of neck rotation. In this instance, the authors consider having the patient lie with the unaffected side down and neck rotation to the affected side.

These concepts reflect the underlying principle of rehabilitation by using residual function, an approach that is common in the rehabilitation of hemiplegia or paraplegia.

Outcome of dysphagia rehabilitation

The authors conducted a retrospective study on the rehabilitation outcome of dysphagia in their university hospital [14]. They treated 19 chronic cases of severe dysphagia due to brainstem disorder (requiring no peroral [NPO] status and tube feeding) with an intensive inpatient rehabilitation program for a long period of several months per patient. The average time from onset of dysphagia was about 200 days and the median of the duration of hospital stay was about 115 days. This study showed that, after the rehabilitation program, 50% of the cases were able to resume a partial oral diet, and 4 cases returned to full oral feeding. In the 8 cases that showed no benefit, their medical condition on admission was unstable because of saliva aspiration (Table 2). It was concluded that rehabilitation or therapeutic exercise are necessary for individuals who have dysphagia due to brainstem disorder even if they need total tube feeding in the chronic phase, particularly for people who did not have an experience of intensive rehabilitation and who did not have saliva aspiration. The authors believe the effectiveness of the rehabilitation resulted from their fine kinematics-based evaluation by videofluorography and the intensive and careful direct therapy exercise

Table 2
Results of inpatient rehabilitaion for tube-fed dysphagia secondary to brainstem disorder in the Department of Rehabilitation, Fujita Health University Hospital, from 1997 to 2005

Patient status on admission	Eating status at discharge		
	Total tube	Partial tube	Oral
Saliva aspiration (7 cases)	6	1	0
Nonsaliva aspiration (11 cases)	2	5	4

Data from Ozeki Y, Baba M, Saitoh E, et al. Rehabilitation for chronic dysphagia secondary to brainstem stroke. Sogo Reha 2008;36(7):573–7 [in Japanese].

provided by speech therapists, nurses, dentists, and rehabilitation resident physicians using videoendoscopic biofeedback. Although the authors' clinical manner mentioned above is not common even in Japan especially in reference to the long term hospital stay rehabilitation, the result is highly useful when considering the indication and effectiveness of dysphagia rehabilitation.

Surgical treatment

Japanese otolaryngologists have taken a major role in dysphagia treatment, not only in structural problems but also in dynamic disorders, by performing reconstructive surgery. In the authors' university, they treat dysphagic patients in collaboration with otolaryngology, and surgical methods are considered when necessary. Surgical methods are often applied to patients who have severe dysphagia due to brainstem disorder when more than 6 months have passed since onset; improvement with therapeutic exercise for more than 3 months is not sufficient; the patient does not have mental problems such as dementia; trunk control is good; and the patient is anxious to take food by mouth. The specific surgical procedure is the combination of bilateral cricopharyngeal myotomy and laryngeal suspension. From 2000 to 2007, the authors applied this surgery to 12 cases. All cases showed some improvement in eating status and 9 cases became able to take all food and drink by mouth, although they needed dysphagia rehabilitation periods for several months after the surgery. Experience with individuals older than 70 years old is insufficient to evaluate their outcomes. Reconstruction surgery was effective for many patients. Surgical methods should be considered for severe dysphagia due to brainstem disorder that does not show any improvement with rehabilitation.

Summary

This article described the features of Japanese dysphagia rehabilitation, particularly where it differs from that in the United States. Many kinds of professionals participate in dysphagia rehabilitation; nurses and dental associates take important roles, and the Japanese insurance system covers that. Videofluorography and videoendoscopy are common and are sometimes done by dentists. Intermittent catheterization is applied to nutrition control in some cases. The balloon expansion method is applied to reduce pharyngeal residue after swallowing. If long-term rehabilitation does not work effectively in dysphagia due to brainstem disorder, the authors consider reconstructive surgery to improve function.

References

[1] Morioka Y, Nakazawa H, Naruse Y, et al. Trends in stroke incidence and acute case fatality in a Japanese rural area. The oyabe study. Stroke 2000;31(7):1583–7.

[2] American heart association. Heart disease and stroke statistics 2007 update. Circulation 2007;115:e69–171.

[3] Kobayashi S. Stroke databank. Tokyo: Nakayama shoten; 2005.

[4] Kameda W, Kawanami T, Kurita K, et al. Lateral and medial medullary infarction. A comparative analysis of 214 patients. Stroke 2004;35(3):694–9.

[5] Sasaki H, Sekizawa K, Yanai M, et al. New strategies for aspiration pneumonia. Intern Med 1997;36(12):851–5.

[6] Oguchi K, Saitoh E, Mizuno M, et al. The repetitive saliva swallowing test (RSST) as a screening test of functional dysphagia (1) normal values of RSST. Japanese Journal of Rehabilitation Medicine 2000;37(6):375–82 [In Japanese].

[7] Oguchi K, Saitoh E, Baba M, et al. The repetitive saliva swallowing test (RSST) as a screening test of functional dysphagia (2) validity of RSST. Japanese Journal of Rehabilitation Medicine 2000;37(6):383–8 [In Japanese].

[8] Tohara H, Saitoh E, Mays KA, et al. Three tests for predicting aspiration without videofluorography. Dysphagia 2003;18(2):126–34.

[9] Suzuki M, Sonoda S, Saitoh E, et al. Effect of dental treatment on activities of daily living in the disabled elderly. Japanese Journal of Rehabilitation Medicine 2003;40(1):57–67 [In Japanese].

[10] Yoneyama T, Yoshida M, Ohrui T, et al. Oral care reduces pneumonia in older patients in nursing homes. J Am Geriatr Soc 2002;50(3):430–3.

[11] Ueda K, Yamada Y, Toyosato A, et al. Effects of functional training of dysphagia to prevent pneumonia for patients on tube feeding. Gerodontology 2004;21(2):108–11.

[12] Shaker R, Easterling C, Kern M, et al. Rehabilitation of swallowing by exercise in tube-fed patients with pharyngeal dysphagia secondary to abnormal UES opening. Gastroenterology 2002;122(5):1314–21.

[13] Hojo K, Fujishima I, Ohkuma R, et al. Balloon catheter treatment methods for cricopharingeal dysphagia. Japanese Journal of Rehabilitation Medicine 1997;1(1):45–56 [In Japanese].

[14] Ozeki Y, Baba M, Saitoh E, et al. Rehabilitation for chronic dysphagia secondary to brainstem stroke. Sogo Rehabilitation 2008;36(6):573–7 [In Japanese].

ELSEVIER
SAUNDERS

Phys Med Rehabil Clin N Am
19 (2008) 939–946

PHYSICAL MEDICINE
AND REHABILITATION
CLINICS OF
NORTH AMERICA

Index

Note: Page numbers of article titles are in **boldface** type.

doi:10.1016/S1047-9651(08)00073-9   *pmr.theclinics.com*

Moving?

Make sure your subscription moves with you!

To notify us of your new address, find your **Clinics Account Number** (located on your mailing label above your name), and contact customer service at:

E-mail: elspcs@elsevier.com

800-654-2452 (subscribers in the U.S. & Canada)
1-407-563-6020 (subscribers outside of the U.S. & Canada)

Fax number: 407-363-9661

Elsevier Periodicals Customer Service
6277 Sea Harbor Drive
Orlando, FL 32887-4800

*To ensure uninterrupted delivery of your subscription, please notify us at least 4 weeks in advance of move.